Medical Tourism in Developing Countries

Bhupinder Chaudhary • Dinesh Bhatia
Mahesh Patel • Sunaina Singh
Sushman Sharma
Editors

Medical Tourism in Developing Countries

A contemporary approach

Springer

Editors
Bhupinder Chaudhary
Department of Hospital Management and Hospice Studies
Jamia Millia Islamia
New Delhi, India

Mahesh Patel
Aster DM Healthcare
Doha, Qatar

Sushman Sharma
Department of Hospital Management
Hemchadracharya North Gujarat University
Patan, Gujarat, India

Dinesh Bhatia
Department of Biomedical Engineering
North Eastern Hill University
Shillong, Meghalaya, India

Sunaina Singh
ADA
Singapore, Singapore

ISBN 978-981-99-8908-9 ISBN 978-981-99-8909-6 (eBook)
https://doi.org/10.1007/978-981-99-8909-6

This Springer imprint is published by the registered company Springer Nature Singapore Pte Ltd.
The registered company address is: 152 Beach Road, #21-01/04 Gateway East, Singapore 189721, Singapore

Paper in this product is recyclable

Preface

We are happy to write the preface for the book entitled *Medical Tourism in Developing Countries: A Contemporary Approach*. This book is a compilation of work by experts from different domains working in the tourism industry, ranging from marketing and economics of medical tourism, regulatory policies and medical ethics, technology as a catalyst for medical tourism and quality management.

The tourism sector being a very diverse, sensitive and intricate area warrants its thorough and flawless planning for its growth and sustenance. The structure should not only be operationally efficient but also safe for its occupants and visitors. This book presents a detailed insight into the world of Medical Tourism and how it has evolved over the past few years since its inception. It has been written in a lucid and simple manner, so as to cater to audiences at various levels. The non-availability of comprehensive resources in this particular area prompted the creation of this resource. The book includes interaction and impact of diverse sectors like Insurance, Accreditation and Information Technology with ever-expanding universe of Medical Tourism.

The book provides insights into the growth and rise of healthcare tourism in developed and developing countries, with a special focus on the latter to cater to audience at various levels. The book would be a boon for people working in the field of Tourism, Healthcare and Hospitality areas. The modern trend of sustainable and community-based tourism approaches has been covered in the book. We believe the book would immensely benefit academicians, government officials, freelance travellers, scholars and researchers working in the field of Tourism and its allied sectors. People working in the field of medical tourism, insurance, policy making, accreditation and quality management would avail additional knowledge from this book.

The salient features of this book are the incorporation of best practices in this sector with reference to segments like patient safety, accreditation, employability, use of technology to enhance customer satisfaction and also make the entire ecosystem credible and efficient. The theoretical aspects have been complemented with relevant case studies to enable readers to establish a linkage. A section of the contents has also been dedicated to the most recent developments globally in the wake of the COVID-19 pandemic, which led to the overhauling of this sector. Finally, this book is expected to provide a holistic insight into the sector of Medical Tourism and how it functions at the micro level.

New Delhi, India Bhupinder Chaudhary
Shillong, India Dinesh Bhatia
Doha, Qatar Mahesh Patel
Singapore, Singapore Sunaina Singh
Patan, India Sushman Sharma

Acknowledgements

Developing this book on medical tourism has been an incredibly enriching and fulfilling journey, and we're filled with immense gratitude as we stand at the completion of this endeavour. This project has been a collaborative effort and this would not have been possible without the dedication, expertise and contributions of numerous individuals and organizations, and it is with deep appreciation that we acknowledge their invaluable assistance.

First and foremost, we extend our heartfelt gratitude to the contributors of this book on medical tourism. Their passion for the subject matter and your meticulous research have been evident throughout the writing process. Their commitment to delivering accurate and insightful information has been instrumental in shaping this book into the valuable resource that it is. Working with them on this project has been an enriching experience, and we commend you for your unwavering dedication to excellence.

We want to acknowledge the support and encouragement of the publishing house in bringing this book to life. Your belief in the importance of educating readers about medical tourism and your commitment to disseminating knowledge have been integral to the success of this project.

We extend our thanks to the constant support of our employers and colleagues for enabling us to complete this challenging task of preparing the assignment in available time.

To the readers, we express our deepest appreciation for your interest in this book on medical tourism. We hope that this work serves as an informative and enlightening resource for you. Your engagement with the material and your pursuit of knowledge contribute to the ongoing conversation and advancement of medical tourism as a global phenomenon.

We express our gratitude to the Almighty God for his kind blessings, wisdom and grace to keep us motivated to complete this assignment. We are wholeheartedly thankful to the support of our family members and well-wishers for allowing us sufficient time to complete the book in time.

As the editors, we must acknowledge that while we have endeavoured to make this book as comprehensive and accurate as possible, the field of medical tourism is continually evolving. New advancements, challenges and opportunities may arise beyond the publication of this book. We welcome feedback from readers to improve future editions.

In conclusion, the completion of this book on medical tourism marks the culmination of a labour of love and dedication from numerous individuals. We are deeply grateful for the opportunity to be part of this endeavour, and we sincerely hope that the insights and information shared in these pages contribute to a better understanding of medical tourism and its impact on global healthcare.

Bhupinder Chaudhary
Dinesh Bhatia
Mahesh Patel
Sunaina Singh
Sushman Sharma

Contents

Chapter 1
Medical Tourism: An Overview on the Cross-Border Care

Kanakavalli K. Kundury, K. C. Shylaja, Namitha, and H. Basavana Gowdappa

Abstract Advancements in the medical care technologies, increasing cost of care, demand and supply mismatch in healthcare services are few of the many contributing factors for the progressive growth of 'Medical Tourism' services worldwide. Along with medical care services, tourism packages are value-added services, as medical tourists will have the opportunity to visit the best tourist attractions in the destination country. As medical tourism services are comprehensive in nature, involving many stakeholders from medical and tourism industries, it is vital to understand the roles of each of the players in the industries. Thus, this book chapter focuses on explaining the concept of Medical Value Travel (MVT), factors influencing the medical tourism services, role of various stakeholders involved, along with possible concerns on the country of origin and destination while delivering the medical tourism services. Considering the significant role of regulatory affairs in offer-

K. K. Kundury (✉)
Department of Health System Management Studies, JSS Academy of Higher Education and Research, Mysuru, Karnataka, India

Special Interest Group in Patient Care Management, JSS Academy of Higher Education and Research, Mysuru, Karnataka, India
e-mail: kanakavalli.dhsms@jssuni.edu.in

K. C. Shylaja
Department of Health System Management Studies, JSS Academy of Higher Education and Research, Mysuru, Karnataka, India

Center for Distance and Online Education, JSS Academy of Higher Education and Research, Mysuru, Karnataka, India

Namitha
Center for Distance and Online Education, JSS Academy of Higher Education and Research, Mysuru, Karnataka, India

H. B. Gowdappa
Special Interest Group in Patient Care Management, JSS Academy of Higher Education and Research, Mysuru, Karnataka, India

Department of General Medicine, JSS Medical College and Hospital, JSS Academy of Higher Education and Research, Mysuru, Karnataka, India

B. Chaudhary et al. (eds.), *Medical Tourism in Developing Countries*,
https://doi.org/10.1007/978-981-99-8909-6_1

ing these services, this book chapter also highlights the blueprint of India's approach in upscaling the Medical Value Travel Services in the country.

Keywords Medical tourism · Wellness tourism · Medical value travel · Cross-border care

Abbreviations

AYUSH	Ayurveda, Yoga, Unani, Siddha and Homeopathy
EHR	Electronic health record
EMR	Electronic medical records
JCI	Joint Commission International
MVT	Medical value travel
NABH	National Accreditation Board for Hospitals
NMWTB	National Medical & Wellness Tourism Board
PPP	Public-private partnership
TPA	Third party administrators
UK	United Kingdom
USA	United States of America
USD	United States Dollar

1.1 Introduction to Medical Tourism

'Medical Tourism' in simple terms is where people travel to other countries for their healthcare needs (CDC 2022; Gaines 2019). Rapid advancements in medical care along with ever-increasing healthcare expenditure are contributing to the popularity of 'Medical Tourism' at an exponential rate (CDC 2022; Sultana et al. 2014). Though the concept of 'Medical Tourism' is not new, these services were opted earlier either due to lack of medical care availability or inaccessibility to quality care (Neil Lunt et al. 2011). Considering the current situations of growing healthcare needs, demand-supply mismatches and long waiting times for treatments, 'Medical Tourism' has become the best destination for healthcare services worldwide (Neil Lunt et al. 2011). Adding to the medical services, tourism services are bonus for medical tourists (Neil Lunt et al. 2011; Zhang et al. 2022).

According to The Medical Tourism Association, 'Medical tourism is where people who live in one country travel to another country to receive medical, dental and surgical care while at the same time receiving equal to or greater care than they would have in their own country, and because of affordability, better access to care or a higher level of quality of care' (Jeayaram Subramanian 2021). This definition makes it clear on the treatments people opt for along with various factors influencing their decision to travel for medical services.

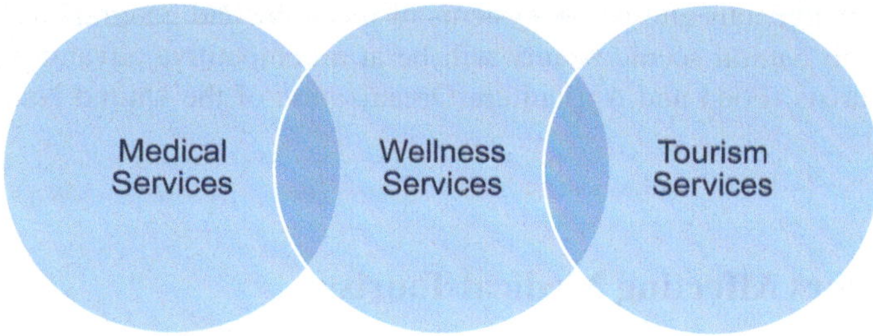

Fig. 1.1 Concept of medical value travel

1.1.1 Medical Value Travel (MVT)

Though 'Medical Tourism' and 'Wellness Tourism' are often used interchangeably, the earlier one focuses on treatments or cure of a disease/condition through cardiac surgery, organ transplantation, etc.; whereas, the latter aims at health rejuvenation or enhancing one's own physical, mental and spiritual purposes through spiritual healing, spas, stress relief, etc. (Kanjanachaiyasit 2019; Ministry of Tourism GoI 2022a) (Fig. 1.1).

Medical Tourism, also often referred to as Medical Value Travel (MVT), is an amalgamation of Medical, Wellness and Tourism services that leads to 'Medical Tourism' services (Neil Lunt et al. 2011; Ministry of Tourism GoI 2022a). This also provides wide access to alternative systems of medicine AYUSH comprising of Ayurveda, Yoga, Naturopathy, Unani, Siddha and Naturopathy services (Ministry of Tourism GoI 2022a; Rudra et al. 2017). Countries across the world are appreciating the concept of Medical Value Travel not only as a reason for improvement or restoration of health conditions but also for the economic impact on the nations hosting these services, for example, India. This is also a rich means to develop the health and tourism industries of one's own country (Ministry of Tourism GoI 2022a; Health and Federation of Indian Chambers of Commerce and Industry (FICCI) 2016).

1.2 Need for Medical Tourism

Every country, either developed or developing, tries to be self-contained in terms of its healthcare requirements (Peabody et al. 2006). However, a few of the basic factors such as cost of care, longer waiting times, and quality of medical care services have been found to influence medical tourism services to other countries (Peabody et al. 2006). Also, a few other issues including availability of procedures, accessibility to trained professionals, alternative medicine systems and advancements with cutting-edge technologies were found to create more opportunities to medical tourism services (Neil Lunt et al. 2011; Indian Institute of Tourism and Travel Management 2011). Adding to this, countries with rich heritage and culture, possessing indigenous alternative systems of medicine and geographical locations enriched with natural scenic beauty will be at a competitive advantage to attract medical tourists (Food and Agriculture Organization of the United Nations 2021) (Table 1.1).

1.3 Factors Affecting Medical Tourism

Medical tourism carries a range of benefits both directly and indirectly depending on the situations of the medical tourist. If the condition of the medical tourist is not so severe where it is needed to be immediately addressed, then he/she can have a better time getting treated in a foreign country. Though medical tourism services provide benefits of affordable care at quality standards and provide travel opportunities, there are certain factors that determine the choices of medical tourists.

The study of medical tourism is an integration of economic, social, cultural, and personal factors. It is a known fact from research that medical tourism contributes to the economic development of the destination countries (Zhong et al. 2021). It helps in creating employment opportunities, improves the existing healthcare infrastructure and improves capital turnover (Zhong et al. 2021). Also, the existing healthcare scenarios of the country of origin, health insurance coverages, standard of living and per capita income are strong social determinants that influence the consumer's decision on medical tourism (Zhong et al. 2021; Johnston et al. 2010b). Often, cultural factors also play a crucial role in opting for medical tourism services. Research shows that individuals would choose their medical tourism destinations which are culturally comparable (Zhong et al. 2021; Johnston et al. 2010b). 'Cultural competence' determines the ability of the healthcare provider to provide culturally congruent services to the patients (Zhong et al. 2021). Cultural orientations and interactions help to strengthen the doctor-patient relationship through effective communication, improve quality of care by reducing medical errors, reduce the stress among highly vulnerable foreign patients and eliminate the tolerance to face cultural differences (Johnston et al. 2010a; Zhong et al. 2021; Vovk et al. 2021).

Though medical tourism services provide a wide range of choices on medical and tourism services to the patients, few of the personal determinants such as confidentiality of information, patient privacy, safety and risk of care influence the patient's decision-making (Johnston et al. 2010a; Vovk et al. 2021). The psychological and emotional strengths of the individuals also impact their decision to choose a medical tourism destination, along with their personality traits and family factors and current state of mind (Zhong et al. 2021).

Though there are many influences on consumer decision-making of medical tourism, the two very important elements of any healthcare experience are the 'Patient' and the 'Provider'. Examining the factors from the 'Patient-Provider' perception is very essential, which influence the individual's decision-making on medical tourism (Neil Lunt et al. 2011; Oberoi and Kansra 2019).

Table 1.1 Need for medical tourism services

Lesser cost of medical care: Cost of medical care beyond one's affordability is the prime reason for opting medical tourism services (Neil Lunt et al. 2011; Simple HT-MTM Health Tourism 2022). As a known fact, medical care in developed countries is very expensive when compared to the costs in the developing countries (World Health Organization (WHO) 2019). Patients could save up to 80% of the treatment costs when travelling outside the residential country for treatment (Shifa External Services International Patients Assistance Shifa International Hospitals Ltd 2021)
No/minimum waiting time: Patients waiting for longer durations to get their treatments might cause them emotional stress and influence them psychologically (Gagliardi et al. 2021; Reichert 2018; Chu et al. 2019). It is quite common that in some countries patients have to wait for a period of one full year or more to get medical services for certain conditions (Taber and Persoskie 2015; Mosadeghrad 2014). So, they may choose to opt for medical tourism services before their medical conditions get aggravated (Mosadeghrad 2014). Often these prolonged waiting for medical services may happen due to unorganized services or lack of trained professionals (Taber and Persoskie 2015). Even then, emergency services would be given high priority rather than the elective services. Among the most developed countries of the world, Britain (60%) and Canada (57%) have the highest number of patients waiting for medical services in the world with a minimum of 4 weeks to get consultation with their doctors (Services 2017). Thus, medical tourism is the choice of the hour for patients to receive prompt treatment, without further deterioration in their health condition (Neil Lunt et al. 2011)
Quality medical care: Though there is an immediate need for treatment, quality of medical care is identified as a significant contributor while choosing the medical care services. In order to facilitate medical tourism services, hospitals across the world get their healthcare facilities accredited by international organizations such as Joint Commission International (JCI); which demonstrates the gold standard for quality in healthcare (Neil Lunt et al. 2011; Chaudhry 2020). Other international accreditation bodies include the Australian Council for Healthcare Standards, the Canadian Council on Health Services and the Society for International Healthcare Accreditation (Alkhenizan 2011). On one hand, this is required for healthcare facilities offering medical tourism services to demonstrate their quality care standards; and on the other hand, this also helps the patients to choose a particular healthcare facility offering quality care in the destination place (Sultana et al. 2014). Quality standards of hospitals help in smoothing of selection process by the individual as they would be assured on safe practices, established treatment protocols, patient monitoring during the process and after care with standards in policies and procedures (Crooks et al. 2010)
Availability of range of procedures: The range of services that are available for medical tourists include cosmetic surgery (breast, face, liposuction), dentistry (cosmetic and reconstruction), cardiac care (by-pass, valve replacement), orthopaedic surgery (hip replacement, knee replacement, joint surgeries), bariatric surgeries (gastric by-pass, gastric banding), fertility/reproductivity treatments (IVF, gender reassignment), organ transplantation services (stem cells, tissues) along with eye surgeries, diagnostics and check-ups (Neil Lunt et al. 2011; Simple HT-MTM Health Tourism 2022). To meet the patient requirements, healthcare facilities are equipping themselves with state-of-the-art facilities and expanding their range of services (Kruk et al. 2018). This product line concept of services makes it convenient for the patients to avail their treatments under one roof (Herzlinger 2016). This plays a vital role in patient choice on medical tourism destinations. If the healthcare facilities in the home country don't provide multitude of services, they would choose the same in the destination that provides comprehensive services (Neil Lunt et al. 2011)

(continued)

Table 1.1 (continued)

Accessibility to trained healthcare providers: If getting treated by the expert is the priority of the patient, then medical tourism presents the best of the choices. The patient can collect the relevant information about the specialist doctors and choose to get their treatment done through them, even if, out of the country of origin (Neil Lunt et al. 2011; Say and Thomson 2003)
Access and affordability to latest advancements: Healthcare facilities offering cutting-edge technologies and advancements in their services, and broad range of quality services, possess the competitive advantage in providing medical tourism services (Herzlinger 2016). These advanced services would captivate the patients coming from other countries. Some countries are also coming up with 'Healthcare Cities', focusing on the state-of-the-art infrastructure, wide range of medical services, quality standards, connectivity to various international airports and collaborations with reputed scientific universities and hospitals. For example, Biomedical city in Singapore, Dubai Health Care City (DHCC) (Neil Lunt et al. 2011; Dubai Healthcare City 2022; Cambridge University 2021)
Opportunity to explore various destinations: Multi-star hotels and various reputed hospitals across the globe are coordinating to offer medical and tourism services to the individuals at the destination countries (Johnston et al. 2010a). These facilities would be providing excellent service experience to the medical tourists from the early steps of counselling to choose the destination country till return back home. They would ensure the medical tourists receive excellent services at every step of encountering with the medical treatments, thereafter visiting tourist attractions; along with customer relationship management post visit (Neil Lunt et al. 2011; Johnston et al. 2010a)
No rigidity of regulatory affairs: Considering the demand for the medical tourism services across the globe, many countries across the world had liberalized their policies such as visa approvals, foreign investments and implementation to encourage this growing business (Richard Smith et al. 2015)

1.3.1 *Patient-Related Factors*

Factors that concern patients include, selection of the country, selection of the hospital and availability of the doctor. While identifying the country of destination, a patient would also consider the economic and political conditions, any natural disasters, social situations and government policies of the nation (Neil Lunt et al. 2011; Oberoi and Kansra 2019). Patients would also collect information on visa approval processes, travel and accommodation arrangements in the destination country. Once the decision on the destination country is made, then identification of a hospital begins. Few factors that influence selection process include cost of care, reputation and location of the hospital, connectivity to international and national airways, quality standards and international accreditations (Oberoi and Kansra 2019). Patients would also consider a range of medical services, care process and post-discharge follow-up as few of the other factors influencing patient's decision. Adding to that, language proficiency in the area, patient engagement and patient relationship management, and proximity to various tourist attractions also are the contributing factors to select the healthcare facility (Oberoi and Kansra 2019). While choosing a medical service, the expertise and reputation of the care provider becomes a key criterion for the patients. Also, depending on the advice of the native physician, a patient would look into international certification of doctors and healthcare teams, safety and quality of medications, service orientation and advancements in medical treatments (Oberoi and Kansra 2019). Few other considerations would also include availability of on-site pharmacies, prescription assistance, availability of doctor on-call and follow-up visits (Oberoi and Kansra 2019). Reviews and ratings on patient engagement and communication from 'first time to contact' till 'real time contact' also create an impact (Oberoi and Kansra 2019).

In identifying and selection of a care provider, often word-of-mouth reference from inner circles and families work as a magic wand for patient decision-making. Adding to these factors, the role of family/friends cannot be considered lighter for the conversion of a potential medical tourist into an active medical tourist. The opinions of the closed ones become vital during this decision process. Also, the previous experiences, references and suggestions of the dear ones become extremely important for decision-making (Alsarayreh et al. 2017; Wang et al. 2020).

1.3.2 Provider-Related Factors

Providers in this context may include the healthcare facility that offers medical care services and/or a doctor who is involved in patient care. World-class infrastructure, internationally certified and accredited healthcare facilities act as efficient marketing tools to convert potential medical tourists to active medical tourists. Infrastructure and amenities determine the advancements of medical services and patient safety (Oberoi and Kansra 2019; Alsarayreh et al. 2017). International certifications and accreditations that support quality of care and patient safety protocols also enhance confidence of medical tourists for confirmed decisions on selected destinations. Information shared by the hospitals in their websites or blogs, language used for communication, professionalism and relationship management strategies by the hospital teams will add support to medical tourist's decision for choosing the hospital (Alsarayreh et al. 2017). These factors not only influence the patient but also ease their anxiety and stress both mentally and physically to visit another nation for their medical care. A combination of these factors from the provider side stimulates medical tourism services (Oberoi and Kansra 2019). Thus, medical tourism being a trendy niche market gets positively influenced by both the patient and provider-related factors.

1.4 Medical Tourism Industry

Medical tourism is a booming industry worldwide with a large number of countries, healthcare organizations and healthcare teams actively participating in these services. It is a comprehensive care which involves many stakeholders from the medical and tourism industries. In few of the countries, medical tourism services are supported and backed up by the government like in Thailand and Malaysia, while in few countries private healthcare organizations are taking an active part (Neil Lunt et al. 2011). However, every nation has its own framework on the execution of these medical tourism services. Because of the hidden possibilities in medical tourism, several interested parties have invested their resources to explore the features efficiently, which has led to the flourishment of this industry in recent years (Kim and Kim 2019). Few of the participants in the medical tourism industry include healthcare organizations, insurance providers, brokers, mass media communicators, information technology providers, travel and accommodation agents, hospitality industry and financers (Neil Lunt et al. 2011; Kim and Kim 2019).

1.4.1 Healthcare Organizations

Healthcare organizations' preparedness in terms of incorporating quality of care standards, documentation of patient information, medication safety and follow-up care would help medical tourists to have a pleasant experience (Kácha et al. 2016). Accreditations from international agencies would add definite value to the services healthcare facilities offer.

1.4.2 The Insurers

Another important role in the process of medical tourism is of insurers. Insurance coverage of the medical services, range of cover, liabilities and premiums should be carefully attended by the medical tourist before finalizing the process (Channel 2021). Also, the identification of network of hospitals and empanelment with the insurance services has to be confirmed on priority. If not, the medical bills would end in huge numbers and the savings on the treatment would get paid back multiple times for the medical expenses (Agency for Healthcare Research and Quality (AHRQ) 2007). Exclusively for medical tourism, health and travel insurance packages are provided considering the health conditions of the patients and travel destinations (Neil Lunt et al. 2011). Identifying the depth of the medical tourism services, health insurance companies across the world started to research cross-border and international medical coverage (Neil Lunt et al. 2011). The aim of the insurance plans is that people can visit any country for their medical treatments mentioned in their policy, where their medical expenses can get reimbursed either fully or partially based on the policy terms and conditions. As an add-on, few of these companies also offer waivers on out-of-pocket expenditures and coverage including the travel expenses of the individual and/or the travel companion. To further strengthen the synergy and enhance policy holder's satisfaction, the insurance companies are also tying up with reputed hospitals and collaborating with renowned physicians across the world (Agency for Healthcare Research and Quality (AHRQ) 2007). In fact, strengthening their network in multiple nations, many of the insurance companies are proposing insurance schemes to many organizations for supporting their employee wellbeing and healthcare through medical tourism.

For example, Aetna, one of the well-known healthcare management companies in America, had made collaborations with Apollo Hospitals, India to establish an insurance plan for Americans to receive healthcare treatment at the hospital. It sends the employees of its client, Serigraph Inc., to Apollo Hospital for specific routine procedures and then to its network of JCI-accredited clinics. This plan includes travel and accommodation along with healthcare services (Medical Tourism Magazine 2022a).

1.4.3 Travel and Accommodation Facilities

Next another important contributor to medical tourism is travel and accommodation. It is obvious that patients and families travelling to other countries for medical services would also focus on logistics such as transportation, accommodation, food services, shopping and tourist activities (Medical Tourism Magazine 2022b). Adding to this, the culture prevailing in the destination country and experience during the service delivery process (before, during and after) also impact the mindset of the individuals. A comprehensive medical tourism destination should position themselves with comfortable accommodations, amenities and services required for a pleasant customer experience (Medical Tourism Magazine 2022b).

It is a fact that hospitals would usually prefer to shorten the length of stay of their patients for cost savings and control the spread of nosocomial infections (Curtis 2008). However, if they are accommodating the medical tourists, hospitals are in great demand to create an ambience that look no less than start hotel and offer standard stay arrangements to satisfy their customers. This creates cost pressures to hospitals, which makes them to collaborate with star hotels in close proximity or at least within the vicinity (Neil Lunt et al. 2011; Medical Tourism Magazine 2022b). This provides an opportunity to hospitality industry to build hotels with attractive infrastructures and amenities that fulfil the comforts of medical tourists. This is thus an appetite-filling strategy for both hospitals and hotels, where both the parties can get into a memorandum of understanding, or house the services in the same building with innovative designs and services working under the same ownership. Few certain provisions that are required for hotels accommodating international patients include adjustable beds, nursing call systems with bedside controls, bathroom facilities with hand railings and facilities fulfilling family needs (Medical Tourism Magazine 2022b). These stay services can also plan for the overall stay of the medical tourists and accompanying family members from the time of pickup from the airport till their departure. They can also plan to arrange for travel log with the local agencies.

1.4.4 The Individuals

It is evident that in this process of medical tourism, there are many people involved from various segments of services. These individuals have their own unique role to play along every step of medical tourist. Medical tourism agents are the individuals or companies who would assist the medical tourist in the selection of a hospital, travel plan, tourism and sightseeing (Khan et al. 2016). They would bring the prospective medical tourist seeking a medical service to interact with a service provider (a hospital or doctor). These agencies would facilitate or develop medical tourism services. While few of hospitals themselves do offer medical tourism services as a separate specialty, few of these get outsourced to an agency. These organizations could be operating in a single country or multinational as well. Medical tourists would look for these agencies to provide information about range and quality of services, safety and ethical practices, and legal issues if any (Khan et al. 2016). So, the excellence of these services depends to a large extent on the professionalism of individuals while encountering medical tourists. Considering the high demand of these services and estimating the future growth demand for trained professionals, various agencies are also coming with certification programs in medical travel profession (Ruka and Garel 2015; Global Healthcare Accreditation 2022). This professional building is required for the standardization of the medical tourism industry by seamless integration of quality, safety and top-notch services throughout the customer touchpoints (Ruka and Garel 2015). In fact, many medical tourism companies across the world are working with healthcare clusters to develop these services and standardize the practices for quality care. The American Medical Association is in the lead to partner with various universities and educational institutions for professional certification of medical travel to promote best practices and better evolution of services.

1.4.5 Information and Technology Services

In this era of digitalization, access and availability to information & technology has already come to the fingertips of the user. Communication channels through mass media, websites, customer reviews and blogs are bringing more transparency in business operations like never before. A prospective medical tourist would use the internet as the first option for information search (Ruka and Garel 2015). So, organizations involved in medical tourism services including the middle man and agencies should ensure to provide reliable, authentic and genuine information in their websites (Ruka and Garel 2015). Also, as excellence in services would be expressed through customer reviews, ensure to maintain the user review blogs and testimonials as an assurance to opt for the services. Along with this, if healthcare organizations have integrated technological advancements like Electronic Medical Record (EMR) systems or Electronic Health Record (EHR) systems and cloud storage systems, that would help in portability of information binding to the legal issues of the destination country (Neil Lunt et al. 2011; Ruka and Garel 2015).

Hospitals can also come up with integration of health services with technology through smart applications that can be accessed from the smartphones of the patients (Ventola 2014). These applications can facilitate direct patient access to their medical information, just a click away, though the patient is accommodated elsewhere outside the healthcare facility (Ventola 2014). Also, as a joint effort, hospitals and hotels can also deploy patient monitoring systems and biosensors as efficient tools for continuous monitoring of patients. But healthcare organizations have to ensure to maintain information confidentiality by having standard security protocols to control patient information flow in the network (Neil Lunt et al. 2011).

1.4.6 Banks and Financial Institutions

In order to execute this process, banks and financial institutions can also collaborate with hospitals and hotels to facilitate the medical expenses of the tourists. Financial strength is required not just for the medical tourists, also for the healthcare facilities and hotels to upgrade their services in meeting the international requirements. Thus, these financial institutions have a huge role to play (Neil Lunt et al. 2011). Investments, loans, shares and debentures are various ways in which these monetarists can support medical tourism services, which have the stamina to produce huge returns in foreign currency (Neil Lunt et al. 2011).

1.5 Concerns Pertaining to Medical Tourism

Though there is lot of information and literature available on medical tourism services, consider the ‘distance’ as a factor, few issues that concern patients are quality, safety and risks associated with the medical services. Standardization of medical tourism regulatory affairs, transparency of information, quality evaluation mechanisms for hospitals and healthcare providers are required to increase the number of medical travellers (Kim and Kim 2019). An element of risk is obvious considering the process of medical tourism; which could include travel risk, health risk, worsening of medical conditions due to international travel and post-discharge care (Kim and Kim 2019).

1.5.1 Patient Satisfaction

Patient satisfaction is of paramount importance to any healthcare facility or provider; also, a very important quality indicator of services provided. Satisfaction of patients on medical tourism services would depend on many confounding factors. Patient clinical outcomes and satisfaction cannot be tagged together and satisfaction on clinical services depends on the type of service they opted for (Neil Lunt et al. 2011). For example, dental treatments and cosmetic surgeries, as patients might also experience certain psychological distresses during the process which could impact their level of satisfaction. Thus, there exists a gap between patient's expectations and satisfaction, as satisfaction is determined by multiple factors.

1.5.2 Clinical Outcomes

Medical tourism aims for good clinical results at affordable costs. However, the immediate results of medical services might be satisfactory, but patient follow-up by doctors is unsure. This leads to the post-service complication redressal by the local physicians along with additional expenses from the patient's pocket (Neil Lunt et al. 2011). Adding to this is the disruption to regular care from the local care provider when medical care is sought abroad. It is important for a patient to go through the complete cycle of medical care stages, pre till post services. Once the destination country is confirmed, then information about the existing climatic conditions and disease ecosystem should be collected. So that the patient can get counselled by the local physician to take measures on pre-existing disease conditions, any medications prior to the travel can be taken as a preparation for the visit. The tourist may also become ill due to a cause not related to the primary reason or might develop side effects or complications related to the treatment, which will be addressed by the attending clinician (Neil Lunt et al. 2011). It is better if patients become aware of any complications further developed or long-term effects of the procedure, if any, might have to be addressed by the medical care system at the home country.

1.5.3 Patient Confidentiality

As continuity of care becomes important in medical tourism, patient data access through cross-border healthcare facilities becomes important, which poses a concern to patient confidentiality of information (Mutalib et al. 2016). This is of greater concern to those people who opt for medical tourism as a solution to get their medical conditions treated confidentially in a foreign country. Patient's details including travel, medical and accommodation information are needed to be accessed by many parties such as travel guides, insurance companies, and healthcare providers (Ruka

1.6.1.2 Other Repercussions

Continuous travel of medical tourism also would create a trend for large numbers to follow the path and encourage citizens to avail low-cost medical services at a foreign nation. While outsourcing the high-cost services would result in reduced revenue generation and also the development of local services (Neil Lunt et al. 2011). These changes would again create pressure for investors in the field of medical technologies. This demand for medical tourism services may also send signals of poor policy-making in the country of origin (Pocock and Phua 2011). Individuals who cannot afford to travel can consider themselves at disadvantageous position for not able to get the treatments either at the source country (due to high costs) or at a foreign nation (unaffordability to care), resulting in the low morale. If planned properly, source country can have policies to collaborate with the healthcare systems in destination country establishing a bilateral system (Neil Lunt et al. 2011; Pocock and Phua 2011). This would create a win-win financial opportunity for both the nations in terms of outsourcing to destination country, resulting in cost savings for the citizens of the home country. Source nations would also build the morale of their citizens as they create concern for the countries' healthcare systems by strengthening the 'collective' medical travel policies (Pocock and Phua 2011).

1.6.1.3 Pressure on Local Healthcare Systems

Export of medical tourism services could also indirectly hint the inefficiency of the existing medical systems which would also create restricted entry barriers for some medical systems. The development of medical tourism can create competitive pressure on the medical systems outsourcing the services to overseas to lower down the treatment costs offered in the country of origin (Horowitz et al. 2007). Medical tourism helps the nation's economy to maximize their competitive advantage in labour costs, technology or capacity.

1.6.2 Implications on the Country of Destination

Medical tourism historically has been from lower to higher-income countries and consists of better healthcare facilities with professionally trained care providers. Many countries in the world are coming with hubs or healthcare cities of medical excellence that attract medical tourists regionally (Dubai Healthcare City 2022). Many countries participate in medical tourism as both exporters and importers or both. Many of the issues are genuine to many of the destination countries, irrespective of the economic development at different magnitudes (Cambridge University 2021).

1.6.2.1 Economic Impacts

Medical tourism will undoubtedly enhance the economic growth of the destination country by bringing in direct foreign exchange (Ruka and Garel 2015). These foreign currencies at the hospital level help in capital formation, clearing of debts or to expand their range of clinical services. Also, the revenue generated from medical tourism through publicly funded healthcare facilities can be reinvested into the national systems (Ruka and Garel 2015). Some destination countries also seek medical tourists in order to develop facilities for better serving of local patients. Destination countries should also confirm if the foreign patients are an addition to the domestic patients using the spare capacity or utilizing the local resources as substitutes (Neil Lunt et al. 2011). It has to be noted that the income generated from medical tourism is not just health income but also tourist income. Nations aiming to promote their medical tourism services can strengthen their countries' private healthcare infrastructure by offering them tax benefits (Neil Lunt et al. 2011).

The hospitality and travel industries also benefit to some extent from increased medical tourists, and taxed income on the revenue thus generated can support the domestic public health system. Few of the costs involved in the preparedness for medical tourism at the destination country include infrastructural investments such as telecommunications and roads, accreditation of healthcare facilities and any other facilities to attract medical tourists (Neil Lunt et al. 2011).

1.6.2.2 Adopting the Best Practices

Medical tourism leads to the diffusion of technologies across the world adopting the best practices. It enhances the ability to purchase and use the best of the latest medical technology. Serving the foreign patients would help in better training of manpower in the destination country and adopt the best practices, thereby enhancing the quality of care to domestic patients (Aluttis et al. 2014). Broadened case-mix would train the staff and enhance the human capital leading to compliance with international standards for care. This also promotes a culture of personal development in enhancing skills and technical knowledge to treat the general public. In this context, there is also a possibility of misusing domestic resources by investing in private hospitals or investments diverted to urban tertiary care centres from rural primary health centres allotted for general public needs (Neil Lunt et al. 2011). There could also be conditional utilization of resources associated with medical tourists than those with the local population, for example high technology dental and reproductive care. It is not sure if the proportion of private or public hospitals serving medical tourists only gets accredited or as well the healthcare facilities catering to the domestic population (Aluttis et al. 2014).

1.6.2.3 Reverse Brain Drain

As medical tourism is a potential revenue-fetching service, taking advantage of this, many healthcare facilities are attracting back their home countries' healthcare workforce force who work overseas (Neil Lunt et al. 2011). These facilities can afford to offer competitive salary packages and working conditions comparable to overseas facilities. This strategy has the dual advantage of convincing the medical tourists to get treated with internationally trained doctors and also potential human resources are brought back home (Ruka and Garel 2015). Uncertainty exists if these trained professionals cater services to international patients or extend it to domestic population as well. Looking at the lucrative situation, there is a possibility of care providers working at public health facilities to migrate to private hospitals serving medical tourism patients, leading to internal brain drain (Neil Lunt et al. 2011).

1.6.2.4 Impact on Health Systems

Considering the benefit of medical tourism, healthcare system could be re-constituted, where foreign patients benefit from sophisticated private hospitals with state-of-the-art infrastructure and advanced medical technology; whereas the local population has access only to basic health resources (Neil Lunt et al. 2011). Also, there is a chance for unequal distribution of healthcare resources to facilities treating domestic people and foreign patients.

As the above sections provide an overview on Medical Tourism Services, the following sections of this book chapter provide a summary of recent strategies to be adopted by the Indian government for facilitating Medical Tourism Services. Similar framework can be adopted by countries with tailor-made modifications to fit their medical requirements.

1.7 Contemporary Approaches in Medical and Wellness Tourism in Developing Countries

India is one of the rapidly developing countries implementing several strategies to promote medical tourism services. Hence, in this section of book chapter, an overview on the contemporary approaches adopted by the Indian government is discussed. As per the report released in January 2022 from The Ministry of Tourism, Government of India, it is stated that India is one of the top-rated destinations for medical tourism services (Ministry of Tourism GoI 2022b). It was ranked in the 7th position with 56 million trips in medical and wellness tourisms with 16.3 billion US dollars of total revenue as estimated by Global Wellness Tourism. Maintaining healthcare facilities with high-end medical services equipped with technological advancements offering medical care at international quality standards at relatively much low cost has made India a much-appreciated destination for medical tourists. One another reason includes the accessibility to integrated indigenous systems of medicine through AYUSH-Ayurveda, Yoga, Unani, Siddha and Homeopathy, focused on traditional therapies. There is surge in the number of medical tourists visiting India from 4.3 lacs in 2016 to 7 lacs in 2019 with an approximate market size of ~5–6 billion USD. India currently consisted of 29 JCI-accredited hospitals located across different parts of the country. These facilities are located in Tier1 cities which have the necessary infrastructural facilities connecting the international airports, roadways and waterways along with the required telecommunication networks.

1.7.1 India's Strategy for Medical Tourism

Identifying the potential of Medical Tourism, otherwise known as Medical Value Travel (MVT), Government of India had aimed to accelerate these services considering it as one of the objectives of Aatmanirbhar Bharat. 'Aatmanirbhar Bharat' which means 'Self-Reliant India' is a phrase used by the Prime Minister of India, Narendra Modi and his government with respect to the country's economic development by being more efficient, competitive and resilient and playing a large role in the world economy. India has come up with a national strategy aiming at facilitating institutional framework, strengthening medical ecosystem and creating a brand with assured quality of services.

Vision Statement
'To position India as a sustainable and responsible medical and wellness tourism destination'.

Mission Statement
'To create a robust framework and synergy amongst the Ministries of Central Government and State Governments and Private Sector for promoting India as a Medical and Wellness tourism destination through a dedicated agency to promote Medical and wellness tourism in India'.

SWOT Matrix
Having confidence in the existing strengths to offer medical tourism and foreseeing the potential opportunities, strategies to face the threats posed and overcoming the weaknesses, India's national strategy for Medical Value Travel is progressing forward (Fig. 1.2).

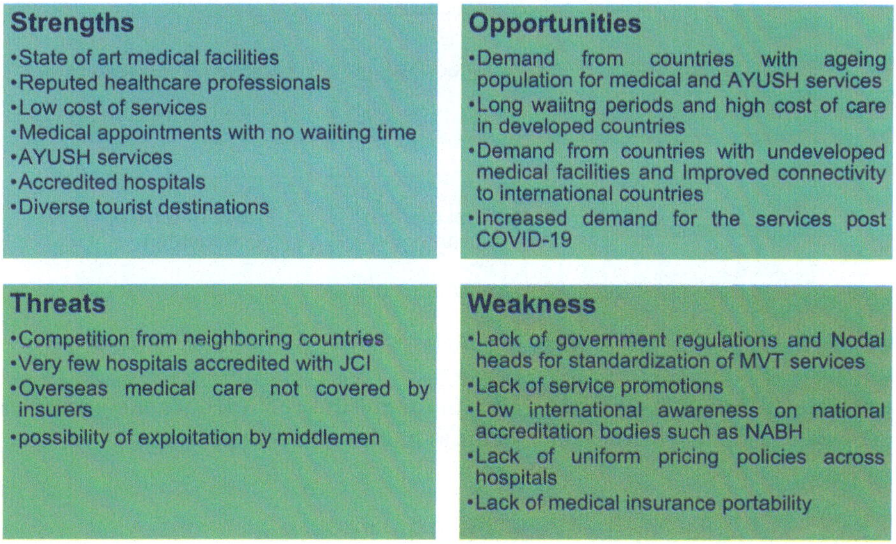
Strengths
•State of art medical facilities
•Reputed healthcare professionals
•Low cost of services
•Medical appointments with no waiiting time
•AYUSH services
•Accredited hospitals
•Diverse tourist destinations
Opportunities
•Demand from countries with ageing population for medical and AYUSH services
•Long waiitng periods and high cost of care in developed countries
•Demand from countries with undeveloped medical facilities and Improved connectivity to international countries
•Increased demand for the services post COVID-19
Threats
•Competition from neighboring countries
•Very few hospitals accredited with JCI
•Overseas medical care not covered by insurers
•possibility of exploitation by middlemen
Weakness
•Lack of government regulations and Nodal heads for standardization of MVT services
•Lack of service promotions
•Low international awareness on national accreditation bodies such as NABH
•Lack of uniform pricing policies across hospitals
•Lack of medical insurance portability

Fig. 1.2 SWOT analysis of India's medical value travel

1.7.2 Stakeholders Involved

Key stakeholders involved in the medical tourism for promotional activities and process standardization include central ministries, state governments, healthcare industry, industry associations, medical tourism facilitators, travel and hospitality industries.

The roles of each of these participating parties are crucial for the success of the national strategy on Medical Value Travel.

India's National Strategy for Medical Value Travel (Fig. 1.3)

1.7.3 'Heal in India': Branding for India's Medical Value Travel

Along with campaigning to India's tourist destinations through 'Incredible India', there is an urgent need to promote its high expertise in modern medical sciences and alternative systems of medicine AYUSH for medical and wellness tourisms. As the best of both the disciplines, the country offers holistic healthcare services under the brand 'Heal in India' with industry partnerships. This brand thus gets promoted as a part of Incredible India on all the government digital platforms and campaigns; thereby getting into arrangements with corporate organizations for collaborating

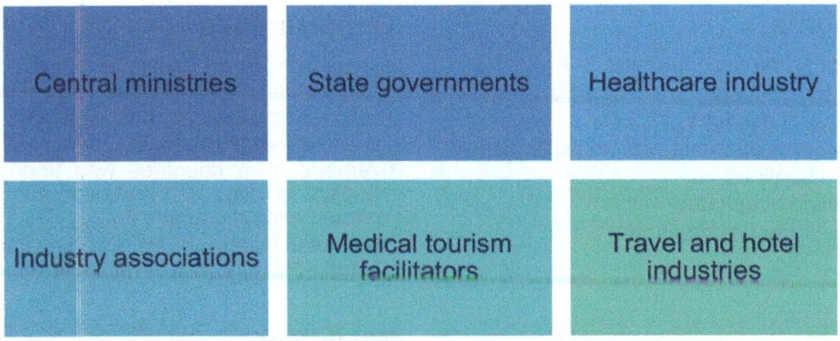

Fig. 1.3 Stakeholders involved in India's medical value travel

with various foreign governments. The Ministry of Tourism will be creating schemes to market and attract Medical and Wellness tourism providers to India.

1.7.3.1 Strengthening the Medical Tourism Ecosystem

Medical Value Travel Ecosystem comprises of hosts of service providers, facilitators, airways, hotels, regulatory authorities and government. Strengthening of linkages and coordination between all these parties, establishing regulatory framework for execution of medical tourism services, defining the roles and responsibilities of individual stakeholders and promoting partnerships are required for marketing of the services.

1.7.3.2 MVT Facilitator Associations

Government is going forward to establish MVT facilitator associations, where the facilitators can get registered as members. With the help of government, these association helps in professional training and capacity building, also assist governments in policy formulations and regulations, and addressal of difficulties encountered by the facilitators. Based upon the performance of the facilitators, they get categorized into Gold, Silver and Platinum categories, which help in transparency with foreign patients and with the other stakeholders.

1.7.3.3 NABH Accreditation

After a considerable number of years of operation, it is mandatory that these facilitators should get themselves accredited with NABH to ensure that certain quality standards in the care delivery are maintained. Also, to make the pre- and post-operative care coordination comfortable, government is also planning to integrate Telemedicine services for consultation and promotion of MVT services.

1.7.3.4 Portability of Health Insurance

Health insurance portability is an important step towards promoting MVT services. Government is planning to establish a framework where joint ventures can be made between MVT industry and Indian insurance companies. To approach foreign insurance companies currently active in the country to include Indian hospitals in their empanelled list of network hospitals. Also, to consider the possibility of including Indian health insurance companies in global markets, thereby operating through the Third Party Administrators (TPAs) can be explored.

1.7.4 Developing Medical Enclaves and Special Wellness Tourism Zones

Establishing exclusive townships for MVT services with world-class infrastructures, imported equipments, state-of-the-art medical advancements and medical care with cutting-edge technologies will provide a competitive advantage to Indian markets. AYUSH system of services can be located at spiritually significant places. These establishments are proposed to operate in Public-Private-Partnership (PPP) modes and long-term debt needs to be further explored. While state governments take the lead on the development of these special zones, central governments provide necessary assistance for infrastructural development. The Ministry of Tourism will also assess and rank the States and Destinations to encourage progressive competitiveness in the development of MVT services.

1.7.5 Organizing the Medical Service Providers

All the medical care providers will be registering their details with the respective portal to make them visible to the source markets. For the standardization of care charges, the healthcare facilities will also be ranked based on the quality-of-care standards and range of services, which helps the international patients to choose hospitals based on the requirements. The registered hospitals should also be publishing the clinical outcomes for various services on their websites with periodic statistical information on number of procedures, mortality and morbidity rates and audit information to benchmark the performance with providers at top destinations. Hospitals may also provide approximate price ranges for various services, to prevent foreign patient exploitation by middlemen. As value-added services, patient assistance can be provided through designated facilitators for addressing their queries on medical expenses, travel, data management and language barriers.

1.7.6 'MVT Portal: One Stop Solution' for International Patients

Medical Value Travel portal will get synergized with the Incredible India website, to support international patients in the entire process of MVT to India. It helps them to search, plan, pre-book and pay services along with post-procedure services. It will facilitate end-to-end mapping of industry players and stakeholders involved throughout the process. The key features of the portal include individual login accounts to every stakeholder; data capturing from international patients, services provided by facilitators and hospitals; capturing industry data for better decision-making and continuous assistance for ensuring strict regulations; capturing feedback and rating the services on user experiences.

1.7.7 Service Accessibility Through Policy Liberalization

India already provides electronic VISA (e-VISA) services to make medical travelling easy. Continuing further this gets liberalized to bring a holistic and transparent process to make MVT a pleasant and comfortable experience. It is also planning for better air-connectivity with several countries, to support the health conditions of foreign travellers seeking intensive medical care to reach their favourite destination, India, with no break journey. Designated helpdesks or MVT lounges at airports would assist the foreign travellers through immigration claims, baggage transfers, hosting till their departure to the next destinations, informing them about Do's and Don'ts during their stay. These helpdesks will be responsible to capture the traveller's complete details along with the information pertaining to their health condition, treatment sought and name of the service provider and facilitator. They will also help the patients to connect with the facilitators or service providers thus eliminating the unorganized third parties.

1.7.8 Governance and Institutional Framework

The National Medical & Wellness Tourism Board (NMWTB) is established by The Ministry of Tourism in 2015 to provide an institutional framework on the promotion of Medical Value Travel services in India including Allopathy and AYUSH systems of medicines in an organized manner. The board focuses on the amalgamation of patient-centric and tourist-centric approach by bringing all the stakeholders onto the platform and acting as a 'One Stop Centre' for the promotion, development, facilitation, networking, regulation and grievance redressal for MVT services in India.

Key functions of the board include:

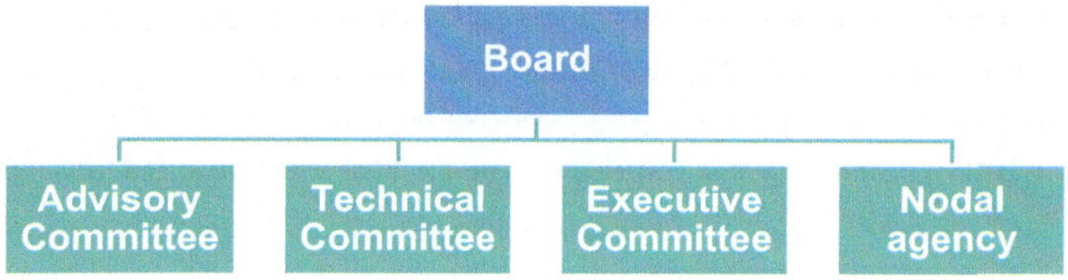

Fig. 1.4 The national medical and wellness tourism board structure

- Providing a common platform for exchange of ideas, strategies and recommendations from all the key stakeholders
- The Board in consultation with the National Accreditation Board for Hospitals (NABH) and other stakeholders develop quality of care standards to ensure the trust and confidence of the medical tourists
- To provide government incentives and subsidies to those facilitators and hospitals abiding by the regulations of MVT and levy penalties on those who violate the same
- Brand building through 'Heal in India' campaign by arranging for seminars, conferences, exhibitions and networking events
- Develop and maintain MVT web portal and databases with details of various stakeholders, hospitals, AYUSH clinics and companies, hotel services, etc.
- Connecting all stakeholders in a retail chain to offer comprehensive MVT services as a complete package
- Coordinating and facilitating any other service with regard to MVT for further promotion and development of this sector

Board Structure (Fig. 1.4)

The advisory committee contain representation from relevant ministries and states potential of conducting MVT. It will also comprise of members representing industry associations, healthcare industry, MVT facilitators, airlines and hotels. The technical team includes experts to sort out grievance issues and quality concerning matters; whereas the executives are responsible for approving various initiatives and implementation of projects. Nodal agency extends its full support to the Board for the implementation of various projects through the funds allotted for the same, and promotes India's brand for MVT services internationally. State governments can also establish a Board focusing on the conduct of MVT services and a dedicated cell in their tourism operations serving the requirements of MVT.

1.7.9 Action Plan-Way Forward

With the above institutional framework and guidelines, the Ministry of Tourism will head forward to a detailed action plan in consultation with concerned central and state ministries; industrial relations and stakeholders for the implementation of the strategy. The plan thus made will be reviewed by the Board for execution thereafter. State governments prepare individualized policies specific to their state and in alignment with the centre policies and propose action plans for the development of MVT. The Ministry extends the required support and guidance for the same.

1.8 Summary and Conclusions

'Medical Tourism' has definite stamina to increase healthcare accessibility and affordability to the world. These services, though are not new to the world, their utility has increased in recent times as never before. Increasing healthcare costs, substandard quality of care, unavailability of specialist doctors, and poor healthcare infrastructures are some of the reasons influencing people to opt these services. As an added benefit to the services, foreign patients after medical procedures also get the opportunity to visit the tourist places in the destination country. Though there are few risks associated with these services for both the participating countries, implementing regulations for standardization of practices would bring in uniformity across. Definite guidelines considering the operational activities of these services give the way forward for Medical Value Travel across the world. Governments of various nations have already drafted policy books for the execution of Medical Value Travel; including medical and wellness services. However, continuous efforts and constant monitoring for the implementation of policies determine the success of the Medical Tourism services.

1.9 Future Directions

Exploring the possibilities associated with medical tourism industry, the below can be considered as an extension to the current work:

- Operational feasibility of regulatory frameworks on medical tourism services can be conducted by comparing the guidelines across various nations.
- As competent and qualified healthcare teams are vital for the success of medical tourism services, recruitment and retention strategies of competent workforce can be studied.
- India having its own indigenous systems of medicines and being the hub of various cultures and traditions, there is a need to explore the avenues for marketing and promotion of medical tourism services worldwide.
- Taking advantage of medical value travel opportunities, India possesses, awareness on NABH accreditation for Medical Value Travel facilitator can be conducted. So that the hospitals located in convenient geographical locations with rich tourist attractions can get their facilities accredited for international visibility.

Acknowledgements We acknowledge the Leaders, JSS Academy of Higher Education and Research and thank them for providing us the opportunity and the resources required for drafting this book chapter. We extend our thanks to Dr. H. Basavana Gowdappa, Leader, Special Interest Group in Patient Care Management, JSS Academy of Higher Education and Research for empowering us to take up this project. We thank our families for all their unconditional support in making this writing happen.

References

Agency for Healthcare Research and Quality (AHRQ) (2007) Questions and answers about health insurance. Report No. AHRQ Publication No. 07-0043. Available from: www.ahrq.gov

Alkhenizan A (2011) Impact of accreditation on the quality of healthcare services: a systematic review of the literature. Ann Saudi Med 31(4):407–416

Alsarayreh A et al (2017) A study of the determinants influencing customer satisfaction in the medical tourism industry in Jordan. Int Rev Manag Mark 7(3):349–356

Aluttis C, Bishaw T, Frank MW (2014) The workforce for health in a globalized context-global shortages and international migration. Glob Health Action 7:23611

Cambridge University (2021) Singapore's biomedical cluster. Lessons from two decades of innovation and manufacturing policy. Available from https://www.ciip.group.cam.ac.uk/

CDC (2022) Medical tourism: travel to another country for medical care: U.S. Department of Health & Human Services. https://wwwnc.cdc.gov/travel/page/medical-tourism

Channel BH (2021) Medical tourism and insurance. Department of Health, State Government of Victoria, Australia. Available from https://www.betterhealth.vic.gov.au/health/healthyliving/medical-tourism

Chaudhry S (2020) Dynamics of medical tourism in India. IP Int J Aesth Health Rejuven 3(2):52–56

Chu H, Westbrook RA, Njue-Marendes S et al (2019) The psychology of the wait time experience – what clinics can do to manage the waiting experience for patients: a longitudinal, qualitative study. BMC Health Serv Res 19:459

Crooks VA, Kingsbury P, Snyder J (2010) What is known about the patient's experience of medical tourism? A scoping review. BMC Health Serv Res 10:266

Curtis LT (2008) Prevention of hospital-acquired infections: review of non-pharmacological interventions. J Hosp Infect 69(3):204–219. https://doi.org/10.1016/j.jhin.2008.03.018

Dubai Healthcare City (2022) Discover Dubai Healthcare City. Available from https://www.dhcc.ae/

Food and Agriculture Organization of the United Nations (2021) Mountain tourism – towards a more sustainable path. World Tourism Organization, Rome

Gagliardi AR, Irish J, Wright FC, Rubin B, Ross H, Green R, Abbey S, McAndrews MP, Stewart DE (2021) The psychological burden of waiting for procedures and patient-centred strategies that could support the mental health of wait-listed patients and caregivers during the COVID-19 pandemic: a scoping review. Health Expect 24(3):978–990

Gaines J (2019) Medical tourism. In: Keystone JS (ed) Travel medicine, 4th edn. Elsevier, Amsterdam, pp 371–375

Global Healthcare Accreditation (2022) Certified medical travel professional. Available from https://www.globalhealthcareaccreditation.com/professionals-home

Health and Federation of Indian Chambers of Commerce and Industry (FICCI) (2016) Medical value travel in India enhancing value in MVT

Herzlinger RE (2016) Why innovation in health care is so hard. Harvard Business Review, Brighton. Available from https://hbr.org/2006/05/why-innovation-in-health-care-is-so-hard

Horowitz MD, Rosensweig JA, Jones CA (2007) Medical tourism: globalization of the healthcare marketplace. MedGenMed 9(4):33

Indian Institute of Tourism and Travel Management (2011) A study of problems and challenges faced by medical tourists visiting India
Jeayaram Subramanian HV (2021) Medical tourism: trade and business opportunities between Oceania and India. https://doi.org/10.4018/978-1-7998-4126-5.ch008
Johnston R, Snyder J, Kingsbury P (2010a) What is known about the effects of medical tourism in destination and departure countries? A scoping review. Int J Equity Health 9:24
Johnston R, Crooks VA, Snyder J et al (2010b) What is known about the effects of medical tourism in destination and departure countries? A scoping review. Int J Equity Health 9:24
Kácha O, McCarthy C, Schuurmans AA, Dobyns C, Haller E, Hinrichs S, Ruggeri K (2016) An approach to establishing international quality standards for medical travel. Front Public Health 4:29
Kanjanachaiyasit Y (2019) Medical tourism–the scoping review. IOSR J Bus Manag 21(3):1–8
Khan MJ, Chelliah S, Haron MS (2016) International patients' travel decision making process- a conceptual framework. Iran J Public Health 45(2):134–145
Kim S, Kim I (2019) Critical success factors of medical tourism: the case of South Korea. Int J Environ Res Public Health 16:24
Kruk ME, Arsenault C, Jordan K, Leslie HH (2018) High-quality health systems in the sustainable development goals era: time for a revolution. Lancet Glob Health 6(11):e1196–e1252
Medical Tourism Magazine (2022a). Insurers changing the game in medical tourism. Available from https://www.magazine.medicaltourism.com/article/insurers-changing-game-medical-tourism
Medical Tourism Magazine (2022b) The role of hotel industry in medical & wellness tourism. Available from https://www.magazine.medicaltourism.com/article/the-role-of-hotel-industry-in-medical-wellness-tourism
Ministry of Tourism GoI (2022a) National strategy and roadmap for medical and wellness tourisrn. In: Medical tourism. Government of India, New Delhi
Ministry of Tourism GoI (2022b) National strategy and roadmap for medical and wellness tourism. Report No.: NT 703/1/2020 NT
Mosadeghrad AM (2014) Factors influencing healthcare service quality. Int J Health Policy Manag 26(2):77–89
Mutalib NSA, Ming LC et al (2016) Medical tourism: ethics, risks and benefits. Indian J Pharm Educ Res 50:2
Neil Lunt RS, Exworthy M, Green ST, Horsfall D, Mannion R (2011) Medical tourism: treatments, markets and health system implications: a scoping review. Directorate for Employment, Labour and Social Affairs, London
Oberoi S, Kansra P (2019) Factors influencing medical tourism in India: a critical review. SAMVAD SIBM Pune Res J XVII:28–37
Peabody JW et al (2006) Improving the quality of care in developing countries, 2nd edn. The World Bank, Washington
Pocock NS, Phua KH (2011) Medical tourism and policy implications for health systems: a conceptual framework from a comparative study of Thailand, Singapore and Malaysia. Glob Health 7:12
Reichert A (2018) The impact of waiting time on patient outcomes: evidence from early intervention in psychosis services in England. Health Econ 27(11):1772–1787
Richard Smith CB, Mirza Z, Beyer P, Drager N (2015) Trade and health: towards building a national strategy. World Health Organization, Geneva
Rudra S, Kalra A, Kumar A, Joe W (2017) Utilization of alternative systems of medicine as health care services in India: evidence on AYUSH care from NSS 2014. PLoS One 12(5):e0176916. https://doi.org/10.1371/journal.pone.0176916
Ruka E, Garel P (2015) Medical tourism. HOPE European Hospital and Healthcare Federation. Available from: www.hope.be
Say RE, Thomson R (2003) The importance of patient preferences in treatment decisions-challenges for doctors. BMJ 327(7414):542–545. https://doi.org/10.1136/bmj.327.7414.542

Services MH (2017) Long waiting times? Medical tourism can save you. Available from: http://www.medhalt.com/blog/long-waiting-time-medical-tourism

Shifa External Services International Patients Assistance Shifa International Hospitals Ltd (2021) 10 reasons why medical tourism is becoming popular around the world. Available from https://shifainternationalpatients.com/blog/10-reasons-why-medical-tourism-is-becoming-popular-around-the-world/

Simple HT-MTM Health Tourism (2022) Medical tourism made simple. Medical tourism benefits and advantages. Available from https://www.health-tourism.com/medical-tourism/benefits/

Song P (2010) Biotech pilgrims and the transnational quest for stem cell cures. Med Anthropol 29:384–402

Sultana S, Momen A, Yasmin F (2014) Factors affecting the attractiveness of medical tourism destination: an empirical study on India. Iran J Public Health 7(43):867–876

Taber JM, Persoskie A (2015) Why do people avoid medical care? A qualitative study using national data. J Gen Intern Med 30(3):290–297

Ventola CL (2014) Mobile devices and apps for health care professionals: uses and benefits. P T 39(5):356–364

Vovk V, Beztelesna L, Pliashko O (2021) Identification of factors for the development of medical tourism in the world. Int J Environ Res Public Health 18(21):11205. https://doi.org/10.3390/ijerph182111205

Wang A et al (2020) Exploring key factors of medical tourism and its relation with tourism attraction and re-visit intention. Cogent Soc Sci 6:1746108

World Health Organization (WHO) (2019) Countries are spending more on health, but people are still paying too much out of their own pockets. Available from https://www.who.int/news/item/20-02-2019-countries-are-spending-more-on-health-but-people-are-still-paying-too-much-out-of-their-own-pockets

World Health Organization (WHO): Europe (2014) Migration and health: key issues refugees and migrants: common health problems. Available from: https://www.euro.who.int/

Zhang D, Yan Y, Liao M et al (2022) How to evaluate surgical tourism service organizations in China: indicators system development and a pilot application. Glob Health Res Policy 7:26

Zhong L, Morrison AM, Coca-Stefaniak JA, Yang L (2021) Medical, health and wellness tourism research-a review of the literature (1970-2020) and research agenda. Int J Environ Res Public Health 18:18

Chapter 2
Amalgamation of Healthcare and Hospitality

Averil Rebello, Divya Rao, N. Shalini, and H. K. Mamatha

Abstract In recent years, the convergence of the healthcare and hospitality sectors has emerged as a transformative trend with the potential to revolutionize medical services. This integration is fueled by a shared commitment to prioritize patient satisfaction and elevate service levels by placing patient experience at the forefront of healthcare delivery. By merging the principles of hospitality with healthcare, this innovative approach aims to create healing environments within medical facilities that promote comfort, trust, and emotional well-being.

Vital elements of hospitality, such as warm greetings, comfortable accommodations, and attentive staff, significantly alleviate the anxiety and stress often associated with medical treatments. This human-centric approach enhances patient satisfaction and contributes to better treatment outcomes. The confluence of hospitality and healthcare benefits patients and creates a positive work environment for healthcare professionals.

Integrating hospitality-driven practices into healthcare improves patient satisfaction and contributes to better treatment outcomes and a more positive healthcare environment for patients and medical professionals. This evolving concept represents a significant step forward in continuously pursuing excellence in healthcare delivery.

Keywords Healthcare and hospitality · Patient satisfaction · Medical tourism

A. Rebello (✉)
Department of Hospital Administration, Yenepoya (Deemed to be University), Mangalore, India
e-mail: averilrebello@yenepoya.edu.in

D. Rao · N. Shalini · H. K. Mamatha
DHSMS, JSSAHER, Mysuru, India

B. Chaudhary et al. (eds.), *Medical Tourism in Developing Countries*,
https://doi.org/10.1007/978-981-99-8909-6_2

2.1 Introduction

Healthcare and hospitality may appear to be two very different industries, but closer examination reveals that they share the same objective, "consumer satisfaction". Additionally, both sectors evaluate customer satisfaction by using a combination of both tangible and intangible elements. In the healthcare realm, a patient's emotional well-being and comfort play a crucial role in the healing process. Thus, the environment and amenities contribute significantly to fostering a positive and supportive atmosphere for recovery. This amalgamation highlights the importance of recognizing the interconnectedness of these seemingly different domains.

The word "hospitality"—as with the word "hospital"—it comes from the Latin word **hospes**, meaning both "host" and "guest." It is interesting to note the fact that these two words share a common linguistic origin and is reflected in the two industries. Whether we experience them as host or guest, hospitals and hospitality spaces have more in common than etymology. Both industries offer an implied promise that whoever walks through the door will be well-cared for.

2.2 Hospitality Bridging Healthcare

De Micco FJ in his book, 'Medical Tourism and Wellness: Hospitality Bridging Healthcare introduces a compelling concept known as Hospitality Bridging Healthcare, often known as H2H services. This innovative approach aims to provide patients or guests a positive and enriching experience that fosters loyalty over the long term. De Micco underscores that the efficiency of the entire procedure depends on the provision of hospitality and medical services. (DeMicco 2017).

One of the most popular niche segments in the hospitality and travel sectors currently is medical tourism. The preplanning of the medical journey, leading up to the arrival at the medical/health/wellness destination initiates a cascade of multiple H2H services creating an overall satisfying experience for the patient/guest. If the performance of this sector is at the highest level throughout the entire process, it can result in customer loyalty. Success of H2H services depends on the cadence and harmony of the healthcare and hospitality sectors.

The H2H model illustrates how hotels and hospitals can collaborate on their service offerings. In order to deliver higher service quality, the model comprises of several approaches to combine the operations of hospitals and hotels.

- First, it suggests combining operations for hotels and hospitals.
- The second method entails offering a comprehensive service package, including accommodation and hospital services, to customers seeking medical attention.
- The third concept involves combining the two entities into a single entity (DeMicco 2017).

In time to come, patients can both enjoy hospitality from the hotel industry and use the technological advancements in their room while receiving medical services offered by expert staff from the hospitals. If hotels collaborate with hospitals to provide service to their patients, the overall patient experience would be improved.

As healthcare facilities increasingly evolve into "medical campuses" becoming hotspots for medical tourism, they are adopting hospitality standards for service excellence and wellness offerings. Many of these facilities either construct hotels or establish affiliations with hotels to accomodate both tourists and patients. In fact, within hospital settings, approximately 75% of the services provided to patients are related to hospitality (De Micco and Guzman 2023).

In order to meet the unmet requirements of some patients and their families, providing a hygienic, complementary, and welcoming setting that delivers quality accommodation, upmarket treatments, and cutting-edge wellness facilities for recovery, H2H develops a fresh and unique business model for entrepreneurs (DeMicco 2017).

H2H strategically combines hotels and hospitals to produce a complete client experience as part of the larger industry of medical tourism, linking medical institutions to hotels and wellness centres.

In Orlando, The Rosen Care model, represents an innovative approach to blending hospitality and healthcare. This patient-centered onsite medical home model is grounded in five key tenets: Access, Quality, Service, Cost, and Innovation (RosenCare 2023).

Another facility in Flushing, New York, is poised to become a milestone for high-caliber healthcare in the community. The Eastern Mirage Medical Center, connected to five-star Eastern Mirage Hotel, will help meet the growing demand from patients for modern medical facilities. This will assist the practices and contribute to the growth of healthcare organizations connected to the center, fostering the development of their respective businesses (Partner 2021).

2.3 Increasing Patient Experience Through H2H Services in Medical Tourism

In the modern world, an increasing number of businesses are moving away from the traditional commodity, goods, and service model to an experience-driven paradigm. B. Joseph Pine II and James H. Gilmore first introduced the term "The Experience Economy" in 1999 recognizing this transformative shift. What some hospitals fail to realize is that patients are customers in an experience economy, where they are charged not just for medical care but for the overall well-being gained by engagement (Pine and Gilmore 2011).

To meet the demands of patients, medical facilities must provide travel, housing, spa services, and even exercise sessions. The aim of the medical care process is changing from transactional care model to a transformational experience, where customers/patients obtain health benefits beyond traditional medical care.

The effectiveness of medical treatment is undoubtedly a key factor in determining medical tourism. Unfortunately, patients and consumers will not view a well-executed treatment that is accompanied by poor customer service as a great source of care.Successful medical tourism requires the alignment of competitive strategies from both healthcare and hospitality teams. The synergy of their essential competencies leads to enhanced success in this field.

Aligning every aspect of medical tourism increases productivity and efficiency. Additionally, a great medical tourism experience combines successful medical treatment with outstanding customer service.

An H2H service involving medical staff, hoteliers, spa professionals, personal trainers, and other well-being facilitators can significantly differentiate the healthcare institution from conventional ones (Li and DeMicco 2015).

2.4 Hospitality Elements Seen in Hospitals

Today, a lot of healthcare facilities want to develop and strengthen their brands. The astute owners and operators of these businesses have realized that the future belongs to those who can create exceptional experiences by fusing the best elements of hospitality and healthcare. The knowledge of hospitality and healthcare is, in fact, the key to success in the rapidly growing field of medical tourism. Some of the elements of hospitality industry now seen in hospitals are: hotel-like rooms and decor, hotels built into medical facilities, family-friendly dining options, hotel-quality food, room service, and common areas.

Moreover, healthcare facilities are offering enhanced service options like concierge services, spas, or therapy centers, hotel-style way finding tools, and entertainment amenities. The incorporation of executive lounges and/or communal lobbies with free Wi-Fi and refreshments, patient-centered controls, and adaptable furniture further exemplifies the fusion of hospitality and healthcare in modern medical facilities (Wu et al. 2013).

2.5 Integrating Wellness in Hospitality (Pierre-Louis 2019)

The introduction of "spas" as a feature of opulent hotels and resorts might be seen as the industry's first step toward incorporating contemporary wellness. The word "spa" has changed over time to refer to locations that offer "renewal for body, mind, and spirit," and hotel spas are now the most prevalent kind of health facility. Hotel spas are described as hospitality establishments with a significant spa component that cater to visitors for whom wellness pursuits are typically not the main reason for vacation. This segment, which makes up about 89% of all wellness tourism travel, is known by the Global Wellness Institute as "secondary wellness tourists."

Hotels have advanced in integrating wellness-oriented products into various aspects of the guest stay, from food and beverage menus to in-room amenities, as wellness products continue to permeate our daily routines. A select few properties, including Westin by Marriott and EVEN hotels by IHG, expressly cater to wellness customers. Even hotels now offer in-room cycling alternatives, yoga mats, and exercise gear.

Also, the growth of wellness has also prompted the creation of a unique category of resort that targets "primary wellness tourists." For many visitors, preserving or improving personal wellness is the primary driving force behind the journey.

Resorts targeting primary wellness tourists usually offer immersive wellness experiences in two formats:

1. Individual Wellness Immersions offering tailored routines that include suggested exercise, professional medical exams, spiritual education, diet or cleanses, and daily spa treatments.
2. Retreat Centers focusing on shared learning experiences and provide group experiences that are frequently guided by internationally renowned health professionals.

2.6 Conclusion

Amalgamation of healthcare and hospitality is the key for a satisfying experience and is very crucial for medical and wellness tourism.It is imperative that healthcare take a lead in fostering a customer experience that not only meets but exceeds customer expectations and win patients' loyalty for years to come.

References

DeMicco FJ (ed) (2017) Medical tourism and wellness: hospitality bridging healthcare (H2H). CRC Press, Boca Raton

DeMicco F, Guzman J (2023) Hotel managers: new career opportunities in hospitality bridging healthcare (H2H). Hospitality Net. https://www.hospitalitynet.org/opinion/4115443.html

Li M, DeMicco FJ (2015) Best "experience" practices in medical tourism. In: IGI Global (ed) Handbook of research on global hospitality and tourism management. Hershey, pp 493–500

Partner Q (2021) Blending healthcare and hospitality to thrive in the post-covid-19 Medical Landscape. Fierce Healthcare. Available https://www.fiercehealthcare.com/sponsored/blending-healthcare-and-hospitality-to-thrive-post-covid-19-medical-landscape. Accessed 17 February 2023

Pierre-Louis A (2019) How to integrate wellness into hospitality for guest satisfaction and owner return. Insights. Available https://insights.ehotelier.com/insights/2019/08/08/how-to-integrate-wellness-into-hospitality-for-guest-satisfaction-and-owner-return/. Accessed 17 February 2023

Pine BJ, Gilmore JH (2011) The experience economy. Harvard Business Press, Cambridge

RosenCare (2023). Available https://www.rosencare.com/. Accessed 17 February 2023

Wu Z, Robson S, Hollis B (2013) The application of hospitality elements in hospitals. J Healthc Manag 58(1):47–62

Chapter 3
Concerns and Considerations in Medical Tourism: An Overview

Kanakavalli K. Kundury, K. C. Shylaja, and Namitha

Abstract Medical tourism services have gained much acceptance in the recent times as they facilitate cross-border care with much ease and access. Though there are immense benefits of these services, as a contrast, there are certain inherent risks associated while operating medical tourism services. Few of the risks include language barriers, sub-standard quality of care, legal and financial issues and medical malpractices. There could be also risks involved in post-treatment care, mental and emotional well-being of patients and attenders, travel hazards, insurance policies and coverages. Individuals should carefully consider the possible risk factors before opting for the services. Therefore, it is crucial for patients to weigh all the potential risks and benefits of medical tourism before deciding whether or not to pursue it as an option for their medical treatment. Thus, this chapter highlights the details of potential risks that are associated with medical tourism services; and possible considerations to be made by the medical tourist before opting for the services.

Keywords Risks · Considerations · Medical tourism · Quality of care · Hazards

K. K. Kundury (✉)
Department of Health System Management Studies, JSS Academy of Higher Education and Research, Mysuru, Karnataka, India

Special Interest Group in Patient Care Management, JSS Academy of Higher Education and Research, Mysuru, Karnataka, India
e-mail: kanakavalli.dhsms@jssuni.edu.in

K. C. Shylaja
Department of Health System Management Studies, JSS Academy of Higher Education and Research, Mysuru, Karnataka, India

Center for Distance and Online Education, JSS Academy of Higher Education and Research, Mysuru, Karnataka, India

Namitha
Center for Distance and Online Education, JSS Academy of Higher Education and Research, Mysuru, Karnataka, India

B. Chaudhary et al. (eds.), *Medical Tourism in Developing Countries*,
https://doi.org/10.1007/978-981-99-8909-6_3

3.1 Introduction to Various Risks in Medical Tourism Services

In recent years, the phenomenon of medical tourism, wherein individuals travel to a foreign country for medical treatment, has gained significant popularity. Nonetheless, individuals should carefully consider various risks and factors before opting for this form of healthcare. These risks and considerations include potential language barriers that could impede communication with medical professionals, the possibility of receiving care of a different quality than that which is available in the patient's home country, legal and financial issues that could hinder obtaining compensation in case of medical malpractice (Al Shamsi et al. 2020). The risks also include limited post-treatment care due to distance or language barriers, cultural differences that may hinder comprehension or adherence to treatment plans, travel-related hazards such as health risks and complications, and the possibility of insurance coverage being invalid in the destination country (Jin et al. 2008).

Moreover, individuals must also consider additional risks, such as medical malpractice, the quality and adequacy of medical facilities and equipment, the credentials of healthcare providers (Rodziewicz et al. 2022; Donabedian 2005). Few other factors to consider also include infection control and sanitation standards, mental and emotional health of the individuals, handling of emergency situations; time differences, if any, that may impact their treatment or recovery (Pope et al. 1995). Thus, it is crucial for patients to weigh all the potential risks and benefits of medical tourism before deciding whether or not to pursue it as an option for their medical treatment.

Patients must also exercise caution with regard to follow-up care and monitoring, as these aspects of medical tourism can carry inherent risks (Crooks et al. 2013). Potential issues include miscommunication with medical providers due to physical distance or language barriers, delays in receiving test results or treatment, and challenges in obtaining remote monitoring and virtual communication tools (Haleem et al. 2021). To address these risks, patients are advised to conduct thorough research on medical providers that offer remote monitoring and virtual communication tools, leverage such tools to remain in communication with their healthcare providers, and identify a local point of contact in the destination country who can assist with follow-up care (Ventola 2014a). To minimise the risks and considerations associated with medical tourism, patients should conduct extensive due diligence on the destination country, medical provider, and treatment options (Khan et al. 2016). They may also wish to obtain a detailed medical report from the medical providers in the destination country, which can be shared with their home-country doctor for follow-up care and monitoring (Bali et al. 2011).

3.2 Quality of Care

Medical tourism can offer patients an exciting opportunity to receive treatment in exotic locales. However, it also carries a significant risk—subpar quality of care (Chen and Wilson 2013; Al-Lamki 2011). The lack of proper accreditation, regulation, and oversight in some foreign medical facilities can pose a threat to the health and well-being of patients (Alkhenizan and Shaw 2011). This includes inadequate technology, equipment, and training standards for healthcare providers, which can directly affect the quality of care received (Mosadeghrad 2014). For instance, a patient may not receive the same level of care they would have received in their home country due to the unavailability of required technology and equipment (National Academies of Sciences, Engineering, and Medicine; Health and Medicine Division; Board on Health Care Services; Committee on Health Care Utilization and Adults with Disabilities 2018).

Quality of care is a critical concern for patients seeking medical tourism, and the lack of continuity of care is one aspect of this risk (Chen and Wilson 2013). Patients may not have access to the same level of follow-up care and monitoring that they would have received in their home country, potentially leading to difficulties in managing any complications that arise during recovery (Brown and Bussell 2011). This lack of access to proper resources and support systems can impede a patient's recovery and overall well-being, leaving them feeling isolated and unsupported (Reblin and Uchino 2008). The transition from a foreign healthcare system back to their home country's healthcare system can also pose challenges in terms of continuing care and managing any complications.

To ensure the best possible care during medical tourism, patients must take charge of their own information research (Khan et al. 2016). This includes investigating potential destinations and providers, seeking out facilities with proper accreditation, board certification, and other qualifications. Reading reviews and testimonials from other patients who have undergone similar treatments, and seeking recommendations from their home-country healthcare providers, can also provide valuable insight into the quality of care patients can expect (Crooks et al. 2010). In addition to this, it is important for patients to understand the follow-up care and monitoring plan post-treatment, and to know how to reach their provider in case of any complications or questions (Crooks et al. 2010). With careful preparation, patients can reduce their risks and ensure the highest level of care possible.

3.3 Language Barriers

Language barriers pose a significant risk in medical tourism, as they can lead to misunderstandings and miscommunication between patients and healthcare providers (Rokni et al. 2017). In addition to difficulty in post-treatment care and monitoring, patients may struggle to understand the risks, benefits, and alternatives of their treatment due to language barriers, leading to a lack of trust between patient and provider (Martin et al. 2005).

To mitigate these risks, patients should thoroughly research potential destinations and providers to ensure that they are fluent in the patient's native language (Squires 2018). Patients may also consider bringing a translator or language interpreter with them on their trip to facilitate communication with healthcare providers (Squires 2018). It is also important for patients to bring their medical records and relevant documents translated into the local language of the destination country to ensure that healthcare providers have all the necessary information to provide appropriate care.

3.4 Legal and Financial Issues

Patients should examine the legal system and healthcare laws of the country of destination as well as the insurance coverage from the healthcare provider in order to address the legal and financial concerns related to medical tourism (Labonté et al. 2018). Patients should also speak with their insurance company to find out what costs are covered and what out-of-pocket costs they might have to pay (Hardee et al. 2005). To make sure they are financially ready for the medical tourism experience, patients must also acquire a precise and comprehensive estimate of all expenditures related to the treatment, including travel and lodging charges (Lunt et al. 2014). Patients might also think about working with a facilitator or consultant for medical tourism who can help them with the financial and legal sides of the process and offer support all along the way (Kim et al. 2019).

It is crucial for patients to examine their insurance coverage and comprehend the services that are covered under and what is not covered, in order to reduce the dangers of both the law and money (Institute of Medicine (US) Committee on the Consequences of Uninsurance 2002). Patients should also be sure to educate themselves with the procedures for pursuing compensation or legal action if something goes wrong, as well as the rules and regulations of the destination countries (Nandimath 2009). In order to cover the costs of medical procedures, travel and lodging expenditures, and other unforeseen costs, patients may also think about getting supplemental travel insurance.

It is best that the patients exercise due diligence in their choice of physician by verifying their credentials and performance record (Lobelo and de Quevedo 2016). It is imperative that patients confirm the accreditation of the facility and the licensure and board certification of the healthcare professionals/ facilities to ensure their safety (Roy 2021).

In addition, seeking advice from dependable healthcare professionals and obtaining feedback from other patients who have undergone the same or similar treatments is essential (Roy 2021). Through these measures, patients can make informed decisions and reduce the risk of unfavourable outcomes. The importance of conducting thorough research cannot be overstated, as it is a crucial factor in ensuring safe and successful medical tourism experience (Sultana et al. 2014).

3.5 Post-treatment Care

Patients must take into account post-treatment care, which is a crucial component of medical travel (Khan et al. 2016). Medical tourists might not have access to the same level of post-treatment monitoring and care as those obtaining care in their own country (Khan et al. 2016). Patients may find it more challenging to recuperate and handle any consequences as a result. Patients might not have the same resources and assistance networks at their disposal as they would if they were receiving care back home (Hardavella et al. 2017).

Another aspect of medical tourism post-treatment care is the time and distance difference between the patient's home country and the destination country (Crooks et al. 2010). Patients may find it difficult to communicate with their healthcare provider for follow-up appointments and check-ups as a result of this (Crooks et al. 2010). Furthermore, if an emergency occurs, patients may struggle to get the assistance they require in a timely manner.

Patients must comprehend the post-treatment follow-up care and monitoring plan in order to reduce the risks connected with that care (Jimmy and Jose 2011). This entails being aware of the timetable for follow-up visits, how to contact the doctor in case of problems or inquiries, and what tools are available to help patients manage their recovery (Jimmy and Jose 2011). In order to ensure that they have access to the necessary follow-up care and monitoring following their treatment, patients should also think about living in the destination country for a while after their treatment (Putsch III and Joyce 1990).

Patients should budget for any additional travel, lodging, and follow-up appointments that may be necessary as well as the cost of post-treatment care. To guarantee continuity of care and to make communication with the physician in the destination country easier, patients should also discuss the treatment and the follow-up plan with their home country's doctor (Putsch III and Joyce 1990).

3.6 Cultural Differences

Cultural differences can also pose significant risks for patients seeking medical treatment abroad (Putsch III and Joyce 1990). These differences can include variations in healthcare practices, customs, and social norms that can create confusion and misunderstandings for medical tourists. For example, patients may not be familiar with the healthcare system and the way in which medical treatments are delivered in the destination country, which can lead to confusion and mistrust (Institute of Medicine (US) Committee 2002). Additionally, cultural differences in communication styles and expectations can also create challenges, as patients may not be able to fully understand or communicate their needs to healthcare providers (Putsch III and Joyce 1990).

Another thing to consider is how people differ in their perspectives about health care and illness. Traditional or alternative medicine may be more common in various cultures, which may not confirm to the patient's views or expectations. Additionally, patients seeking medical care abroad may encounter difficulties due to cultural variations in views regarding pain management and end-of-life care (Putsch III and Joyce 1990).

To assuage the risks associated with cultural differences, it is crucial for patients to research the destination country's healthcare system and customs. Patients should also familiarise themselves with the communication styles and expectations in the destination country, as well as any cultural differences in attitudes towards healthcare and illness (Schouten and Meeuwesen 2006). Additionally, patients should consider hiring a translator or cultural liaison to assist with communication and cultural understanding (Schouten and Meeuwesen 2006; Ladha et al. 2018).

3.7 Travel Risks

Travel risks are a significant consideration for patients seeking medical treatment abroad. These risks can include physical hazards such as illness, injury, and accidents that can occur during travel (Roupa et al. 2012). Additionally, patients may also be at risk for theft, crime, and other security issues. Furthermore, there are risks related to the destination country's political stability and natural disasters (Roupa et al. 2012).

Another phase of travel risks in medical tourism is the potential for delays or cancellations of flights and other transportation (Grépin et al. 2021). These issues can disrupt treatment plans and make it difficult for patients to access the medical care they need. Additionally, patients may also face challenges related to travel insurance and reimbursement for any medical expenses incurred during travel (Grépin et al. 2021).

To lessen travel risks, it is important for patients to research the destination country and plan their travel accordingly. This includes researching any travel warnings or advisories issued by the government and familiarising oneself with the destination country's political stability, crime rate and natural hazards. Additionally, patients should also purchase travel insurance that covers medical expenses and emergency evacuation in case of an emergency (Neil Lunt et al. 2011).

Patients must plan their budgets and consider the financial implications of medical travel (Lunt et al. 2014). This includes the costs associated with travel, lodging, transportation, and food. Patients should also factor in other expenses associated with travel, such as travel insurance and visa fees. It is advised that patients carefully plot their travel routes and make sure they have enough time following the treatment before flying home (Lunt et al. 2014). This can also help patients enjoy their experience of medical tourism more and stay out of debts.

It is imperative for patients to understand the potential impact of travel on their pre-existing medical conditions and to take necessary precautions to ensure a comfortable trip (Lunt et al. 2014). Patients should ensure they have the required medical documentation with them and communicate with their doctor in their home country about their travel plans to seek advice on managing their medical concerns while travelling. By taking these necessary measures, patients can help minimise any health-related risks during their medical tourism experience.

3.8 Insurance Coverage

Insurance coverage is an important consideration for patients seeking medical treatment abroad (Neil Lunt et al. 2011). Many insurance plans do not cover medical treatments received outside of the patient's home country, which can result in significant out-of-pocket costs for patients. Additionally, patients may also face challenges related to reimbursement for any medical expenses incurred during travel.

Another crucial factor of insurance coverage in medical tourism is the potential for substandard care (Neil Lunt et al. 2011). Some medical providers may not have the same standards of care as providers in the patient's home country, which can lead to poorer outcomes and increased costs for patients. Additionally, patients may also face challenges related to follow-up care and access to specialists after returning home.

To relieve the risks associated with insurance coverage, it is critical for patients to study in detail their insurance plan and understand what it covers (Institute of Medicine (US) Committee on the Consequences of Uninsurance 2002). This includes identifying any exclusions or limitations related to medical treatments received outside of the patient's home country (Institute of Medicine (US) Committee on the Consequences of Uninsurance 2002). Additionally, patients should also consider purchasing additional travel insurance to cover medical expenses and emergency evacuation (Institute of Medicine (US) Committee on the Consequences of Uninsurance 2002; Neil Lunt et al. 2011).

Patients should also research the destination country's healthcare system and providers to ensure that they meet the standards of care in the patient's home country. Additionally, patients should consider discussing their insurance coverage and follow-up care plans with their home country doctor and the medical tourism provider (Neil Lunt et al. 2011).

Patients should also know the cost of the medical treatment and budget accordingly. They should also research the destination country's healthcare system and providers to ensure that they meet the standards of care in the patient's home country (Neil Lunt et al. 2011). Additionally, patients should consider discussing their insurance coverage and follow-up care plans with their home country doctor and the medical tourism provider before making any decision (Khan et al. 2016).

3.9 Communicating with Home-Country Doctors

Communicating with home-country doctors is an important consideration for patients seeking medical treatment abroad (Neil Lunt et al. 2011). Due to the distance and time difference, it can be difficult for patients to stay in contact with their home-country doctors and keep them informed about their treatment and progress. Additionally, patients may also face challenges related to follow-up care and access to specialists after returning home (Schouten and Meeuwesen 2006).

Another part of communicating with home-country doctors in medical tourism is the potential for language barriers. Patients may not speak the language of the destination country, which can make it difficult for them to communicate with medical providers and understand their treatment plans (Ladha et al. 2018). Additionally, patients may also face challenges related to cultural differences in healthcare, which can lead to misunderstandings and poor outcomes.

Patients should make plans in advance and establish a strategy for updating their home-country doctors about their treatment and progress in order to minimise the hazards involved with doing so. Before travelling to the destination country, they should review their treatment options and post-operative care with their doctor in their home country. To facilitate communication with medical professionals in the destination country, patients should also think about travelling with a translator or using translation apps (Panayiotou et al. 2019).

Additionally, patients should be prepared to deliver any pertinent medical documents and test results from the destination nation to their home country's doctor (Bali et al. 2011). Additionally, patients should think about talking with their home country doctor and the medical tourism provider about their insurance coverage and follow-up care plans.

Patients must also be aware of the time difference and make appropriate plans. Patients should think about planning their consultations and follow-up care so that they can consult with their local physician at a convenient time (Neil Lunt et al. 2011). Patients might also think about contacting their home-country doctor via video conferencing or other technology.

Before embarking on medical tourism, patients must take into account the cultural and language barriers they may face in the destination country. Differences in culture and language can cause misunderstandings between the patient and the healthcare provider, leading to poor communication and inadequate treatment (Squires 2018). It's essential for patients to get relevant information and familiarise themselves with the customs and practices of the destination country, as well as any language barriers they may encounter (Squires 2018). This can help prevent any misunderstandings and ensure the patient receives the best possible care.

3.10 Medication and Prescriptions

The issue of medication and prescriptions is a crucial aspect that patients must consider when seeking medical treatment abroad. Patients may encounter difficulties bringing all their medications with them or finding the same medications in the destination country (Jimmy and Jose 2011). They may also face challenges in understanding the different dosage and administration instructions for their medications in the destination country.

Patients must be aware of the potential risks associated with counterfeit or expired medications when purchasing them from unregulated sources. Quality and effectiveness issues may also arise when taking medications in the destination country (Jimmy and Jose 2011).

Patients must make advance plans and discuss their pharmaceutical requirements with their home country doctor before departing for the destination country in order to reduce the hazards associated with medications and prescriptions (Zheng et al. 2021). They should buy enough medication to last them for the entire trip, and they should think about taking a copy of their prescriptions and a note from their doctor back home.

Patients should also check whether their prescriptions are offered in the destination nation and, if necessary, make plans to get them. They should also talk about their prescription requirements with the medical tourism provider and any local healthcare professionals they will consult while travelling. It is crucial for patients to be informed of the rules and restrictions that apply to prescription drugs and medications in the destination country (Neil Lunt et al. 2011). They should familiarise themselves with and abide by the importation, possession, and other legal requirements for drugs and prescriptions in the destination country.

3.11 Medical Malpractice

Medical malpractice poses a significant risk for patients seeking medical treatment abroad, as it involves a failure by medical professionals to provide appropriate care, resulting in harm or injury to the patient (Pandit and Pandit 2009). This risk is compounded by factors such as a lack of oversight, unfamiliarity with local laws and regulations, and cultural differences in healthcare.

Patients who seek medical treatment abroad must consider the potential for inadequate or substandard care, which can lead to poor outcomes and complications (Chen and Wilson 2013). Additionally, they may face challenges related to the lack of transparency and accountability in the destination country's healthcare system, which can make it difficult to hold medical providers accountable for any harm or injury caused (Chen and Wilson 2013).

To mitigate the risks associated with medical malpractice, it is essential for patients to thoroughly research and carefully select reputable medical providers and facilities in the destination country (Dahlawi et al. 2021). This includes checking for accreditation, certification, and licensing of the medical providers and facilities, as well as reading reviews and testimonials from other patients. Patients should also engage in open communication with their medical tourism provider and any local medical providers they will be seeing in the destination country to discuss their concerns and questions (Dahlawi et al. 2021).

Patients must also ensure they understand and comply with the laws and regulations related to medical malpractice in the destination country. Conducting research on the destination country's laws and regulations is crucial to ensure compliance (Crooks et al. 2013). Moreover, obtaining travel insurance that covers medical malpractice and any other potential risks associated with the medical treatment they are seeking is highly recommended. Patients should also be aware of cultural differences in healthcare and how they may affect their treatment. Communication with the medical provider and the medical tourism provider is critical to understanding how these cultural differences may impact the patient's treatment (Ladha et al. 2018).

In addition, patients must understand the importance of follow-up care and seek medical attention if they experience any complications or adverse reactions to their treatment (Brown and Bussell 2011). It is essential to keep their home-country doctor informed of their treatment and progress and seek their advice regarding the management of their medical conditions after returning home. Obtaining a detailed medical report from the destination country's medical providers can be useful for follow-up care and shared with their home-country doctor (Bali et al. 2011).

3.12 Medical Facilities and Equipment

When patients seek medical treatment abroad, medical facilities and equipment present a significant risk and consideration (Neil Lunt et al. 2011). Patients may face a higher risk of receiving inadequate care due to the lack of oversight, unfamiliarity with local laws and regulations, and cultural differences in healthcare. One of the most significant risks associated with medical facilities and equipment in medical tourism is the potential for inadequate or substandard care, which may result in poor outcomes and complications (Chen and Wilson 2013). Additionally, patients may encounter challenges related to the lack of transparency and accountability in the destination country's healthcare system, making it difficult to ensure that the facilities and equipment meet appropriate standards.

Patients must do extensive research and choose recognised healthcare practitioners and facilities in the destination country in order to reduce the hazards related to medical facilities and equipment (Blandford et al. 2014). This includes looking into the medical facility's accreditation, certification, and licensure as well as reading reviews and patient comments. Patients should also think about talking with the medical tourism provider and any local healthcare professionals they will be seeing in the destination nation about their worries and inquiries.

3.13 Healthcare Provider Credentials

It is crucial for patients to check the credentials of their healthcare providers before enlisting their services (Neil Lunt et al. 2011). This is especially true when it comes to medical tourism, when patients can obtain treatment from professionals who lack the necessary credentials or licences in their native country. The licence, board certification, and other pertinent credentials of a physician can be checked by patients. Additionally, patients can look into the provider's credentials, experience, and history of disciplinary actions and malpractice claims (Neil Lunt et al. 2011). Patients may assist in ensuring they receive top-notch care from licenced and experienced professionals by taking the time to check a healthcare provider's qualifications.

3.14 Communicating with the Hospital/Clinic Staff

Patients seeking medical care overseas should be aware of the challenges while communicating with hospital or clinic workers. Patients may experience communication difficulties with the hospital or clinic staff due to linguistic and cultural obstacles (Putsch III and Joyce 1990). This may result in misunderstandings, poor communication, and undesirable results.

The possibility of receiving an incorrect diagnosis or inadequate care when speaking with hospital or clinic employees in medical tourism is one of the major risks (Ladha et al. 2018). Ineffective communication between patients and hospital or clinic staff regarding their symptoms or medical history may result in the wrong diagnosis and course of therapy. The hospital or clinic staff may also give instructions or advise that the patients are unable to comprehend, which can result in problems and subpar results (Schouten and Meeuwesen 2006).

To allay the risks associated while communicating with hospital/clinic staff, it is important for patients to choose reputable medical providers in the destination country that can provide translation services. Patients should also consider bringing a translator or a family member who can speak the local language to the appointment (Schouten and Meeuwesen 2006). Additionally, patients should consider discussing their concerns and questions with the medical tourism provider and any local medical providers they will be seeing in the destination country.

It is imperative for patients to acquaint themselves with the cultural nuances that underpin healthcare communication. Cultural disparities may potentially impact communication with hospital or clinic staff (Ladha et al. 2018). To this end, patients are advised to discuss their queries and apprehensions with the medical provider and the medical tourism provider, in order to comprehend how the cultural differences may influence communication with hospital/clinic staff (Ladha et al. 2018).

3.15 Infection Control and Sanitation

Infection control and sanitation are important risks and considerations for patients seeking medical treatment abroad. Patients may be exposed to different types of infections and diseases in the destination country, and the level of infection control and sanitation may not be the same as in their home country (Chen and Wilson 2013). This can lead to poor outcomes and complications.

The possibility of hospital-acquired infections is one of the most serious risks associated with infection control and sanitation in medical tourism (Chen and Wilson 2013). Pathogens such as bacteria, viruses, and fungi could cause severe complications, extended hospital stays, and even death.

Patients must also be aware of a hospital's compliance with infection control practices and sanitation protocols. Patients should also review the facility's infection control and sanitation policies and inquire about the protocols in place (Chen and Wilson 2013). Accreditation (national or international) of healthcare facilities, in this context, is an assurance for the medical tourist in selecting the hospital at the destination country (Jones et al. 2014).

3.16 Mental and Emotional Health

Patients who seek medical treatment overseas must take their mental and emotional health into account. Numerous mental and emotional health problems might result from the strain of travelling and being in a strange setting (Kirmayer et al. 2011). Furthermore, patients may feel anxious and uncertain about the medical care they want to get. Patients should think about getting assistance from a mental health professional both before and after their medical treatment to lessen these risks (Kirmayer et al. 2011). Patients should look into and select healthcare organisations and institutions that place a strong emphasis on mental and emotional health and have the resources necessary to handle any problems that may develop. Additionally, it is crucial for patients to let their doctor and the medical tourism provider know about any issues they have with their mental and emotional health (Bishop and Litch 2000). To address these situations, it is indeed a good practice for healthcare facilities to provide patient counselling services as a value addition to their medical tourism packages, to assist the medical travellers with their anxiety or stress, if any (Kirmayer et al. 2011).

3.17 Time Differences and Emergency Situations

Patients must take into account time variations and how they may affect their care when travelling for medical treatment overseas (Helble 2011). Time zone differences can interfere with arranging visits, receiving test results, and receiving follow-up care from medical professionals. In order to ensure timely communication with their medical providers, patients should be aware of the time difference between their home country and the destination country and plan appropriately (Helble 2011). This can entail changing their sleep patterns and being accessible at odd hours.

Patients must be prepared for unforeseen emergencies that may occur while travelling for medical treatment (Neil Lunt et al. 2011). Patients should familiarise themselves with the emergency medical services available in the destination country to ensure appropriate measures are in place. This may entail obtaining travel insurance that includes emergency medical evacuation and medical treatment coverage. Patients should also ensure that they have unrestricted access to critical medical information, such as their medical history, current medication list, and contact information for their healthcare providers. Patients are advised to contact local emergency services in the event of an emergency and seek prompt medical attention (Helble 2011).

3.18 Follow-up Care and Monitoring

Follow-up care and monitoring are essential risks and considerations for patients who are considering medical tourism (Neil Lunt et al. 2011). One of the most significant risks associated with follow-up care is the potential for miscommunication between the patient and the medical provider. This can occur when the patient is not able to communicate with the medical provider due to distance or language barriers (Steinberg et al. 2016).

The potential for delays in receiving test findings or therapy is a risk linked with follow-up care. This may happen if the healthcare provider is abroad and is unable to process test results or administer treatment promptly. If the patient develops difficulties or requires more care after coming home, this could be extremely challenging.

Patients may look into healthcare companies that provide remote monitoring and virtual communication solutions in order to reduce the dangers related to follow-up care (Haleem et al. 2021). In order to stay in touch with their doctor and guarantee that they get timely information on their treatment and test results, patients can also think about using virtual communication technologies, such as teleconferencing or messaging (Haleem et al. 2021).

In case of an emergency, patients should also have a dial-in numbers handy, including those for emergency services, their medical provider, and their doctor back home (Ventola 2014b). Patients should also think about getting a thorough medical report from the destination country's healthcare providers, which they may then give to their primary care physician for follow-up treatment.

Though few of these risks get identified prior to the initiation of medical tourism services, few risks might suddenly pop up leading to contingent situations. Medical tourism facilitators, agents, financiers and facilities have a plan of action drafted for addressing these potential risks (Neil Lunt et al. 2011). However, the level of preparedness and commitment in identifying and eliminating these risks depicts the quality of services. Hence, all the participants of the medical tourism industry should thus be drafting strategies for identification and addressing the anticipated risks and; also implementing and updating the same on a continuous basis for better patient experience (Neil Lunt et al. 2011).

3.19 Summary and Conclusion

While medical tourism can offer patients access to a wider range of treatments and lower costs, it is important to be aware of the risks and considerations involved. Patients should make a sound decision in identifying the service provider at the destination country prior to the initiation of medical tourism services. Also the medical traveller should be aware of existing laws of the land in the destination country, language and cultural barriers, insurance coverages and follow-up care services before final selection of the hospital. By being aware of these risks and considerations, patients can make an informed decision about whether or not to pursue medical tourism and can take steps to mitigate potential risks.

3.20 Future Directions

The current work highlighted various risks that are frequently associated with medical tourism services along with possible considerations the medical tourist had to make to mitigate the risks. Future works can also include to study the preparedness of each of the stakeholders of medical tourism industry, in identifying and addressing the potential risks. As this cross-border care involves a wide magnitude of services, it is very much important that each of the service providers should have a plan of action in dealing with the anticipated potential risks and unforeseen situations as well. This preparedness will help in creating a positive and comfortable experience for the medical traveller.

Acknowledgements We acknowledge the Leaders, JSS Academy of Higher Education & Research and thank them for providing us the opportunity and the resources required for drafting this book chapter.

References

Al Shamsi H, Almutairi AG, Al Mashrafi S, Al Kalbani T (2020) Implications of language barriers for healthcare: a systematic review. Oman Med J 35(2):e122. https://doi.org/10.5001/omj.2020.40

Alkhenizan A, Shaw C (2011) Impact of accreditation on the quality of healthcare services: a systematic review of the literature. Ann Saudi Med 31(4):407–416. https://doi.org/10.4103/0256-4947.83204

Al-Lamki L (2011) Medical tourism: beneficence or maleficence? Sultan Qaboos Univ Med J 11(4):444–447

Bali A, Bali D, Iyer N, Iyer M (2011) Management of medical records: facts and figures for surgeons. J Maxillofac Oral Surg 10(3):199–202. https://doi.org/10.1007/s12663-011-0219-8

Bishop R, Litch JA (2000) Medical tourism can do harm. BMJ 320(7240):1017. https://doi.org/10.1136/bmj.320.7240.1017

Blandford A, Furniss D, Vincent C (2014) Patient safety and interactive medical devices: realigning work as imagined and work as done. Clin Risk 20(5):107–110. https://doi.org/10.1177/1356262214556550

Brown MT, Bussell JK (2011) Medication adherence: WHO cares? Mayo Clin Proc 86(4):304–314. https://doi.org/10.4065/mcp.2010.0575

Chen LH, Wilson ME (2013) The globalization of healthcare: implications of medical tourism for the infectious disease clinician. Clin Infect Dis 57(12):1752–1759. https://doi.org/10.1093/cid/cit540

Crooks VA, Kingsbury P, Snyder J et al (2010) What is known about the patient's experience of medical tourism? A scoping review. BMC Health Serv Res 10:266. https://doi.org/10.1186/1472-6963-10-266

Crooks VA, Turner L, Cohen IG, Bristeir J, Snyder J, Casey V, Whitmore R (2013) Ethical and legal implications of the risks of medical tourism for patients: a qualitative study of Canadian health and safety representatives' perspectives. BMJ Open 3(2):e002302. https://doi.org/10.1136/bmjopen-2012-002302

Dahlawi S, Menezes RG, Khan MA, Waris A, Saifullah NMM (2021) Medical negligence in healthcare organizations and its impact on patient safety and public health: a bibliometric study. F1000Res 10:174. https://doi.org/10.12688/f1000research.37448.1

Donabedian A (2005) Evaluating the quality of medical care. Milbank Q 83(4):691–729. https://doi.org/10.1111/j.1468-0009.2005.00397.x

Grépin KA, Ho T, Liu Z et al (2021) Evidence of the effectiveness of travel-related measures during the early phase of the COVID-19 pandemic: a rapid systematic review. BMJ Glob Health 6:e004537

Haleem A, Javaid M, Singh RP, Suman R (2021) Telemedicine for healthcare: capabilities, features, barriers, and applications. Sens Int 2:100117. https://doi.org/10.1016/j.sintl.2021.100117

Hardavella G, Aamli-Gaagnat A, Frille A, Saad N, Niculescu A, Powell P (2017) Top tips to deal with challenging situations: doctor-patient interactions. Breathe 13(2):129–135. https://doi.org/10.1183/20734735.006616

Hardee JT, Platt FW, Kasper IK (2005) Discussing health care costs with patients: an opportunity for empathic communication. J Gen Intern Med 20(7):666–669. https://doi.org/10.1111/j.1525-1497.2005.0125.x

Helble M (2011) The movement of patients across borders: challenges and opportunities for public health. Bull World Health Organ 89(1):68–72. https://doi.org/10.2471/BLT.10.076612

Institute of Medicine (US) Committee on the Consequences of Uninsurance (2002) Care without coverage: too little, too late. National Academies Press, Washington, p 3. Available from https://www.ncbi.nlm.nih.gov/books/NBK220636/

Institute of Medicine (US) Committee (2002) The future of the public's health in the 21st century. National Academies Press, Washington, p 5. Available from https://www.ncbi.nlm.nih.gov/books/NBK221227/

Jimmy B, Jose J (2011) Patient medication adherence: measures in daily practice. Oman Med J 26(3):155–159. https://doi.org/10.5001/omj.2011.38

Jin J, Sklar GE, Min Sen OV, Chuen LS (2008) Factors affecting therapeutic compliance: a review from the patient's perspective. Ther Clin Risk Manag 4(1):269–286. https://doi.org/10.2147/tcrm.s1458

Jones G, Brooks J, Garton T, Aplin S (2014) Implementing a ward accreditation programme to drive improvements in infection prevention. J Infect Prev 15(4):128–132. https://doi.org/10.1177/1757177413520056

Khan MJ, Chelliah S, Haron MS (2016) International Patients' travel decision making process- a conceptual framework. Iran J Public Health 45(2):134–145

Kim S, Arcodia C, Kim I (2019) Critical success factors of medical tourism: the case of South Korea. Int J Environ Res Public Health 16(24):4964. https://doi.org/10.3390/ijerph16244964

Kirmayer LJ, Narasiah L, Munoz M, Rashid M, Ryder AG, Guzder J, Hassan G, Rousseau C, Pottie K, Canadian Collaboration for Immigrant and Refugee Health (CCIRH) (2011) Common mental health problems in immigrants and refugees: general approach in primary care. CMAJ 183(12):E959–E967. https://doi.org/10.1503/cmaj.090292

Labonté R, Crooks VA, Valdés AC, Runnels V, Snyder J (2018) Government roles in regulating medical tourism: evidence from Guatemala. Int J Equity Health 17(1):150. https://doi.org/10.1186/s12939-018-0866-1

Ladha T, Zubairi M, Hunter A, Audcent T, Johnstone J (2018) Cross-cultural communication: tools for working with families and children. Paediatr Child Health 23(1):66–69. https://doi.org/10.1093/pch/pxx126

Lobelo F, de Quevedo IG (2016) The evidence in support of physicians and health care providers as physical activity role models. Am J Lifestyle Med 10(1):36–52. https://doi.org/10.1177/1559827613520120

Lunt N, Smith RD, Mannion R et al (2014) Implications for the NHS of inward and outward medical tourism: a policy and economic analysis using literature review and mixed-methods approaches. NIHR Journals Library, Southampton. Available from https://www.ncbi.nlm.nih.gov/books/NBK263147/

Martin LR, Williams SL, Haskard KB, Dimatteo MR (2005) The challenge of patient adherence. Ther Clin Risk Manag 1(3):189–199

Mosadeghrad AM (2014) Factors influencing healthcare service quality. Int J Health Policy Manag 3(2):77–89. https://doi.org/10.15171/ijhpm.2014.65

Nandimath OV (2009) Consent and medical treatment: The legal paradigm in India. Indian J Urol 25(3):343–347. https://doi.org/10.4103/0970-1591.56202

National Academies of Sciences, Engineering, and Medicine; Health and Medicine Division; Board on Health Care Services; Committee on Health Care Utilization and Adults with Disabilities (2018) Health-care utilization as a proxy in disability determination. National Academies Press, Washington, p 2. Available from https://www.ncbi.nlm.nih.gov/books/NBK500097/

Neil Lunt RS, Exworthy M, Green ST, Horsfall D, Mannion R (2011) Medical tourism: treatments, markets and health system implications: a scoping review. Directorate for Employment, Labour and Social Affairs, London

Panayiotou A, Gardner A, Williams S, Zucchi E, Mascitti-Meuter M, Goh AM, You E, Chong TW, Logiudice D, Lin X, Haralambous B, Batchelor F (2019) Language translation apps in health care settings: expert opinion. JMIR Mhealth Uhealth 7(4):e11316. https://doi.org/10.2196/11316

Pandit MS, Pandit S (2009) Medical negligence: coverage of the profession, duties, ethics, case law, and enlightened defense - a legal perspective. Indian J Urol 25(3):372–378. https://doi.org/10.4103/0970-1591.56206

Pope AM, Snyder MA, Mood LH (1995) Nursing health, & environment: strengthening the relationship to improve the public's health. National Academies Press, Washington, p 3. Available from https://www.ncbi.nlm.nih.gov/books/NBK232401/

Putsch RW III, Joyce M (1990) Dealing with patients from other cultures. In: Walker HK, Hall WD, Hurst JW (eds) Clinical methods: the history, physical, and laboratory examinations, 3rd edn. Butterworths, Boston. Available from https://www.ncbi.nlm.nih.gov/books/NBK340/

Reblin M, Uchino BN (2008) Social and emotional support and its implication for health. Curr Opin Psychiatry 21(2):201–205. https://doi.org/10.1097/YCO.0b013e3282f3ad89

Rodziewicz TL, Houseman B, Hipskind JE (2022) Medical error reduction and prevention. In: StatPearls. StatPearls Publishing, Treasure Island. Available from https://www.ncbi.nlm.nih.gov/books/NBK499956/

Rokni L, Avci T, Park SH (2017) Barriers of developing medical tourism in a destination: a case of South Korea. Iran J Public Health 46(7):930–937

Roupa Z, Zikos D, Vasilopoulos A, Diomidous M (2012) Common health risks, required precautions of travelers and their customs towards the use of travel medicine services. Mater Soc 24(2):131–134. https://doi.org/10.5455/msm.2012.24.131-134

Roy CG (2021) Patient safety functions of state medical boards in the United States. Yale J Biol Med 94(1):165–173

Schouten BC, Meeuwesen L (2006) Cultural differences in medical communication: a review of the literature. Patient Educ Couns 64(1-3):21–34. https://doi.org/10.1016/j.pec.2005.11.014

Squires A (2018) Strategies for overcoming language barriers in healthcare. Nurs Manag 49(4):20–27. https://doi.org/10.1097/01.NUMA.0000531166.24481.15

Steinberg EM, Valenzuela-Araujo D, Zickafoose JS, Kieffer E, DeCamp LR (2016) The "Battle" of managing language barriers in health care. Clin Pediatr 55(14):1318–1327. https://doi.org/10.1177/0009922816629760

Sultana S, Haque A, Momen A, Yasmin F (2014) Factors affecting the attractiveness of medical tourism destination: an empirical study on India- review article. Iran J Public Health 43(7):867–876

Ventola CL (2014a) Social media and health care professionals: benefits, risks, and best practices. P T 39(7):491–520

Ventola CL (2014b) Mobile devices and apps for health care professionals: uses and benefits. P T 39(5):356–364

Zheng SQ, Yang L, Zhou PX, Li HB, Liu F, Zhao RS (2021) Recommendations and guidance for providing pharmaceutical care services during COVID-19 pandemic: a China perspective. Res Social Adm Pharm 17(1):1819–1824. https://doi.org/10.1016/j.sapharm.2020.03.012

Chapter 4
Significance of Accreditation on Medical Tourism

Jawahar S. K. Pillai and Ramkrishna Mondal

Abstract Traveling to foreign countries for medical treatment is becoming more common. There are numerous opportunities for ethical providers and practitioners in the frontiers of globalized healthcare and medical tourism. Patient care quality encompasses everything a healthcare institution does, from how they care for their patients to ensuring effective, efficient, and fair service delivery and adherence to occupational safety. Because the quality of patient care in hospitals can only be judged after treatment, international patients frequently choose their hospitals abroad depending on their accreditation status. Accreditation ensures cost-effective healthcare and allows patients to make informed decisions about which hospitals they prefer for their abroad treatment. Despite the medical tourism industry's tremendous growth, just a few criteria exist to assure that these institutions provide high-quality, competent international healthcare. Accreditation fills a significant regulatory void in various nations. Patients should seek treatment only at certified foreign healthcare centers. Standards should be set to guarantee that medical tourism clients make informed decisions. Accreditation of medical tourism companies is required. Continuity of care must become an essential component of cross-border care. Medical tourism companies should set restrictions on liability waiver forms. Medical tourism companies must guarantee that they follow appropriate patient privacy and confidentiality legislation. Medical tourism is one of India's fastest-growing industries, and the country is known as a global medical tourism hotspot. India is a popular medical tourism destination because of its high-quality healthcare at a low cost. This sector has enormous potential to grow its services with more investments in building, infrastructure, technology, and services to offer a seamless experience for overseas patients.

Keywords Medical tourism · Quality · Standards · Certification · Accreditation · Healthcare

---

J. S. K. Pillai (✉) · R. Mondal
Department of Hospital Administration, All India Institute of Medical Sciences, Bhubaneswar, Odisha, India

B. Chaudhary et al. (eds.), *Medical Tourism in Developing Countries*,
https://doi.org/10.1007/978-981-99-8909-6_4

4.1 Introduction

Medical tourism is one of the fastest-increasing types of international and domestic tourism (Arunmozhi 2013). Health problems and disorders are likely to affect people of all ages and backgrounds. Medical care and health maintenance are crucial for people of all states, communities, and jobs. Health problems and disorders are likely to affect people of all ages and backgrounds. Medical care and health maintenance are crucial for people of all states, communities, and jobs. A growing number of patients are traveling across borders to access superior healthcare services that are now available in developing countries. Better connectivity and more relaxed medical visa policies have made it easier than ever for people to go outside of their own country to receive superior care at hospitals all around the world. An increased transnational focus on redefining patient treatment outcomes, safety, and quality care of patients and hospital staff has led stakeholders and healthcare provider establishments to advocate for standardized processes for evaluating healthcare organizations based on Standard Operating Procedures (SOPs) through a global standards-based accreditation process. Accreditation increases patients' confidence and trust in their choice of hospitals for abroad treatment since accreditation ensures that member healthcare facilities follow and offer quality services, ensuring the best benefits for the patients. Accreditation is a quality indicator that ensures healthcare organizations not only follow evidence-based practices (EBP), but also care about access, cost-effectiveness, efficacy, and unrivaled quality of service. Accreditation bridges the gap of patient expectation—service mismatch or eliminates the grey extents of inadequacy and insufficiency and eventually institutes best standards, flawless service, professional accountability, and clinical excellence (Alkhenizan 2011). Accreditation is a voluntary method in which healthcare institutions adhere to the standards established by an external certifying agency to ensure standardization, reduce associated risks, and optimize clinical excellence and service delivery. Patients from other countries travel to their home countries for treatment as part of inbound medical tourism. The third sort of medical tourism is intra-bound, in which patients from their nation travel to a center of excellence in another state. In other words, intra-bound tourism occurs when patients travel to another state, city, or region within the country (Mothiravalley 2012). Rising medical treatment expenses in the United States are fueling a drive to outsource medical care. Estimates of the number of Americans flying abroad for treatment range from 50,000 to 500,000. Standard operations, such as heart bypass, can cost up to $13,000 in Thailand, compared to $113,000 in the United States. Knee replacement surgery in the United States might cost $48,000, whereas it costs $13,000 in Singapore (Source: Med One Blog, cited on 31 August 2017; https://www.medonegroup.com/aboutus/blog/cost-of-american-health-care). Medical tourism is a new service that has emerged to advise patients on the best facility available in the country for their illness, make all trip arrangements, teleconference with physicians, and provide medical data. The Joint Commission International (JCI) accredits hospitals globally in response to the increase in medical travel. Although statistics from hospitals outside the United

States are scarce, first-hand accounts of high-quality healthcare are plentiful. A primary advantage of medical tourism is that it allows uninsured and underinsured individuals or self-insured public, municipal, and private institutions to get surgery.

4.2 Medical Tourism and the Globalization of Healthcare

The nature of the global healthcare community in the twenty-first century is rapidly becoming clear. The Indian term "Vasudhiva Kutumbakam" will be the G20 slogan in 2023. Citizens are no longer required to remain in their home nations to meet their healthcare needs. Patients have evolved into global customers. Hospitals are multinational enterprises with a desire to be present in numerous countries. When cost is the primary motivator, it is not difficult to envision a not-too-distant future that includes dollar-saving surgery outsourcing and pocketbook-saving medical tourism. In Singapore, health plan members may be singing the blues. Seniors may become ill in Malaysia or incur medical expenses in Costa Rica. Outside of the United States, demand for and access to medical care is rapidly increasing.

Outside of the United States, demand for and access to medical care is rapidly increasing. It was predicted that approximately 750,000 Americans traveled for medical care in 2007 (Deloitte Center for Health Solutions 2008). Rising medical costs in the United States and throughout the world, combined with connections to international providers through expatriates, immigrants, travelers, retirees, and deployed military personnel and families, have paved the way for greater comfort in seeking medical care outside one's own country. Historically, businesses such as Aetna have insured travelers who needed emergency care abroad, as well as expatriate workers and retirees (Aetna Global Benefits 2008). CIGNA Envoy (2008) have a firsthand understanding of foreign medical access issues. Medical tourism and global healthcare sourcing are two developing trends in seeking medical care overseas (Mydans 2002). Medical tourism may be termed client-active from the perspective of the patient because it is pursued by an individual client. As illustrated, the mobility of individuals between countries is not just a North American phenomenon; impulses to return to one's home country for medical care in a familiar culture and setting persist for several generations and the global map depicts travel patterns and reveals a distinct pattern of the majority of international medical travelers (McKinsey and Company 2008). The Asian nexus is the most popular medical tourism location. Quality disparities continue to be a source of concern in the developing global healthcare market. Accreditation is a component of the solution. To that end, the JCI has accredited more than 100 facilities in 34 countries ranging from Austria and Bangladesh to Turkey and the United Arab Emirates. The United States is not alone in its desire for global reach. Accreditation programs in the Australian and Canadian healthcare systems are expanding into the worldwide medical arena. The Australian Council on Healthcare Standards (ACHS) specifically joined the worldwide arena in 2004 when it began accrediting facilities in the Middle East. The ACHS standards are divided into four categories: safe blood management, infection control, fall prevention, and continuity of care between healthcare professionals (ACHSI 2011). Medical tourism is not a new phenomenon; historical evidence shows that individuals traveled for health cures as early as the middle third millennium B.C. (Kevan 1993). Modern medical tourism, on the other hand, is a globalized commodity that may be found within larger international medical trade frameworks such as the World Trade Organization's (W.T.O.) General Agreement on Trade in Services (GATS) model, as underlined by Cattaneo (2009). Medical tourism is classified as Mode 2 trade consumption. Medical tourism, however, is not the sole Mode 2 consumption. Temporary visitors from other countries; long-term residents; common borders; and outsourced patients are examples of patient mobility (Bertinato et al. 2005; Rosenmoller et al. 2006). Medical tourism often involves out-of-pocket treatment costs and is mostly driven by individual consumers who choose to travel for a variety of reasons, including cost, privacy, accessibility, or treatment availability (Lunt et al. 2011).

However, according to Johnston et al. (2010) and Lunt and Carrera (2010), more specific statistics for judging quality, particularly treatment results, are required (Lunt and Carrera 2010). When patients travel for medical reasons, they trust unfamiliar structures; yet, evidence from the United Kingdom suggests that, even when available, patients should be able to easily use outcome data when determining which private provider to use (Mannion and Davies 2005). According to research, a healthcare provider's public image and reputation, which is heavily influenced by the medical profession's voice, has a greater impact on markets than consumer exit (Hibbard 2008). Medical tourism markets have seen associations with well-known medical centers through franchising. There has recently been an increase in developing nation provider accreditation, which several governments, notably India, Thailand, Singapore, and Malaysia, actively support (Shetty 2010; Pocock and Phua 2011). Though low cost is a key trade driver, it cannot be achieved at the expense of quality (Herrick 2007). There is a significant literature vacuum regarding quality and accreditation, even though there are numerous indications against which healthcare quality can be judged. Adequate infection control techniques emphasize the importance of following protocols and consulting with specialist microbiologists if postoperative infection rates surpass safe ranges.

Connell (2006) and Herrick (2007) hypothesized that the inherent risks are increased because air travel is included in the equation, increasing the risk of deep vein thrombosis (DVT)—a common complication following any operation; the risk of DVT occurring, leading to pulmonary embolism increases from the tenth postoperative day (Williams 1995). Medical tourism is estimated to be a \$60 billion sector in 2006, with revenue increasing year by year until it reaches \$100 in 2012; nevertheless, market size and breadth are challenging to determine (Crone 2008). Ehrbeck et al. (2008) estimate 60–80,000 medical tourists. Youngman (2009) argues that the total number might be five million; however, his estimations include cross-border travel, which will only sometimes involve movement outside of an individual's natural environment. Recent mainstream media articles have focused on "North-South" travel, which is defined as travel from more-developed to less-developed countries. Cattaneo (2009), like Reinhardt (in Herrick 2007), believes that Mode 2 trading can increase competitiveness in domestic markets. Chinai and Goswami (2007) discussed the potential negative effects on allocative efficiency in India, claiming that insufficient regulation may result in an internal "brain drain" when healthcare professionals are lured from the public to the private sector and away from rural areas, which require lower technology interventions as a priority. Many governments, on the other hand, encourage the sector, claiming that it benefits their economy (Shetty 2010; Pocock and Phua 2011). Indeed, Bukonda et al. (2003) questioned whether developing-world hospital certification made the best use of scarce resources. According to Pomey et al. (2004), doctors do not appreciate certification programs because they believe self-assessment is more suitable; however, nurses and health managers were more favorable. According to Mihalik et al. (2003), certification is a necessary investment. Nandraj et al. (2001) investigated public perceptions of certification programs in India, which officials were considering implementing. Turner (2011) proposes that medical tourism workers be accredited as well and that care arrangements be limited to internationally accredited facilities to assist in ensuring quality. According to Herrick (2007), Horowitz et al. (2007), Carabello (2008), and York (2008), the JCI had recognized 100–120 institutions by 2008, and the number had tripled by 2011, with 329 in 2011. The Middle East countries that obtained the most accreditations included Turkey, Saudi Arabia, and the United Arab Emirates. It may be more cost-effective for some countries to outsource accreditation to foreign sources and benefit from economies of scale. Furthermore, because accreditation can necessitate advanced technical skills (Walshe 2009), Mode 3 trade could bridge skill shortfalls.

Accreditors may begin to accredit facilitators who only arrange care for medical tourists at recognized facilities in the future, as Turner (2011) suggests. The value of international accreditation for medical tourism in particular, and the poor world in general, remains to be shown. Bukonda et al. (2003) examined how individual organization certification expenses were unsustainable in poor countries. However, Mihalik et al. (2003) considered accreditation to be a necessary investment. However, there may be some cases when accreditation is done primarily to obtain a badge that allows providers to display their quality credentials and compete in whichever health markets they operate in. This viewpoint contrasts with another, which sees continual learning as a means of enhancing patient safety and healthcare quality. Both are not mutually exclusive. Chen et al. (2003) warn that there can be significant heterogeneity among accredited providers, which may be common to all healthcare systems. They also discovered that accredited hospitals outperformed non-accredited hospitals in several quality metrics. Accreditation implies, at the very least, that staff is willing to participate in quality improvement activities.

Even for Americans who have medical insurance, the exorbitant expense of healthcare can be disastrous. As a result of the lack of professional relationship development, sentiments of loyalty to any one physician are diminished. In an Iranian study, many positive and negative aspects of Iran's medical tourism business were discovered using the diamond of advantage, strategic challenges were highlighted, and numerous potential solutions for addressing them were proposed. The study suggests that increased public-private cooperation, aggressive marketing, improved infrastructure, international accreditation of healthcare facilities, and human resource development could strengthen the country's medical tourism economy. Jabbari (2012) suggests that traveling for surgery is appealing to a large number of people. Campbell (2019)—a study aimed at identifying the individual features of healthy travelers—highlights the associated causal variables for seeking health treatment in Turkey. The majority of visitors came from Europe (44%), followed by North America (28%). Lower costs, physician knowledge, responsiveness, and familiarity or interest in Turkey were the primary factors driving patients to the location (pull factors). Health visitors visiting Turkey were largely pleased with the outcomes of their treatments and the care provided by their doctors, with many expressing a desire to return. A study analyzing the influence of accreditation on quality in basic and secondary healthcare settings in Kerala (Ozan-Rafferty 2014) suggests that if accreditation is to bring entrenched quality, structural and procedural features of healthcare facilities must be changed. A healthcare facility's structural improvement cannot guarantee patient pleasure. The certification process must be viewed as a tool for the holistic and continual transformation of the overall infrastructural and interpersonal dimensions of a healthcare facility. Joseph (2021)—a study to discover possible methods in attracting medical tourists to JCI-accredited hospitals in Saudi Arabia and to measure the usefulness of marketing mix on Saudi Arabian Medical tourism—concluded that marketing mix plays an important role in attracting medical tourists to the K.S.A. and making it one of the most desirable destinations for global medical tourism (Reddy 2017).

4.3 An Overview of Medical Accreditation

"Accreditation is a formal process to ensure delivery of safe, high-quality health care based on standards and processes devised and developed by health care professionals for health care services," according to ISQua. It is also a public acknowledgment of a healthcare organization's achievement of requirements of national healthcare standards. It provides patients with the certainty that rigorous safety and quality of care standards are in place. Accreditation demonstrates that a hospital or clinic is committed to providing high-quality services to its patients. It is proof that the organization's services were granted. Most hospitals will prominently show accreditation information on their websites. Local medical boards or equivalent authorities will need doctors to be licensed. Using a recognized hospital or clinic, on the other hand, significantly enhances the likelihood that your doctor is fully licensed (Accreditation date: 2022). In the United States, hospital accreditation began nearly 100 years ago as an assessment mechanism for surgical training. It grew into a bigger, professionally driven institutional assessment and development framework that is currently present in over 50 nations. Several worldwide initiatives have become available across national lines since the turn of the century. Most accrediting schemes analyze a hospital's conformity with established criteria across the board, but others also provide certification of specialized services. ISO certification often employs standard 9004 (non-specific to healthcare) or 15,189 (specific to medical laboratories) to assess quality management systems. Several countries have regulatory systems in place to ensure that necessary national standards are met, similar to voluntary accreditation programs. Accreditation and similar external assessment systems add value to medical tourism by providing accurate, independent certification of a hospital's compliance with approved organizational norms. The published findings' criteria, methodology, and level of detail differ between programs but are more consistent within ISQua-accredited programs (Shaw 2015). Many worldwide accrediting schemes are run by commercial companies and corporations. Furthermore, poorer countries that often provide medical tourism services may require more access to the certification process or participating would put them in financial jeopardy. Accreditation can also be used as a marketing strategy by hospitals or governments seeking a piece of the lucrative medical tourism sector (Hall 2013; Tomislav 2022). Providers aiming to sell their services to patients in other countries, on the other hand, have offset the disadvantages of linguistic dissimilarity and asymmetric information by capitalizing on the high complementarity between medical and non-medical tourism services (Chung-Ping and Loh 2019).

4.3.1 Global and National Accreditation of Healthcare Institutions

The concept of hospital accreditation dates back to the 1860s, when Florence Nightingale devised a method for collecting and reviewing hospital statistics, thereby reinforcing the assurance of healthcare quality. The findings of her investigation revealed a significant gap in death rates among hospitals (Sheingold 2014). Dr. Earnest Codman, who created the "result system," which enabled healthcare institutions to follow the patients they treated and receive feedback on whether their treatment was beneficial, was another pioneer in healthcare accreditation. The American College of Surgeons (ACS) proposed the Hospital Standardization Programme in 1919, which garnered a remarkable response from the medical community (Dastur 2012). Their "Standard of Efficiency" document is regarded as the first blueprint of hospital accrediting criteria. In 1924, the American College of Surgeons released the hospital standardization program, which foreshadowed the principles of quality and safety (Roberts 1987). The Joint Commission on Accreditation of Hospitals (JCAH) was established in 1951, and the "Standard of Efficiency" was renamed a "Hospital Accreditation Program" (Chuang 2019). The Joint Commission on Accreditation of Hospitals (JCAH) became the Joint Commission on Accreditation of Healthcare Organizations (JCAHO) in 1987. JCAHO-accredited hospitals were deemed suitable for treating patients because they provided superior care. JCAHO was renamed Joint Commission and later Joint Commission International (JCI) in 2007. Another accreditor, Accrediting Canada, created and released "Qmentum," a revolutionary accrediting approach in 2008 that combined clinical appraisal tools with a structured evaluation system (Tomasich et al. 2020). Accreditation of healthcare institutions in India dates back to 2005 when the National Accreditation Board for Hospitals and Healthcare (NABH) was established to assure the quality and safety of healthcare services by pursuing evidence-based medical therapy.

Quality standards for hospitals and other medical institutions were first proposed in the United States in 1917 with the American College of Surgeons' "Minimum Standard for Hospitals." Following World War II, greater global trade resulted in the establishment of the International Standards Organization (ISO) in 1947. Accreditation began formally in the United States in 1951, with the formation of the Joint Commission on Accreditation of Healthcare Organizations (JCAHO). In the 1980s, the same was exported to Canada and Australia. Accreditation programs are proliferating throughout developing countries. Other systems, including certification and licensing, are utilized around the world to govern, improve, and promote healthcare providers and organizations. The Saudi Central Board for Accreditation of Healthcare Institutions (CBAHI) was established in 2005 on the advice of the Saudi Council of Health Services. CBAHI was founded to develop and execute quality standards in all health sectors throughout the Kingdom of Saudi Arabia (CDS 2000). CBAHI (n.d.) ISQua is a non-profit organization founded in 1985 to drive continuous improvement in healthcare quality and safety worldwide through education, research, collaboration, and the transmission of evidence-based information. ISQua delivers internationally recognized healthcare standards principles. ISQua has already recognized several sets of healthcare standards used in Australia, Canada, Egypt, and England, as well as the Joint Commission International standards used in the United States. December 2007 (ISQUA) Saudi Aramco established the Saudi Medical Services Organization Standards in 1994. To be accepted as referral healthcare institutions for Aramco personnel, private and governmental hospitals have to meet Aramco standards. The Makkah Regional Council for the Development of Health Services was created in 2001. One of the key outcomes of this council was the creation of the Makkah Region Quality Program (MRQP) in 2003, which required governmental and private hospitals in the Makkah region (57 hospitals) to meet established requirements. These criteria were developed by JCAHO and ARAMCO guidelines. Saudi Arabia's minister of health founded the CBAHI in October 2005. CBAHI intends to begin the accreditation process in 2010. Several private and public hospitals were accredited by various international accreditation bodies, including JCI, Accreditation Canada, and The Australian Council on Healthcare Standards (ACHS). The majority of ISQua principles were not met or only partially met by the majority of CBAHI standards. The development of CBAHI standards is outlined, along with a defined method for revising the standards. Furthermore, each CBAHI standard lacks quantitative aspects. To enable developing countries to examine, compare, and improve local accreditation programs, there is a need to encourage assessments of local accreditation programs in other countries. Greenfield (2009), Alkhenizan (2010) and Mason et al., drawing on framing theory, analyzed the content of 66 medical tourism Websites from around the world, and the results showed that medical tourism Websites largely promote the benefits of medical procedures while downplaying the risks, and relatively little information regarding the credibility of these services appears; additionally, the presentation of benefits/risks, credibility, and Website interactivity were found to differ by racial group (Mason 2011). The reproductive tourism business should adopt safe and responsible medical procedures in the best interests of consumers, health professionals, and legislators (Smith 2010) Accreditation is well-established on a global scale. Accreditation is defined in the same way by the three largest and oldest organizations: JCAHO, The Canadian Council on Health Services Accreditation (CCHSA), and ACHS. Standards, indicators, surveyors, surveys, accreditation reports, and results are all common features in the organizations. The establishment of ISQua and The Agenda for Leadership in Programs in Healthcare Accreditation (ALPHA) initiative, on the other hand, has inspired increased comparability. The fact that no link has been established between accreditation and quality in patient care is a weakness. According to the order in the "Health Policy Report 2002," external assessment in the form of accreditation will become a reality in the Danish healthcare sector: Accreditation is required for all hospitals in all counties and within 2006 the Copenhagen Hospital Corporation (Frølich 2002).

4.3.2 Accreditation of Healthcare Institutions

The World Health Organization (WHO) stated that patient safety is a major global public health priority. A person traveling by plane has a one in a million probability of getting wounded, but a patient in healthcare has a one in 300 chance of being damaged. According to WHO estimates, there are 421 million hospitalizations worldwide each year, with about 42.7 million adverse events occurring in patients during these hospitalizations. Furthermore, according to recent data, patient injury is the 14th leading cause of illness and mortality worldwide (Jabarkhil et al. 2021). Healthcare services that are safe, patient-centered, and of high quality are required for medical care systems to be strengthened. They discovered an urgent need for global standardization of therapeutic care and medical processes. This approach results in the assignment of a grade or score to a healthcare organization, indicating the degree of conformance to the required standards. Accreditation is an accreditor's acknowledgment and endorsement of a hospital or medical care organization's achievement of accreditation criteria, as confirmed by a third-party peer appraisal on the level of performance of this institution undergoing Accreditation against set standards. Scrivens (1995) *defined accreditation as "a process used for assessing the quality of an organization's performance that is centered on a system of independent third-party peer appraisal using standards...an assessment of compliance with standards is conducted by health service personnel on behalf of an independent body." Concerns about the quality and safety of patient care provided abroad have also arisen, according to* Scally and Donaldson (1998), "*due to a lack of well-planned clinical governance measures and quality guarantee measures in provider organizations, envisioned to reassure the quality of care delivered to tourists.*" Accreditation, according to Shaw (2015), is a system in which "competent external peer assessors assess a health care organization's conformity with prescribed and defined performance criteria." According to Pomey et al. (2004), the accreditation procedure includes "a self-assessment, institution visits, and the compilation of a report about the assessed institution, and then awarding international appreciation to the assessed institution." In contrast to licensure, which is a one-time process, accreditation stresses continuous improvement techniques and accomplishment of ideal quality criteria rather than adherence to nominal norms intended to assure public safety. Accreditation of healthcare institutions is defined as "an official procedure to ensure the provision of safe, high-quality health care based on standards and processes developed and designed by medical professionals for medical care services, and is an acknowledgment of achievement by a healthcare organization in meeting the requirements of national healthcare standards" (ISQua). Following proper training, certified body-appointed assessors are assigned for hospital evaluation. They undertake a verification evaluation using facility rounds, stakeholder interviews, document verification, and inspection of hospital services in accordance with the certified organization's requirements.

4.3.3 The Need for Accreditations

Patients seeking standardized healthcare services abroad prioritize the quality of care provided by healthcare institutions over cost-effectiveness or shorter treatment wait times in comparison to their native country. This quality of care is a major difference when choosing overseas healthcare institutions, as it varies greatly from one medical care center to another and from nation to country. Accreditation motivates the implementation of model healthcare administration systems and practices that improve service delivery and quality, resulting in improved inpatient satisfaction and care. This standardization approach, as verified by accreditation, is a risk-reduction and quality-optimization technique that can considerably improve quality treatment and patient experience while also increasing patient volume (Rawlins 2001). There has recently been a large influx of tourists in need of medical care in growing medical tourism nations. When the medical tourism market becomes more competitive, accreditation will no longer be the main distinction in selecting healthcare establishments. The international medical tourism industry was valued at $54.4 billion in 2020 and is expected to reach $209.9 billion by 2027, growing at a CAGR of 21.1% (Hari Krishnan and Chandrasekhar 2020). The Indian Medical Tourism market is also expected to develop dramatically, from US$3 billion in 2015 to US$9 billion by the end of 2020 (Ministry of Tourism) (David 2017). With the increase in medical tourism, healthcare organizations will need to improve and differentiate their services with an evidence-based framework focusing on enhanced patient experience, superior healthcare outcomes, and outstanding follow-up care. Quality in healthcare is critical since it is directly related to patient safety. As we all know, quality is determined by either regulation or market demand. Regulation has been ineffective in most developing nations due to a shortage of healthcare providers, and governments must be flexible. Quality has taken a back place in such conditions. Accreditation represents the framework for a hospital's quality governance and is based on the highest standards. India is not only building several state-of-the-art hospitals, but it is also seeing a growth in demand for quality as well as medical tourism. In 2006, India launched its accreditation system by ISQua requirements. In research, Gyani (2014) depict the route to accreditation in India and discuss the issues encountered by hospitals as well as the benefits provided for the business and patients.

4.3.4 International Accreditation Agencies: Accreditor of Accreditors

The worldwide Society for Quality in Health Care (ISQua) and the United Kingdom Akkreditering Forum (UKF) are worldwide accreditation bodies that are known as "the accreditor of accreditors." These organizations support global accreditation organizations such as Joint Commission International (JCI), Australian Council on Healthcare Standards (ACHS), Accreditation Canada, Trent Accreditation Scheme Malaysian Society for Quality in Health, NABH, and Saudi Arabia's Central Board for Accreditation of Healthcare Institutions (CBAHI). They ensure that accreditation is not a one-time certification process, but rather a continual quality improvement program facilitated by accrediting institutions. ISQua and UKAF are international organizations that evaluate accreditation agencies and provide criteria in healthcare safety and patient care for hospitals and other patient care facilities.

4.3.4.1 ISQua (International Society for Quality in Health Care)

ISQua is an impartial worldwide healthcare umbrella organization that provides accreditation to organizations. It is in charge of reviewing and evaluating the standards of international, national, and regional accrediting authorities to continuously improve the quality and safety of patient care in hospitals and other healthcare institutions. ISQua did not survey or accredit individual hospitals or clinics on their own.

4.3.4.2 UKAF (The United Kingdom Akkreditering Forum)

UK Accrediting Forum Limited is an independent accreditation institution for healthcare companies. UK Accrediting Forum Limited is an independent, neutral, and pioneer in the field of accreditation; like ISQua, UKAF has never surveyed or accredited hospitals on its own.

4.3.5 Accreditation Bodies

4.3.5.1 Joint Commission International (JCI)

JCI Accreditation is currently held by 958 healthcare facilities worldwide and is regarded as the gold standard in global patient care and a benchmark of global standards on quality, patient confidence, and security. JCI is the world's largest and oldest standards-setting and accreditation body. It evaluates and reviews healthcare institutions to ensure that they provide safe, efficient, and effective patient care. JCI accreditation is expected to take between 12 and 24 months. This includes establishing a realistic period and explaining the importance of taking a consistent, comprehensive approach to Accreditation. Accredited organizations must conduct a baseline assessment, determine the gap between their performance and JCI requirements, and revise their policies and procedures to guarantee JCI compliance. JCI accreditation is regarded by foreign patients, particularly medical tourists, as the highest ranking in worldwide patient care and a symbol of global patient confidentiality and security norms. JCI accreditation is regarded by medical insurance companies around the world as a need for patient coverage for treatments in other countries. Among Asia's critical medical tourist destinations, India has the second highest number of Joint Commission International recognized health institutions (Hari Krishnan and Chandrasekhar 2020).

4.3.5.2 Australian Council on Healthcare Standards (ACHS)

ACHS is an independent, non-profit organization dedicated to improving healthcare quality, and it is an accredited accreditor of Australian and international healthcare providers. The International Society for Quality in Health Care (ISQua) has acknowledged ACHS for its institutional structure, accreditation procedures, and assessor training. ACHS now accredits 1450 health institutions worldwide.

4.3.5.3 National Accreditation Board for Hospitals and Healthcare Providers (NABH)

To establish India as the most favored medical tourism destination, more than only treatment cost competitiveness is required. Because quality of care is the most important distinction, we need additional recognized institutions to further improve the global medical tourism arena. The more globally approved hospitals a place has, the more prominent it will be on the international medical tourism map. It helps to position India as a source of high-end medical treatment that is of high quality, standard, and safe, and it boosts global medical travelers' confidence in our safe and high-grade patient care. The National Accreditation Board for Hospitals and Healthcare Providers (NABH) was formed to develop and implement an accreditation scheme for Indian healthcare institutions. It plays an important role in the Quality Council of India (QCI). It was established to strengthen the healthcare system and sustain constant quality enhancement, patient care, and patient safety against predetermined criteria. NABH offers healthcare facilities with the required foundation for quality assurance and improvement. These guidelines require constant monitoring of sentinel incidents and propose thorough remedial action plans that will lead to quality consciousness in all aspects of patient care. There are currently 716 NABH-accredited hospitals in India (Nahai 2010). NABH was founded to strengthen healthcare systems and encourage continual quality improvement and patient safety. The board has full functional autonomy and is backed by all stakeholders, including industry, consumers, and government. NABH is an Institutional Member of the International Society for Quality in Healthcare (ISQua) Accreditation Council and a founding member of the Asian Society for Quality in Healthcare (ASQua). NABH accreditation is in high demand among SAARC/ASIAN countries. To that end, NABH has formed NABH International, with the Philippines serving as the first international target.

4.3.6 About Medical Tourism and Facilitator

Medical tourism is a tourist institution or resort that intentionally promotes its healthcare services and conventional tourist facilities to attract travelers. International medical tourism refers to cross-border travel by people seeking medical services, either to reduce prices at home or to obtain excellent care from medically advanced countries. A Medical Tourism Facilitator is an organization that manages and coordinates all aspects of patient care and treatment while traveling overseas. Medical tourism companies and facilitators are critical to the medical tourism business since they assist patients in participating in medical tourism. The following are the reasons:

- Medical care was unavailable in their respective countries.
- Expensive healthcare costs.
- Some therapies, such as fertility treatments, may be illegal in the patient's home country.
- Technological advancements and higher standards of care in many countries.
- Shorten healthcare wait times.

Various factors to consider when selecting a medical tourism destination include

- Extensive cultural heritage and tourism potential.
- Access to advanced medical equipment and expertise.
- A reputation for traditional medicines and therapies such as Ayurveda, Homoeopathy, Unani, Naturopathy, and Yoga, as well as Panchakarma.
- Wellness tourism: several tourist destinations for tourist attractions.
- Affordably priced, high-quality healthcare.

- Procedures are available.
- Religious and cultural compatibility.
- The political climate.
- Credentials of healthcare providers, such as the NHS.
- A vacation package is available in addition to therapeutic care.

Accreditation and standardization of hospitals are critical components of any well-organized society. The academic community has characterized it as an external assessment and self-assessment procedure based on set standards to accurately assess performance and implement action plans to improve. Due to some unethical scenarios, medical tourism needs a significant presence of healthcare accreditation. The patient must conduct research and observe that a lack of accreditation may have serious effects, not only in terms of the outcome of the therapy but also in terms of the quality of the service.

4.3.7 Advantages of Accreditation in Medical Tourism

Accreditation in medical tourism provides healthcare organizations with evidence of independent third-party quality assessment against prescribed standards or healthcare criteria, ensuring that international medical tourists are assured of consistent healthcare treatment practices regardless of the geographical location of the healthcare institution where they seek treatment. Most medical tourists are risk-averse, and institution accreditation is viewed as a risk-mitigation element in their cross-border treatment decision-making. The accreditation process includes surveys and reviews conducted by experienced professional peers who use a variety of measures to diagnose issues in advance, correct them, and ensure continual improvement. The accrediting procedure offers follow-up action for the faults detected and assures continuous quality based on the survey recommendations. The evaluation procedure is normally performed every 2–4 years. Accreditation provides various benefits to healthcare institutions and medical tourists, some of which are listed below:

(a) Accreditation continuously enhances the quality of patient care and promotes modern treatment facilities based on accreditation bodies' findings and endorsements.
(b) Reduces treatment risks and errors while identifying gaps through adequate monitoring at various phases.
(c) Consistently promotes patient-centered policies and standards to enhance superior patient care and satisfaction.
(d) Provides a systematic approach to the hospital's working environment involving clinical and support staff.
(e) Ensures that patient care and service delivery are designed to deliver better treatment results.

(f) Applies global standards of excellence in patient-centric services to improve the quality and outcomes of medical tourism treatment.
(g) Ensures patient profile privacy and treatment record confidentiality.
(h) Accreditation can also be utilized for marketing purposes by healthcare facilities, medical travel facilitators (MTF), and governments of rising medical tourism locations to attract profitable medical tourism business and therefore increase international patient inflow.

4.3.8 Evidence of the Impact of Accreditation

What are some of the advantages of gaining international accreditation for hospitals? In terms of evidence, the study sends a mixed message. According to Brubakk et al. (2015), "the review did not find evidence of hospital accreditation and certification being linked to measurable changes in quality of care as measured by quality metrics and standards." Hussein et al. (2021) discovered 76 empirical studies that satisfied their criteria for assessing the impact of international accreditation on hospitals or clinics in a more extended review of over 17,000 papers. Furthermore, Shawan (2021) discovered quantitative results demonstrating that pursuing accreditation positively impacted the majority of the 12 outcomes examined in an investigation of the King Fahd Hospital of the University of Saudi Arabia. These were as follows:

1. The average length of stay.
2. The percentage of people that practice hand hygiene.
3. The incidence of nosocomial infections.
4. The proportion of outliers in radiology reporting.
5. The prevalence of pressure ulcers.
6. The portion of patient identification that is correct.
7. The essential lab reporting component.
8. The rate of bed occupancy.

Furthermore, the qualitative research indicated that the stakeholders involved in the certification process viewed it favorably; however, the impact on revenues from increased occupancy was not quantified. Guastello and Jay (2019) discovered that after implementing this "patient and family engaged care" PCC model, patient satisfaction and experience scores increased in numerous hospitals. Aside from better clinic standards and outcomes, the research finds inconsistent support for the benefits of international health accreditation.

This raises the fundamental topic of accreditation's role in giving brand value to the healthcare system perhaps hospital executives and owners hope that accreditation will offer instant prominence to any medical establishment that achieves approval. The certification procedure addresses all aspects of hospital care, including clinical outcomes and safety, as well as cleanliness and environmental effects. Hospitals seeking accreditation in developing markets are looking for outside solid support for their brand. As a result, the hospital brand's contribution is primarily reliant on affiliations with other companies. As a result, conducting research on worldwide accreditation and branding by healthcare facilities is critical. The impact of global healthcare branding on a facility's capacity to attract customers is still little understood. The literature contains hints that there may be some effects on customer decision-making (Guiry and Vequist 2010).

Consumers are not always aware of all worldwide healthcare accreditation attempts. The application of American standards in other nations is one of the most visible examples of this behavior that many people are unaware of, including many in the US healthcare community. The writers will look at the delayed implementation of American accrediting standards in private and governmental hospitals in Mexico. As a result, Mexico has served as a massive "experimental" model for determining whether foreign accreditation (however silently) influences the country's hospital branding. From 2009 to 2019, revenues from American medical tourists increased by around 120%, while GHA accreditations increased by 180%. In comparison, JCI accreditation of facilities increased by 50% over the same 10-year period. Although this study falls under the "correlation is not causation" category, the findings show that greater quality could be a driver of increasing medical tourism in a country. The preferences of medical tourists may be influenced by an overall macro effect of international accreditation. However, many other reasons could be at work here, such as shifting demographics in the United States and regulatory changes in the American healthcare system. The authors sampled five publicly listed healthcare systems with a "flagship" hospital(s) that received the JCI certification standard to further investigate whether international accreditation had a favorable influence on attracting foreign medical tourists. Because their financials were accessible for review (convenience sample), the following financial ratios were examined both before (including the fiscal year in which accreditation was received) and after (in aggregate) international accreditation approval. The financial ratios are expected to improve in post-accreditation reporting years if the accreditation influences medical tourists' decision-making. The ratios were set to reflect the predicted effects of a growth-oriented strategy centered on investment in international accreditation. If this were more than a symbolic gesture, the healthcare system would be expected to get a greater number of overseas patients following accreditation, resulting in higher operating margins, more prosperous earnings, and maybe bigger debt as a result of the investment. Only a subset of the financials for all years, both pre and post-accreditation, were available for these systems. Based on the convenience sample available, a standard of at most five (5) years before and post-accreditation was employed. The financial measures of the systems were analyzed both before and after accreditation (including the accreditation approval year). According to Erhun et al. (2020), there are two important variations between these systems: (1) patient numbers (which are greater in India) and (2) utilization of mid-tier providers (which is also higher in India). These operational discrepancies, coupled with the other constraints highlighted in this work, which may vary greatly between the nations surveyed, are further reasons to believe that more empirical research on this topic is required.

4.4 Emergence of Medical Tourism in India

Individuals generally sought medical aid from their native country or relocated to more developed countries for medical treatments that were unavailable in their own country. However, it is now being seen that people are seeking medical care in places other than their native country. This is how the relevance of medical tourism became recognized. India, Thailand, Puerto Rico, Argentina, Cuba, Singapore, Malaysia, Taiwan, Mexico, and Costa Rica are major medical tourism destinations. Complex surgeries and dental operations, kidney dialysis, organ transplants, joint replacement, cardiac surgery, dental surgery, cosmetic surgeries, hereditary problems, and psychiatry are among the procedures for which medical tourism is used (Thoke 2017). The rapid rise of the private sector in the 1980s and the establishment of a corporate health sector in the 1990s were the result of deliberate policy choices to foster these segments. This was accomplished through varying subsidies in the form of cheap land, discounts on equipment and drug imports, placing these institutions on government panels and making them a part of government insurance structures, and providing trained personnel and practicing physicians through state-supported medical education (Reddy 2010). The National Health Policy designated urban medical facilities as service production units equal to production units and, as such, critical sources of foreign exchange revenues. The form of care for the poor themselves shifted from broad-based to primary-level care (Reddy 2010).

According to projections, India will take 2.5% of the medical tourism business in 2012, with foreign revenue of $ 2.3 billion, and will receive approximately 1.1 million health tourists globally. Medical tourism is expanding rapidly all over the world. India is the world's second most popular destination for medical tourism. Medical treatment in India is highly affordable, as it charges 20% less than any other foreign country for healthcare services. Other factors, in addition to the lower cost of treatment, are leading to an increase in foreign health tourist traffic in India. Today, Indian clinical and paramedical skill is well recognized, and JCI accreditation to select hospitals in India has proven to be a boon to the Indian medical system, assisting in garnering international patients' trust in India's hospitals and experts. They do not have to wait long in India, and they do not have to spend extra money for their treatment. The cost of healthcare per capita in Korea is $720, while it is $94 in India. As a result, India offers them 20% less expensive therapy than the United States, United Kingdom, Singapore, and Thailand. In the instance of medical care, India was shown to be more cost-effective than Thailand. For example, CABG in India costs $4400 versus $14,250 in Thailand (From www.ijbmi.org).

A medical tourist is someone who comes to indulge/lure oneself into a healthy and pure environment, study the practice of yoga and meditation, refresh themselves at spas, or preserve their appearance by traveling to Cosmetic Surgery Clinics. It is optional for them to come for surgery or treatment to be considered medical tourists. Going to China for acupuncture and acupressure treatment for backache is an example of former traveling to Kerala for ayurvedic treatment for the full body medical tourism in India is at an all-time high. Health tourists can now swiftly and easily access any type of medical institution. Several private investors and pharmaceutical businesses have expressed interest in providing services to health tourists. According to statistics, India will welcome approximately one million health tourists by the end of 2012, with a compound annual growth rate (CAGR) of 28.09% over 2007. A health tourist in India spends less money on procedures than in other developed and poor countries. Various sources in 2010 and 2011 exhibit cost comparisons of India with other countries, clearly demonstrating the gap (Malhotra and Dave 2022).

4.4.1 The SWOT and TOWS Matrix Analysis of Medical Tourism in India

The SWOT (strengths, weaknesses, opportunities, and threats) and TOWS analysis have been stated as follows in terms of medical tourism in India (Tables 4.1 and 4.2).

4.4.2 Main Issues and Challenges Concerning Medical Tourism

The following are the key difficulties facing medical tourism: Dunn (2011):

1. *Lack of infrastructure*—Some hospitals and healthcare centers, particularly those in rural areas, lack infrastructure and other facilities. Patients attend hospitals and healthcare centers to seek medical and healthcare treatment; thus, good facilities, clean drinking water, efficient service, the availability of electricity and civic amenities, and so on are essential.
2. *Lack of trust*—Illnesses, diseases, and health concerns frequently instill fear and vulnerability in people's minds. When they go to the hospital or a healthcare facility, they usually feel anxious. The key constraints have been noticed in terms of environmental circumstances, diet and nutrition supply, a lack of suitable services, inefficiency in dealing with patient needs, and ineffective communication.
3. *Lack of insurance*—The medical tourism business in the country is facing some challenges in terms of insurance and allied services. These include insufficient insurance coverage, an underdeveloped insurance market, insurance fraud, and foreign corporations refusing to reimburse.
4. *Difficulties in upgrading the medical tourism sector*—The government may make a substantial contribution to the medical tourism sector's upgradation. Nonetheless, the sector is encountering substantial obstacles and setbacks that have shown to be important issues that must be addressed.
5. *Training and development programs*—The people who work in medical and healthcare facilities undoubtedly have the necessary qualifications. The primary

Table 4.1 SWOT analysis: medical tourism in India (Adapted from Dawn 2011)

Strengths	Weakness
1. Good service at a reasonable price 2. A large pool of qualified doctors 3. A high concentration of advanced healthcare facilities 4. Hospitals and doctors' international reputation 5. Extensive range of travel places and experiences 6. Indian doctors have a high level of trust 7. Alternative medical treatments such as Yoga, Homeopathy, and Ayurveda 8. Use of cutting-edge technology 9. High rate of success 10. Increasing scarcity of qualified medical personnel and specialists in underdeveloped nations	1. There is minimal government support or initiative to promote medical tourism 2. Lack of collaboration among business participants 3. Customer perception of an unsanitary country 4. There is no effective hospital certification and regulating framework 5. Inconsistent pricing policies among hospitals 6. Inadequate infrastructure in government-assisted institutions and a high demand for healthcare in the country
Opportunities	**Threats**
1. Increased demand for healthcare services from the United States and the United Kingdom 2. A fast-paced lifestyle raises the desire for wellness tourism and alternative treatments 3. Supply shortages in national health systems in the United Kingdom and Canada 4. Demand from poor countries' healthcare facilities 5. Lowering the competitive cost of international travel 6. Growth in GDP and Forex 7. Market entry of foreign players 8. Medical treatment costs more in developing countries than in developed countries	1. Intense rivalry from Thailand, Malaysia, and Singapore 2. The lack of international accreditation is a significant impediment 3. Insufficient investment in health infrastructure 4. The entry of new foreign players into the market 5. A lack of government funding for medical tourism promotion 6. Demand

Table 4.2 TOWS matrix for Indian medical tourism (Adapted from Dawn 2011)

Internal factors	Strengths (S)	Weakness (W)
External factors	SO strategies or maxi-maxi	WO strategies or mini-maxi
Opportunities (O)	• Affordable costs in India can maintain and increase the demand from underdeveloped countries • International reputation, high success rate, qualified doctors, and increasing shortage of competent staff in developed countries can increase demand for medical tourism from developed countries • Alternative cures are available in India for fast-paced lifestyle • Confidence in Indian doctors and advancement in the medical field can meet the shortage of supply in national health systems of developed countries • Foreign players can take advantage of the latest technology	• GDP earned from medical tourism should be reinvested to promote medical tourism, to improve health conditions and infrastructure in healthcare • Coordination should be maintained between the players of the medical tourism industry to face competition from foreign players and take advantage of reduced competitive costs and price differences • Proper accreditation should be done to increase demand for healthcare services and to take benefit of the shortage of supply in developed countries • Uniform pricing policy should be maintained to the benefit from fast-paced life and demand from underdeveloped countries
Threats (T)	ST strategies or maxi-mini	WT strategies or mini-mini
	• Reduced cost, vast pool of doctors, alternative cures, and confidence in Indian doctors can face competition from already developed countries in the medical tourism area • A strong presence and international reputation can face the problem of lack of accreditation • A high success rate and the latest technology can be beneficial for foreign players • Vast tourism destinations could be developed with government support • The government took advantage of the increasing shortage of competent staff in developed countries and alternative cures available in India	• Uniform pricing policy should be adopted to face strong competition from medical tourism developed countries • Proper accreditation and regulation systems should be implemented • The government should invest in infrastructure to promote medical tourism • The government should be invested in improving unhygienic conditions in the medical industry • The players in the medical tourism industry should be coordinated to face competition from foreign players

goal of training and development programs is to increase individuals' skills and talents.

6. *Other issues*—Other issues that have arisen as a result of the development of infrastructure in the medical tourism sector within the country include a lack of availability and approachability, a lack of capital and resources, a lack of awareness and community participation, a lack of rural sector involvement, a lack of concern for sustainability, complicated visa procedures, a lack of good language translators, and a lack of airport facilities.

The tourist business is expanding globally, and India accounts for a considerable portion of global tourism receipts and traffic. The World Travel and Tourism Council (WTTC) estimates that the tourism industry will provide approximately 40 million employment by 2019. Although India accounts for only 1.24% of international tourism receipts and 0.59% of international tourist flow, its contribution must be recognized. Another important impediment to the development of medical tourism in India is the government's partial stance toward corporate and public hospitals. The government must pay attention to the function of corporate hospitals as a source of foreign exchange income, a provider of high-quality medical facilities and technology, and a medium for meeting the needs of foreign patients. In the future, the government may be forced to provide them with even more extravagant subsidies and exemptions for their development. This would put a strain on government finances and subsidies. Despite having enormous tourism potential, India's percentage of global visitor arrivals is substantially lower. The reasons for this are a lack of proper infrastructure, appropriate lodging facilities, security measures, and a qualified and skilled crew. To address the issue of insufficient capacity and meet the gap of around 150,000 rooms in the accommodation sector, the government must invest INR 600 billion over the next five years. The high service tax is another reason. A tourist must pay money to use tourism-related services because the sales tax on these services is twice as expensive as in any other developed country. In their union budget for 2011–2012, the government doubled the service tax on flights, making air travel more expensive. Similarly, independent eateries must pay an additional 10% tax for air conditioning in a country where temperatures can reach 48–50 °C. Insurance firms can play an important role in promoting medical tourism by preventing insurance fraud. They should provide the victim with proper insurance coverage and reimburse them in full. The major obstacles include:

1. Marketing and raising awareness about cutting-edge facilities in India.
2. Fierce competition from low-cost options from Thailand, Malaysia, Singapore, Turkey, and South Korea.
3. There has to be greater cohesion among the industry's major participants.
4. An inconsistent price structure, a lack of transparency in billing, and outrageously high margins to trade to refer patients.
5. A lack of trust among international patients as a result of low hygiene knowledge, unsanitary food handling, a lack of acceptable hospitality services, disparities in service pricing, and industry standards. Rethinking government policies

on regulations, taxation, land reforms, long-term investor-friendly policies, and instability concerning terrorism and communal tensions.
6. Key bottlenecks in insurance and allied services include insufficient insurance coverage, an underdeveloped insurance market, insurance fraud, and offshore corporations denying reimbursement.
7. India's infrastructure suffers from a lack of access, a lack of finance, a lack of community participation and awareness, a lack of rural sector participation, a lack of concern for sustainability, difficult visa procedures, a lack of professional language interpreters, and bad airport facilities.
8. Quality accreditations for Indian hospital providers, training and development courses for medical staff, and a lack of a customer-oriented approach are some specific challenges with developing medical tourism in India.
9. In the Indian environment, information and communication technology (I.C.T.) and I.C.T.-enabled services such as online reservations, as well as I.C.T.-enabled healthcare and allied services, are comparably low.

According to the most recent FICCI research, the country's capacity in the Medical Value Travel (MVT) industry is predicted to reach $9 billion by the end of 2020. Support for the industry in the form of incentives and new programs will go a long way toward assisting the sector's recovery following the pandemic. The industry requires tax breaks, duty relaxation or reductions to import medical equipment, infrastructure development, particularly transportation, and collaboration among all critical public and private partners. Anecdotal evidence suggests that American and British surgeons notice more major issues in patients who travel abroad for therapy. This is hardly surprising given the considerably increased dangers of medical tourism versus care at home. Whole-genome sequencing may provide additional issues, necessitating greater consideration of the ethics of genetic testing in A.R.T. Diagnostic laboratories must report their findings following internationally recognized accreditation criteria (ISO 15189). More research is needed to determine the effect of A.R.T. on early embryo epigenetic reprogramming. The legal environment of assisted reproduction is changing, yet it remains diverse and frequently conflicting. Cross-border reproductive care is encouraged in Europe and abroad due to a lack of legal harmonization and unequal access to infertility treatment (Harper 2013).

4.5 Ethics and Regulatory Oversight of Medical Tourism

The tragic story of a 31-year-old man exemplifies the negative aspects of the medical tourism movement. The tragic example of a 31-year-old Swedish woman who traveled to Gdansk, Poland, after viewing a web advertisement, exemplifies the negative aspects of the medical tourism movement (Niechajev 2012). The Ethical concept should apply not only to physicians/surgeons but also to the travel and insurance industries, as well as the companies that make those products (van Heijningen 2010; Nahai 2010). The World Health Assembly, the World Health

Organization's (WHO) governing body, established guiding principles on human organ transplantation in 1991. These principles forbid the exchange of money as well as other commercial transactions in this field. In December 2004, the United Nations General Assembly issued a resolution on the problem of "preventing, combating, and punishing trafficking in human organs." Many experiences are similar to those of Swedish women who have witnessed or heard of various tragedies or disasters as a result of medical procedures in foreign countries. The agreement was to call for legislation prohibiting lay people from trading or acting as intermediaries or brokers in medical treatments abroad. Medical tourism enterprises must be regulated by legislative bodies such as the federal and provincial or state governments. Legislation must be drafted to regulate the practices of businesses that incorporate features of both travel agencies and healthcare facilities, just as legislation is used to ensure the accreditation of hospitals and clinics, the licensing of healthcare professionals, and the accreditation of travel agencies. Medical tourism firms not only arrange travel to other countries, but they also help to coordinate health treatments. Medical tourism organizations should be limited to arranging health services at hospitals and medical clinics that have undergone international accreditation when creating international networks of healthcare providers. ISQua, the "accreditor of accreditors," accredits organizations such as Joint Commission International, Accreditation Canada, and the Malaysian Society for Quality in Health. Recognizing the multiple organizations involved in national and international accreditation, medical tourism enterprises should limit their marketing and provision of global health services to facilities accredited by recognized international accreditation agencies. Licenses are required for medical tourism organizations that arrange care at unaccredited international healthcare facilities. Some of the proposed standards for medical tourism accreditation and regulatory monitoring are as follows:

1. Medical tourism businesses must go through accreditation reviews, which are subject to external evaluation and accreditation.
2. Medical tourism enterprises must arrange care exclusively at accredited international medical institutions and should be limited to organizing health services at hospitals and clinics accredited by ISQua in healthcare-accredited organizations.
3. Standards must be established to ensure that medical tourism clients make informed choices; there must be a legal obligation to promote informed patient choices, which is a critical ethical and legal standard; and comprehensive discussions about the risks and benefits of medical procedures must take place before deciding whether to seek treatment abroad.
4. Continuity of treatment must become an essential component of international medical travel. Pre-travel assessment and treatment, patient care monitoring, and post-operative care are all critical components of foreign medical travel.
5. Medical tourism organizations should be banned from using the release of liability documents, which should be standardized and limited in scope.
6. Medical tourism organizations must adhere to relevant legal norms governing patient privacy and confidentiality.

7. Medical tourism companies must restrict the health treatments they sell and arrange, and they must be legally liable for providing safe and effective care.
8. Medical tourism agency representatives should have training and certification to perform this function competently and professionally.
9. Patients going for care should have medical travel and complications insurance included in their healthcare plans.
10. Medical tourism businesses should be required to contribute to compensation funds. These funds would be established to reimburse clients for damages incurred when medical tourism providers fail to meet contractual obligations.

Before joining the global healthcare networks developed by medical tourism organizations, hospitals, and clinics wishing to attract overseas patients need to undergo international accreditation evaluation. As healthcare grows more global, regulatory standards must likewise become more global in reach. Accreditation bodies can help guarantee that medical tourism agencies satisfy reasonable standards, and hospitals, healthcare systems, and healthcare professionals frequently address sensible practice quality standards in healthcare. As healthcare increasingly crosses national borders, efforts to improve healthcare quality must consider the expansion of medical tourism corporations and their role in promoting the globalization of health services. Turner (2011) Regulation of the medical tourism and public health sectors overlaps, generating concerns about how to ensure patient safety, economic growth, and health equity. The case of Guatemala examines how regulatory problems provided by medical tourism should be addressed in countries aiming to promote this industry, as well as how it contributes to the ongoing privatization of healthcare institutions globally. This tendency has the potential to undermine efforts to achieve Universal Health Coverage targets while worsening existing imbalances in the worldwide distribution of health and wealth (Labonté 2018).

4.6 Conclusion

Medical tourism is a subset of health tourism in which patients go from one nation to another for medical treatment. It is critical to upgrade infrastructure, technology, facilities, civic amenities, and other facilities in hospitals and healthcare centers to assure development and advancement in the medical tourism sector. The twin key constituents for building improved, safer, and healthier healthcare facilities are quality maximization and risk minimization, which can only be accomplished through the accreditation of healthcare institutions, which necessitates appropriate forms of an organizational framework designed to quantify patient care quality, analysis and isolate risks and mitigate real concomitant patient care concerns. Accreditation is viewed by global medical tourists as an attestation of quality or "endorsement of excellence" for determining the sincerity and service excellence supplied by medical tourism-focused healthcare institutions. Accreditation by worldwide standards guarantees that healthcare organizations establish sensible, prudent practice methods. Accreditation does not guarantee that problems will never emerge, but it helps reduce the likelihood of errors and encourages a desire to learn from them continuously. Accreditation protects international patients from the lack of control and guidelines, as well as international legislation, in the medical tourism industry, which could otherwise increase the hazards involved with overseas treatment. Accreditation is widely regarded as a risk-mitigation technique, a tool for performance evaluation, and an organizational instrument for examining strengths and areas for improvement, and it offers critical stakeholders an objective, unbiased external examination and review. Several studies have found that international hospital accreditation has an effect on clinical standards as well as bed occupancy rates. India provides extremely low-cost services to both Indians and foreigners. India has well-trained health practitioners, fluent English-speaking medical personnel, and a good staff of herbal, natural, allopathic, and alternative medicine systems. According to data, India received approximately one million health tourists by the end of 2012, with a compound annual growth rate (CAGR) of 28.09% over 2007. A health tourist in India spends less on procedures than in other developed countries. The Indian government can play a big role in establishing India as a top health tourism destination. Tourists should be provided a faster visa or visa on arrival to travel with ease and receive instant approval. The biggest disadvantage of hospital accreditation is that it is a purely voluntary process. Everyone understands the importance of accreditation, but in most countries, accreditation is still voluntary. Only a few countries have made accreditation compulsory or legal.

Accreditation, once overcome, has the potential to severely impact medical tourism. To facilitate medical tourism, supporting infrastructures such as transportation, lodging, and communication and information channels must be built. Individuals working in these fields must have the necessary skills, certifications, and experience to provide medical care. It is vital to provide accommodations for those seeking medical visas. As a result, it can be stated that some of the aspects that should be considered to promote medical tourism effectively include the recruitment of skilled, experienced, and qualified individuals in hospitals and healthcare centers, the provision of technology, infrastructure, facilities, and civic amenities, the creation of a warm environment, and paying adequate attention to the needs and problems of the individuals. Governments can create a separate portal displaying hospitals' accreditation status, packages, and so on to stimulate medical tourism.

References

ACHSI (2011) Members list. www.achs.org.au/memberorglist/#HONGKONG. Accessed July 2011

Aetna Global Benefits (2008) Aetna global benefits about products. http://www.aetnaglobalbenefits.com/about/index.html. Accessed 12 December 2008

Alkhenizan A (2010) Assessment of the accreditation standards of the Central Board for Accreditation of Healthcare Institutions in Saudi Arabia against the principles of the International Society for Quality in Health Care (ISQua). Ann Saudi Med 30(5):386–389

Alkhenizan A (2011) Impact of accreditation on the quality of healthcare services: a systematic review of the literature. Ann Saudi Med 31(4):407–416

Arunmozhi T (2013) Types of tourism in India. Int J Curr Res Acad Rev 1(1):84–88

Bertinato L, Busse R, Fahy N (2005) Cross-border health care in Europe. Denmark: policy brief, WHO on behalf of the European Observatory on Health Systems and Policies. www.euro.who.int/document/e87922.pdf. Accessed January 2012

Brubakk K, Vist GE, Bukholm G, Barach P, Tjomsland O (2015) A systematic review of hospital accreditation: the challenges of measuring complex intervention effects BMC Health Services Research 15(1) https://doi.org/10.1186/s12913-015-0933-x

Bukonda N, Tavrow P, Abdallah H (2003) Implementing a national hospital accreditation program: the Zambian experience. Int J Qual Health Care 14(1):7–16

Campbell CA (2019) Plastic surgery medical tourism in Colombia: a review of 658 international patients and 1,796 cosmetic surgery procedures. Plast Reconstr Surg Glob Open 7(5):e2233

Carabello L (2008) A medical tourism primer for US physicians. Med Pract Manage 23(5):291–294

Cattaneo O (2009) Trade in health services what's in it for developing countries? Policy Research Working Paper 5115. The World Bank Poverty Reduction and Economic Management Network International Trade Department. http://papers.ssrn.com/sol3/papers.cfm?abstract_id_1503809. Accessed January 2012

CBAHI (n.d.) Central Board for Accreditation of Healthcare Institutions (CBAHI). Retrieved from www.cbahi.org

CDS (2000) External quality mechanisms for health care: summary of the ExPeRT project on visitatie, accreditation, EFQM and ISO assessment in European Union countries. Eur Found Qual Manage ISO Int Qual Health Care 12:169–175

Chen J, Rathore S, Radford M (2003) JCAHO accreditation and quality of care for acute myocardial infarction. Health Aff 22:243–254

Chinai R, Goswami R (2007) Medical visas mark growth of Indian medical tourism. Bull World Health Organ 85(3):164–165

Chuang S (2019) An international systems-theoretic comparison of hospital accreditation: developing an implementation typology. Int J Qual Health Care 31(5):371–377

Chung-Ping A, Loh RE (2019) International accreditation, linguistic proximity, and trade in medical services. Soc Sci Med 238:112403

CIGNA Envoy (2008) CIGNA envoy. http://www.cignaenvoy.com/ciebpublic/

Connell J (2006) Medical tourism: sea, sun, sand and surgery. Tour Manag 27:1093–1100

Crone R (2008) Flat medicine? Exploring trends in the globalization of health care. Acad Med 83(2):117–121

Dastur F (2012) Hospital accreditation: a certificate of proficiency for healthcare institutions. J Assoc Physicians India 60:12–13

David SN (2017) National accreditation board for hospitals and healthcare providers (NABH) standards: a review. Curr Med Issues 15(3):231

Dawn SK (2011) Medical TOURISM in India: issues, opportunities and designing strategies for growth and development. Int J Multidiscip Res 1(3):185–202

Deloitte Center for Health Solutions (2008) Medical tourism consumers in search of value. Deloitte and Touche, Washington

Ehrbeck T, Guevara C, Mango P (2008) Mapping the market for medical travel. The McKinsey Quarterly. www.mckinseyquarterly.com/Mapping_the_market_for_travel_2134#. Accessed January 2012

Erhun F, Kaplan R, Narayanan V, Milstein A et al (2020) Are cost advantages from a modern Indian hospital transferable to the United States? Am Heart J 224:148–155. https://doi.org/10.1016/j.ahj.2020.04.009. PMID:32402701

Frølich A (2002) Akkreditering af hospitaler. En gennemgang af internationale erfaringer [Accreditation of hospitals. A review of international experiences]. Ugeskr Laeger 164(38):4412–4416

Greenfield D (2009) Developing the evidence base for accreditation of healthcare organizations: a call for transparency and innovation. Qual Saf Health Care 18:162–163

Guastello S, Jay K (2019) Improving the patient experience through a comprehensive performance framework to evaluate excellence in person-centered care. BMJ Open Qual 8(4):e000737. https://doi.org/10.1136/bmjoq-2019-000737. PMID:31673646

Guiry M, Vequist DG (2010) The role of personal values in determining U.S. medical tourists' expectations and perceptions of healthcare facility service quality: an exploratory investigation. J Tour Challenges Trends 3(2):115. https://link.gale.com/apps/doc/A253305990/HRCA?u=txshracd2623&sid=HRCA&xid=a1c12c10

Gyani GJ (2014) The National Accreditation Board for Hospital and Health Care Providers accreditation program in India. World Hosp Health Serv 50(1):9–12

Hall C (2013) Medical tourism - the ethics, regulation, and marketing of health mobility, 1st edn. Routledge, New York, pp 39–41

Hari Krishnan PK, Chandrasekhar KS (2020) Accreditation of hospitals: assuring quality health care for medical tourism in India. PJAEE 17(7). ISSN 1567-214x

Harper J (2013) Current issues in medically assisted reproduction and genetics in Europe: research, clinical practice, ethics, legal issues, and policy. Eur J Hum Genet 21(2):S1–S21

Herrick D (2007) Medical tourism: global competition in health care. NCPA policy report, vol. 304. National Centre for Policy Analysis, Dallas. Available at www.ncpa.org/pub/st304. Accessed January 2012

Hibbard J (2008) What can we say about the impact of public reporting? Inconsistent execution yields variable results. Ann Intern Med 148:160–161

Horowitz M, Rosensweig J, Jones C (2007) Medical tourism: globalization of the healthcare marketplace. Medscape Gen Med 9(4):33

Hussein M, Pavlova M, Ghalwash M, Groot W (2021) The impact of hospital accreditation on the quality of healthcare: a systematic literature review. BMC Health Serv Res 21(1):1. https://link.gale.com/apps/doc/A681621870/HRCA?u=txshracd2623&sid=bookmark-HRCA&xid=d0da22ff

Jabbari A (2012) Medical tourism in Iran: issues and challenges. J Educ Health Promot 1:39

Jabarkhil AQ, Tabatabaee SS, Jamali J, Moghri J (2021) Assessment of patient safety culture among doctors, nurses, and midwives in a public hospital in Afghanistan. Risk Manag Healthc Policy. 19;14:1211–1217. https://doi.org/10.2147/RMHP.S292193.

Johnston R, Crooks V, Synder J, Kingsbury P (2010) What is known about the effects of medical tourism in destination and departure countries? A scoping review. Int J Equity Health 9(24):1–13

Joseph S (2021) Impact assessment of accreditation in primary and secondary public health-care institutions in Kerala, India. Indian J Public Health 65:110–115

Kevan S (1993) Quest for cures: a history of tourism for climate and health. Int J Biometeorol 37(2):113–124

Labonté R (2018) Government roles in regulating medical tourism: evidence from Guatemala. Int J Equity Health 17:150

Lunt N, Carrera P (2010) Medical tourism: assessing the evidence on treatment abroad. Maturitas 66:27–32

Lunt N, Smith R, Mannion R, Green S, Exworthy M (2011) Implications for the NHS of inward and outward medical tourism. Available www.hsr.nihr.ac.uk/projects/09_2001_21.asp. Accessed June 2011

Malhotra N, Dave K (2022) An assessment of competitiveness of medical tourism industry in india: a case of Delhi NCR Internat J Global Busin Comp 17(2):215–228. https://doi.org/10.1007/s42943-022-00060-0

Mannion R, Davies H (2005) Taking stock of social capital in the production of health care. J Health Serv Res Policy 10(3):1–3

Mason A (2011) Framing medical tourism: an examination of appeal, risk, convalescence, accreditation, and interactivity in medical tourism websites. J Health Commun 16(2):163–177. https://doi.org/10.1080/10810730.2010.535105

McKinsey and Company (2008) Effectively characterizing medical travel: current and potential state. http://www.mckinseyquarterly.com/Health_Care/Strategy_Analysis/Mapping_the_market_for_travel_213_4. Accesssed 10 August 2009

Mihalik G, Scherer M, Schreter R (2003) The high price of quality: a cost analysis of NCQA accreditation. J Health Care Finance 29:38–47

Mothiravalley V (2012) Medical tourism in India (with special reference to Mangalore). Retrieved from Educational and Research Institute, Chennai. http://shodhganga.inflibnet.ac.in/bitstream/10603/120158/2/thesis.pdf

Mydans S (2002) The perfecting Thai vacation, sun sea, and surgery. The New York Times, Travel Section, p 3

Nahai F (2010) Don't bargain on safety. In: Media planet: plastic surgery, 1st edn. Elsevier, Amsterdam

Nandraj S, Khot A, Menon S (2001) A stakeholder approach towards hospital accreditation in India. Health Policy Plan 16:70–79

Niechajev I (2012) A plea to control medical tourism. Aesthet Plast Surg 36(1):202–206

Ozan-Rafferty ME (2014) In the words of the medical tourist: an analysis of Internet narratives by health travelers to Turkey. J Med Internet Res 16(2):e43

Pocock N, Phua K (2011) Medical tourism and policy implications for health systems: a conceptual framework from a comparative study of Thailand. Singapore Malaysia Glob Health 7:12

Pomey M, Contandriopoulos A, Francois P (2004) Accreditation: a tool for organizational change in hospitals? Int J Qual Health Care Includ Leadership Health Serv 17:113–124

Rawlins R (2001) Hospital accreditation is important. BMJ 322(7287):674

Reddy S (2010) Medical tourism in India: progress or predicament? Econ Polit Wkly 17(20):69–75

Reddy L (2017) Evaluating medical tourism prospects of Joint Commission International Accredited Hospitals in the Kingdom of Saudi Arabia. Health Sci J 11:8

Roberts JS (1987) A history of the Joint Commission on Accreditation of Hospitals. JAMA 258(7):936–940

Rosenmoller M, McKee M, Baeten R (2006) Patient mobility in the European Union: learning from experience. Eur Observ Health Syst Policies 61(11):1014

Scally G, Donaldson LJ (1998) The NHS's 50 anniversary. Clinical governance and the drive for quality improvement in the new NHS in England. BMJ 4;317(7150):61–5. https://doi.org/10.1136/bmj.317.7150.61

Scrivens E (1995) Accreditation: what can we learn from the Anglophone model? Health Policy 34:193–204

Shaw C (2015) Chapter 37: hospital accreditation and medical tourism. In: Handbook on medical tourism and patient mobility. Edward Elgar Publishing, Cheltenham

Shawan DA (2021) The effectiveness of the Joint Commission International Accreditation in Improving Quality at King Fahd University Hospital, Saudi Arabia: a mixed methods approach. J Healthc Leadership 13:47. https://link.gale.com/apps/doc/A654634771/HRCA?u=txshracd2623&sid=bookmark-HRCA&xid=b7a19afe

Sheingold BH (2014) The history of healthcare quality: the first 100 years 1860-1960. Int J Afr Nurs Sci 1:18–22

Shetty P (2010) Medical tourism booms in India, but at what cost? Lancet 376(9742):671–672

Smith EB (2010) Reproductive tourism in Argentina: clinic accreditation and its implications for consumers, health professionals, and policy makers. Dev World Bioeth 10:59–69

Thoke S (2017) An overview of the medical tourism industry in India and its growth potential in Marathwada Region of Maharashtra. KRSCMS Manage J 7:1–13

Tomasich F, Oliveira AV, Oliveira AJ, Correia MITD (2020) The history of quality and safety of the surgical patient: from the initial standards to the present day. Rev Col Bras Cir 47. https://doi.org/10.1590/0100-6991e-20202650

Tomislav M (2022) Medical tourism accreditation. https://www.news-medical.net/health/Medical-Tourism-Accreditation.aspx

Turner L (2011) Quality in health care and globalization of health services: accreditation and regulatory oversight of medical tourism companies. Int J Qual Health Care 231:1–7

Van Heijningen I (2010) Europe works on standards to enhance patient safety. ISAPS News 4(3):6

Walshe K (2009) Pseudoinnovation: the development and spread of healthcare quality improvement methodologies. Int J Qual Health Care 21(3):153–159
Williams J (1995) Risk management in surgery. In: Vincent C (ed) Clinical risk management enhancing patient safety. BMJ Publishing Group, London, pp 137–151
York D (2008) Medical tourism: the trend toward outsourcing medical procedures to foreign countries. J Contin Educ Health Prof 28(2):99–102
Youngman I (2009) Medical tourism statistics: why McKinsey has got it wrong. Int Med Travel J. Available at www.imtjonline.com/articles/2009/mckinsey-wrong-medical-travel/

Chapter 5
An Overview of Healthcare Accreditations in Medical Tourism

Kiran Hegde, K. C. Shylaja, and Kanakavalli K. Kundury

Abstract Medical tourism (MT) is an amalgamation of healthcare and tourism industries. Medical tourism is gaining importance in recent years due to various additional services and benefits associated with MT packages. In order to meet the expectations of the medical tourist and create a delightful patient experience, the stakeholders such as hospitals, insurers, facilitators, and agents are more focused in offering 'quality services'. As 'Quality' is the core criteria for any healthcare service, analysing the current medical tourism market, hospitals across the world are going for accreditation of their services to create a positive impression in the minds of medical tourists. An accredited healthcare facility is, of course, an eye catcher to the medical tourist in selection of the hospital. To facilitate this certification process, there are many organizations worldwide to offer healthcare accreditation. While few of these bodies accredit the healthcare facilities, few others will accredit the accrediting organizations. Thus, the present book chapter focuses on various healthcare accreditation bodies operating nationally and internationally.

K. Hegde
Department of Hospital Administration, SDM College of Medical Sciences, Dharwad, Karnataka, India

K. C. Shylaja
Department of Health System Management Studies, Center for Distance and Online Education, JSS Academy of Higher Education and Research, Mysuru, Karnataka, India

K. K. Kundury (✉)
Department of Health System Management Studies, JSS Academy of Higher Education and Research, Mysuru, Karnataka, India

Patient Care Management, JSS Academy of Higher Education and Research, Mysuru, Karnataka, India
e-mail: kanakavalli.dhsms@jssuni.edu.in

B. Chaudhary et al. (eds.), *Medical Tourism in Developing Countries*,
https://doi.org/10.1007/978-981-99-8909-6_5

Keywords Medical tourism · Accreditation · Medical value travel · Healthcare quality

Abbreviations

ACHS	Australian Council on Healthcare Standards
ACSQHC	Australian Commission on Safety and Quality in Health Care
CBA	Conformity assessment body
CBAHI	The Central Board for Accreditation of Healthcare Institutions
CPR	Cardiopulmonary resuscitation
GHA	The global healthcare accreditation
HCO	Healthcare organizations
HOP	Hospital orientation program
IAP	International accreditation program
ISQua	The International Society for Quality in Healthcare
ISQua EEA	The International Society for Quality in Health Care External Evaluation Association
JCAH	Joint Commission on Accreditation of Hospitals
JCAHO	Joint Commission on Accreditation of Healthcare Organizations
JCI	Joint Commission International
MT	Medical tourism
MTCC	Medical travel care continuum
MVT	Medical value travel
NABH	National Accreditation Board for Hospitals
NSQHS	National safety and quality health service
SAT	Self-assessment tool
UK	United Kingdom
UKAF	UK Akkreditering forum
USA	The United States of America
USD	United States dollar
VBT	Value-based care

5.1 Introduction to Medical Tourism and Healthcare Accreditation

5.1.1 Medical Tourism

Medical tourism is an amalgamation of medical and tourism industries, where the medical tourist can travel from the country of origin to the destination country for medical services (Neil Lunt et al. 2011). Adding to the medical services, the medical tourist can also visit the tourist places in the destination country (CDC 2022). Though the word 'Medical Tourism' is not new to the world, its potential is getting better recognition with its exponential growth in recent times (Malhotra and Dave 2022).

It is a known fact that the cost of medical care, waiting time for services, availability and accessibility of healthcare in the source country are few of the many reasons why individuals prefer medical tourism (Johnston et al. 2010). Taking advantage of these reasons, countries across the world, market their medical services, offering value addition with their tourism services; as a comprehensive 'Medical Value Travel' (Health and Federation of Indian Chambers of Commerce and Industry (FICCI) 2016).

While medical tourism appears to be operationally very feasible, it demands various preparations, both pre-and-post the services, from the provider and the medical tourist side (Neil Lunt et al. 2011). Few of the common requirements from both the parties include requirement of state-of-the-art healthcare infrastructural facilities in meeting the expectations of foreign tourists, superior hospitality services and top-notch quality of medical care with national or international accreditation (Sultana et al. 2014). These preparations would make the healthcare facilities ready to provide quality medical care services whereas the same would help the medical tourist in right selection of the hospital in the destination country. Considering the increasing demand for quality in healthcare services, many hospitals offering medical tourism would get their services accredited with several national and international certifications (Khan et al. 2016). Thus, the role of accreditation is becoming very significant for standardization of medical practices across the world (Frank et al. 2020).

5.1.2 Healthcare Accreditation

"Healthcare Quality" has become a definite prerequisite to the evolving medical tourism industry, as it facilitates standardized practices adopting patient-centric approaches (Institute of Medicine (US) and National Academy of Engineering (US) Roundtable on Value and Science-Driven Health Care 2011). It is a potential tool in marketing of services, assuring quality care and gaining patient satisfaction (Institute of Medicine (US) and National Academy of Engineering (US) Roundtable on Value and Science-Driven Health Care 2011). It also acts as a firewall in facing intense competitive pressures (Wardhani et al. 2019). As defined by NABH international, "Accreditation is self-assessment and external peer review process used by healthcare organizations to accurately assess their level of performance in relation to established standards and to implement ways to improve the healthcare system continuously" (Mate et al. 2014; National Accreditation Board for Hospital and Healthcare Providers (NABH) International 2023). 'Quality' incorporates the institutions preparedness for patient care, the care delivery process, their practice to offer effective, efficient, equitable and safe healthcare services to all. Accreditation for Health Care Organizations (HCOs) is a third-party assessment for the degree of conformity to established global benchmarking standards (National Accreditation Board for Hospital and Healthcare Providers (NABH) International 2023). This accreditation certificate of a healthcare facility is, of course, important for providing regular day-to-day services to the patients of a community, but gains vital importance while serving foreign patients in respect of medical tourism (Neil Lunt et al. 2011). As the medical travellers cannot experience the quality of services before the treatment, these accreditations certify the quality-of-care standards in a hospital; thus, making it promising for international patients to select the overseas hospitals (Turner 2011). Accreditation also justifies that the cost-effective medical care doesn't mean substandard care, rather superior care at affordable cost; thus, assuring the medical travellers throughout the process of care (G20 India Health Track 2023).

5.2 Benefits of Accreditation in Healthcare Facilities

Accreditation is a detailed process of aligning the medical care services with the pre-determined standards, to facilitate uniformity in care management practices (Young and Smith 2022). Going through the process of accreditation, a healthcare facility would re-define its existing systems and might re-engineer its processes to fit into the requirements of the accreditation standards (Frank et al. 2020). This activity, though appears complex and tedious, brings out fruitful results to both the healthcare facility and also immensely benefits patients (Frank et al. 2020) (Table 5.1).

Table 5.1 Benefits of accreditation (National Accreditation Board for Hospital and Healthcare Providers (NABH) International 2023)

Patients	Providers
• Patients get well informed about the hospital services • Diagnosis and treatment modalities can be done with no/less errors • Patients receive treatment from the team of authorized and well-trained service providers including doctors, nurses and para-clinical professionals in a patient safety environment • Uniform and continuous care can be provided to patients from the team of multidisciplinary certified professionals • Medication safety can be assured through well-drafted guidelines and its implementation • Patient-centric approaches are followed in the hospitals by zero or reduced numbers of medication safety issues and adverse drug reactions • 'Quality of care' is emphasized on day-to-day practices, yielding to reduced medical errors • Increased patient awareness on their rights and responsibilities, in terms of information and education on their healthcare • Patient participation in healthcare gets promoted through informed consent forms, and enhanced disease awareness through education in their own language • Improved communication between doctor-patient; and also, among the team of care providers • Create and maintain a conducive environment for better treatment outcomes to patients and service outcomes to staff • Continuous quality improvement leading to zero repeat investigations, reduced length of stay of patients; thus, cost savings for patients	• Healthcare facilities can demonstrate their commitment in providing patient-centric practices • Enhanced quality in care leads to increased patient satisfaction and build public confidence • Improved standards of care, ethical practices, professional conducts can be observed • Helps to create patient safety environment and sustainability in quality practices • Skill building and knowledge upgradation with continuous professional training to the staff • Efficient systems in preventing and documenting adverse events for timely actions • Staff training at all levels for personal and patient safety including CPR, disaster drills • Employee welfare activities for their physical and mental well-being • Standardized practices in documentation to maintain transparency in record keeping • Incorporating 'Quality' as a mantra in doing things right during day-to-day operations • Competent and stable workforce trained and focused at better productivity • Creating a culture of quality for continuous quality improvement through periodic internal audits • Proper control and monitoring mechanisms would result in reduced wastage, optimum stocks of supplies; leading to better investment of finances • Image building of the hospital leading to more patient footfall with word-of-mouth publicity and increased revenue

5.3 Impact of Hospital Accreditation on Medical Tourism Services

Considering the favourable conditions for medical tourism with increased disease burden and raising cost of services, medical tourism global market was estimated at ~115 billion USD in 2022 and it is estimated to grow around ~286 billion USD by

2030 (Neil Lunt et al. 2011). Identifying the deeper demand of these services, nations across the world have initiated concrete efforts involving all the stakeholders in order to provide a holistic service experience to the foreign travellers (Neil Lunt et al. 2011).

Out of all the facilities that are required for provisioning medical tourism services, hospital selection by the patient plays an important role (Naghipour et al. 2019). A medical tourist's experience gets greatly influenced from the hospital they have selected for availing the medical services, in which, hospital accreditation plays a significant role. Accreditation gives assurance to the patient on the quality of services and justifies the 'Value-Based Care (VBC)' (Alkhenizan and Shaw 2011). Hospitals certified with several national and international accreditation bodies position themselves as the hospitals with quality care and patient safety practices (Jha 2018). Along with this image, accredited hospitals also should showcase their medical outcomes, which reflects their transparency and commitment in services on the global medical tourism platforms (Greenfield et al. 2012). This information portrayed by the hospitals helps in building confidence among the foreign patients; and helps in image building leading to more patient footfall from other countries (Bahadori et al. 2016).

5.4 Evolution of Accreditation Systems

Inception of healthcare accreditation systems began in the 1850s with Florence Nightingale establishing a protocol for collecting and analysing hospital statistics to assure quality of services (Chun and Bafford 2014). Later in 1914, Dr. Earnest Codman introduced 'End Result System', a post-treatment follow-up process to obtain patient feedback on the effectiveness of the care (Chun and Bafford 2014). The origin of accreditation process actually began in USA by the American College of Surgeons in 1917 with a program of 'minimum standards for hospitals' (Chun and Bafford 2014). This program aimed at assessing and identifying selected hospitals for surgical training. This was modified in 1951 as a 'multidisciplinary program of standardization', leading to the establishment of the independent Joint Commission on Accreditation of Hospitals (JCAH) (Wadhwa and Huynh 2022). In 1987, this was renamed as the Joint Commission on Accreditation of Healthcare Organizations (JCAHO) (Wadhwa and Huynh 2022). This was one of the hallmarks of accreditation systems, through with either directly or indirectly, subsequent national accreditation programs are derived. Identifying the growing emphasis for quality healthcare, in 2007, JCAHO was renamed again as the Joint Commission and then to the Joint Commission Accreditation (JCI) which has its standards developed by healthcare professionals worldwide (Wadhwa and Huynh 2022). In 1999, the International Society for Quality in Healthcare (ISQua) was established as an organization providing approvals for other accreditation bodies (ISQua 2015).

5.5 Various Healthcare Accreditation Bodies

Considering the need and requirement for standardization of medical care services and enhanced patient safety through quality care procedures, there were several healthcare accreditation bodies functioning worldwide. While few of these bodies directly assess the quality of care delivered by healthcare facilities across their nation, against the established standards; few others help to train these accreditation bodies in the formulation of international patient care standards (Kruk et al. 2018).

5.5.1 The International Society for Quality in Health Care (ISQua) and the UK Akkreditering Forum (UKAF) (International Society for Quality in Health Care (ISQua) 2023; UK Akkreditering Forum Limited 2023)

The International Society for Quality in Health Care (ISQua) is a not-for-profit organization aimed to promote quality in healthcare. In 1999, ISQua launched its International Accreditation Program (IAP) as the only program that accredits the accreditors and provides worldwide recognition for organizations meeting international standards. The program provides services such as accreditation of healthcare external evaluation organizations, accreditation of international healthcare standards and accreditation of training programs for training of assessors and auditors. ISQua is responsible for the assessment and evaluation of standards of accreditation agencies worldwide for quality and patient safety practices. These accredited agencies in turn accredit hospitals and healthcare facilities for meeting the required standards.

The UK Akkreditering Forum Limited is also a self-regulating accreditation authority which accredits several accreditation bodies and training institutes worldwide, currently operating in more than 25 countries. UKAF follows a novel approach to accreditation by benchmarking its standards through measurable evaluation of Conformity Assessment Body (CBA). Their objectives are well defined to measure annual performance of CBAs in determining their service excellence. Thus, ISQua and UKAF will not be surveying or accrediting individual hospitals or healthcare facilities; but they 'accredits the accreditors' worldwide.

These organizations ISQua and UKF are well-accepted and respected international organizations by many accreditation bodies worldwide such as The Joint Commission International (JCI), The Australian Council on Healthcare Standards (ACHS), The Accreditation Canada, The Trent Accreditation Scheme, The Malaysian Society for Quality in Health, The National Accreditation Board for Accreditation for Hospitals & Healthcare Providers (NABH) and The Central Board for Accreditation of Healthcare Institutions (CBAHI), Saudi Arabia and other healthcare accreditation agencies. Basing on the principles, quality is a continuous process and accreditation is not a one-time activity, ISQua and UKF assess the accreditation agencies for developing/promoting benchmarking standards in providing patient-centred healthcare institutes worldwide.

Among many of the accreditation systems worldwide, few of them would be focusing on nationwide accreditation of healthcare organizations while few of these bodies certify the healthcare organizations internationally; while few other accreditation systems are exclusively made to meet the standard of medical travel or medical tourism.

5.5.2 *The Australian Council on Healthcare Standards (ACHS) (The Australian Council on Healthcare Standards (ACHS) n.d.)*

The Australian Council on Healthcare Standards (ACHS) is a long-standing, autonomous and not-for-profit organization, which takes a leadership role across Australia in providing The National Safety and Quality Health Service (NSQHS) standards program to the Australian healthcare facilities. It is mandatory for major of the healthcare organizations to get certified by NSQHS standards from the Australian Commission on Safety and Quality in Health Care (ACSQHC).

These NSQHS standards developed by ACSQHC focus on implementing safe and standard systems that improve the quality of health services in Australia. There are a total of ten NSQHS standards developed which are essential to achieve safe and quality healthcare services (Table 5.2).

Few reasons of why the NSQHS standards are selected are to have standardized care delivery practices across the nation, to impact the safety and quality of health of a large number of patients, to fill the existing knowledge gap between what is currently being practised and the essential standards and encourage evidence-based achievable practices. Due to the varying capacities of healthcare facilities and care delivery models, NSQHS standards were designed to provide reasonable flexibility by dividing the standards into ***Core*** and ***Developmental standards*** (Greenfield et al. 2015). Core standards are the standards which are essential to patient safety and quality practices; whereas Developmental actions are aspirational targets that include activities that enhance patient safety and quality of care.

Table 5.2 National safety and quality health service (NSQHS) (Greenfield et al. 2015)

1. Clinical governance for safety and quality in health service organisations
2. Partnering with consumers
3. Preventing and controlling healthcare associated infections
4. Medication safety
5. Patient identification and procedure matching
6. Clinical handover
7. Blood and blood products
8. Preventing and managing pressure injuries
9. Recognising and responding to clinical deterioration in acute health care
10. Preventing falls and harm from falls

Assessment of these standards is done against three-point rating scale *'Not Met' (standards required were not met), 'Satisfactorily Met' (standards required are satisfactorily complied)* and *'Met with Merit' (actions required are outstandingly met with higher level achievements and are clearly evident)* (Greenfield et al. 2015). These ratings are used to assess the level of respective actions in each standard. Participating healthcare organizations would obtain membership under the ACHS NSQHS standards program, for three years during which the healthcare organizations would be working towards applying, achieving and maintaining accreditation. During the first year, the healthcare organization enrolled as a member would prepare for the survey measuring their existing practices against the NSQHS standards as a pre-survey and submits the data. Internal self-assessment is conducted by the member organizations on the pre-determined three-point rating scale and rate the existing practices accordingly. In the second year, member organizations produce a plan of action with respect to the unmet standards and submit the quality improvement plan. In the third year, members update the action plan against the unmet action standards of NHQHS and an updated quality improvement plan is also submitted. Member organizations also submit a progress report periodically to the ACHS authorities. The accreditation authorities will then review the progress reports and provide the member organizations the feedback which is necessary for them to improve their standards. The accreditation survey occurs once the healthcare organization is found to be ready for external assessment. This onsite survey by ACHS NHQHS team includes progress review and assessment of the member organizations in the form of staff interviews and document verifications against the NSQHS standards. Advanced Completion (AC) surveys are also conducted by ACHS team along with the onsite survey, in case, if there are any Core Actions in Not-Met criteria. This facilitates the healthcare organizations to correctly address the problems before the completion of the survey report to suggest for accreditation. Once found satisfactory, ACHS will award the healthcare organization, full accreditation for the complete 3-year period. The healthcare organization can then renew the accreditation thereafter as per the procedure.

5.5.3 The Central Board for Accreditation of Healthcare Institutions (CBAHI) (The Central Board for Accreditation of Healthcare Institutions (CBAHI) n.d.)

The Central Board for Accreditation of Healthcare Institutions (CBAHI) is a non-profit organization established from the Saudi Health Council, which is authorized to accredit all the healthcare facilities in Saudi Arabia. The core objective of CBAHI is to establish quality healthcare services and patient safety standards for all healthcare facilities to be complied with. It is mandatory to obtain CBAHI accreditation systems for all the hospitals including public and private healthcare facilities of the country, for inception of new hospitals or renewal of operating license. Thus, there can be nationwide practice of quality care in compliance with the set standards of CBAHI. It offers its accreditation programs for all the healthcare facilities and its ancillary services.

CBAHI standards are certified by the International Society for Quality in Health Care (ISQua) from the International Accreditation Program (IAP). As a requirement of accreditation pathway, the hospitals have to register with CBAHI as a first step towards attaining accreditation. CBAHI provides Hospital Orientation Program (HOP) periodically across various locations throughout the year free of charge (The Central Board for Accreditation of Healthcare Institutions (CBAHI) 2022). It is a good opportunity for the participating hospitals to get aware about CBAHI standards, accreditation policies and survey processes. Once they are oriented, the hospitals will be provided with Self-Assessment Tool (SAT) from CBAHI, which helps them to self-assess their compliance with the accreditation standards (The Central Board for Accreditation of Healthcare Institutions (CBAHI) 2022). This provides the hospitals in time estimations for internal assessments and preparations required before they approach for survey visit by accreditation team. SAT helps the hospitals for conducting periodic internal audits and submit the reports to CBAHI teams for better understanding of the healthcare organizations preparedness and commitment to get accredited (The Central Board for Accreditation of Healthcare Institutions (CBAHI) 2022). Once both the parties are found satisfactory in achieving compliance with the standards, then an onsite survey can be scheduled. If the hospitals want to, there is also a provision that they can apply for a mock survey, before the real survey. For this mock survey to be not interpreted as an 'open-exercise', the healthcare organization can go for a maximum of 2 mock surveys within 2 years period before they go for the real survey (The Central Board for Accreditation of Healthcare Institutions (CBAHI) 2022). Before going to the real onsite survey, the required documents have to be submitted to the accreditation team along with the application forms.

5.5.4 *Joint Commission International (JCI) (Joint Commission International 2023)*

JCI, headquartered in Illinois, United States, is a not-for-profit organization, which accredits healthcare facilities in and around Asia, Europe, the Middle East, and South America. It is one of the oldest and worldwide 'gold standard' in accreditation which has benchmarking standards focusing on quality of care, patient safety and security and confidentiality. This is one of the pioneer international accreditation agencies which is still considered as a hallmark of healthcare accreditation. JCI accreditation of any healthcare facility is assured to operate with international gold standards, delivering safe, effective and efficient patient care. Since 1994, JCI has accredited over 400 healthcare facilities (private and public) in over 80 countries. This accreditation body accredits healthcare organizations, ancillary services and also provides continuum of care. JCI develops its standards with the inputs and information from healthcare organizations, subject experts, scientific literatures, industry guidelines, technical advisory panels and other key stakeholders. According to JCI 7th edition, the following are the standards for academic medical centres (Joint Commission International n.d.) (Fig. 5.1):

Section I: Accreditation Participation Requirements (APR)
1.Accreditation Participation Requirements (APR)
Section II: Patient-Centered Standards
2.International Patient Safety Goals (IPSG)
3.Access to Care and Continuity of Care (ACC)
4. Patient Centered Care (PCC)
5.Assessment of Patients (AOP)
6.Care of Patients (COP)
7.Anesthesia and Surgical Care (ASC)
8.Medication Management and Use (MMU)
Section III: Health Care Organization Management Standards
10.Quality Improvement and Patient Safety (QPS)
11.Prevention and Control of Infections (PCI)
12.Governance, Leadership, and Direction (GLD)
13.Facility Management and Safety (FMS)
14.Staff Qualifications and Education (SQE)
15.Management of Information (MOI)
Section IV: Academic Medical Center Hospital Standards
16.Medical Professional Education (MPE)
17.Human Subjects Research Programs (HRP)

Fig. 5.1 JCI standards

JCI ***standards*** focuses on the expected performances and organizational structures required to perform the standards. International Patient Safety Goals from JCI are the standards that primarily focus on the areas of patient safety during the care procedures in any healthcare facility (Joint Commission International n.d.). These practices are evaluated for their compliance with the established standards during the on-site survey. Standard's ***intent*** gives a detailed explanation of the standards and their intention towards better patient care practices (Joint Commission International n.d.). These intents provide information on the true essence of these standards, their implications in the overall requirement of accreditation and give a deeper understanding of the expected goals.

Measurable elements (MEs) are the goals that can be measured and scored during the on-site survey (Joint Commission International n.d.). These measurable elements of each of the standards are assessed for their full compliance against the set goals and scores are assigned basing on the healthcare facilities' adherence to those practices. These MEs help the facilities in analysing their current standards and highlight the grey areas for improvement. They also bring in more clarity among the healthcare staff and administration by educating them about the preparedness for the accreditation process.

Till date, there are 953 healthcare facilities across the world which are currently accredited by JCI (JCI Accredited Organizations n.d.). Considering the inception time for accreditation till the certification, it would approximately take 1–2 years' time for a healthcare organization to get certified with JCI. Accreditation process with JCI includes baseline assessment, gap identification between current practices and JCI standards, formulation of strategies and implementation of the same to fill the gaps; measurement of performance to ensure the compliance with JCI standards.

The standards set by JCI include the organizations' preparedness to apply for accreditation in terms of the requirements or prerequisites to get themselves certified. Also contains patient care and treatment-related standards and also defines organizations' management standards and clinical systems. Core intents of these standards are in meeting international patient safety goals, access to care, assessment of care processes, infection control practices, education, information management systems, management of human resources, facility management practices, healthcare organizations leadership and management. The accreditation obtained by JCI is valid for 3 years duration and the organizations should apply for re-accreditation 6–9 months before the due date.

JCI is of the accreditations worldwide, which patients opting for medical tourism would look into while selecting the healthcare facilities in the destination country. As JCI comprises of standards which are internationally acceptable, it creates an assurance for patients with respect to quality of care. Though JCI certification creates a confidence in the minds of the patients about the quality of services, it should be noted that it is that particular healthcare facility which should give the patients 'quality guarantee' but not the certification. In spite of this, international medical tourists would still prefer the hospital accredited with JCI to a non-accredited facility.

5.5.5 Global Healthcare Accreditation (GHA) (Global Healthcare Accreditation 2020)

The Global Healthcare Accreditation program is a self-governing accrediting body that sets standards and validates professional norms for medical travel or medical tourism programs, nationally and internationally. It is a globally recognized authority in accreditation of healthcare facilities which emphasizes on workplace safety, health and well-being with specialization in medical and wellness travel. As medical tourist experiences many concerns with respect to selection of hospital, healthcare quality and professionalism of healthcare providers, GHA certification for medical value travel is a complete assurance for the consumers of these services.

The GHA accreditation process helps the healthcare organizations to enhance their customer satisfaction along the medical travel care continuum by gap identification, efficiency building, performance enhancement and adopting the best practices. This is executed through continuous self-assessment for quality improvement by the healthcare facility. This betterment in quality reflects in the best experiences of the travelling patients, leading to better healthcare outcomes.

GHA contains a multi-disciplinary team which includes insurers, employers, healthcare professionals and leading administrators of the medical travel industry. Through this team, GHA can identify the existing gaps in the medical travel and challenges faced by the medical tourists, so that appropriate standards can be established to promote quality patient experience.

5.5.5.1 The Uniqueness of GHA (Global Healthcare Accreditation 2020)

GHA standards are certified by The International Society for Quality in Health Care External Evaluation Association (ISQua EEA), which was found in 2018 by the International Society for Quality in Health Care to deliver external evaluation services. ISQua EEA is an external evaluation agency that offers services to health and social organizations and to the bodies that develop national and international standards.

The standards developed by GHA are deeply reviewed from the global patient service programs; also, the respective domain areas of the stakeholders of the medical travel industry. GHA also ensures that the organizational productivity not only focus on best clinical outcomes but also on business performances that impact the medical travel programs. GHA's multi-disciplinary advisory board helps to offer better patient experience, minimize organizations' risk management, improve employee benefits and facilitation of medical travel. As an addition to this, GHA standards are also made in alignment with the needs of medical tourists under different circumstances. It also helps its client base and stakeholders with workshops, summits and focused group discussions to promote networking and strengthen the connections between the participating parties.

5.5.5.2 Care Continuum (Global Healthcare Accreditation 2020)

GHA's care continuum starts with the selection of hospital by medical tourists and continues till post-discharge follow-up care. Figure 5.2 represents the critical components of the Medical Travel Care Continuum (MTCC).

The Medical Travel Care Continuum (MTCC) is a core component of Global Health Accreditation (GHA) program. MTCC is an integrated approach comprising of broader range of services offered to medical travel patients. It illustrates the entire care continuum that is to be managed for ensuring good clinical outcomes, excellent patient experience and efficient business practices that impacts the healthcare organizations' performance. The team of MTCC comprising of consultants, facilitators and surveyors critically examine each of the components of MTCC, considering the uniqueness of these elements in each healthcare organization. The team also offers customized services for each of the healthcare facilities depending on its speciality services and patient base.

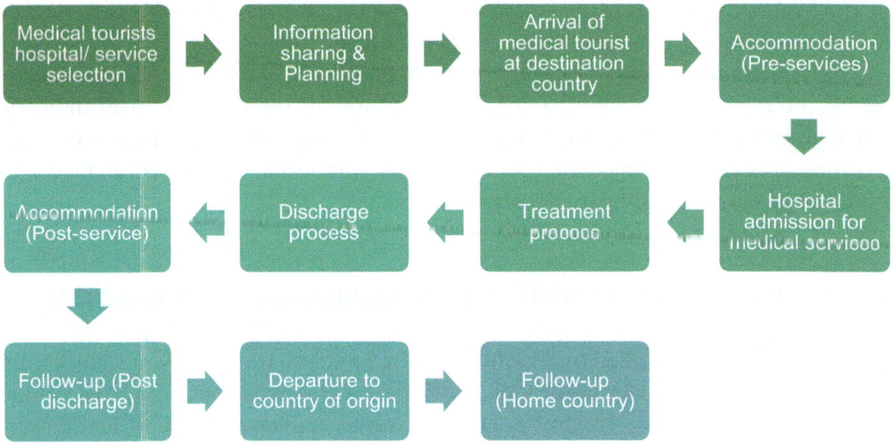

Fig. 5.2 Medical travel care continuum (MTCC)

5.5.5.3 GHA's Core Competencies and Standards (Global Healthcare Accreditation 2020)

GHA Program standards are made around the core competencies such as The Patient Experience, Sustainable Business Processes and The Patient Focused Clinical Processes (Fig. 5.3). Each competency comprises of various sections containing standards, organized in chapters that define structures, processes and outcomes to be achieved for excellence in the competent area. Patient experience standards focus on assessing the patients' overall experience of medical travel services with respect to cultural competencies, patient communication and education, patient advocacy and travel facilities. Sustainable business processes are aimed at marketing of medical tourism services, finances and ethical business practices, vendor management and leadership management which are vital for the healthcare organizational sustenance and performance. Patient-focused clinical processes aim at infection control practices, patient safety and care management for better clinical outcomes.

Thus, Global Health Accreditation (GHA) adopts a three-dimensional approach towards achieving success in clinical outcomes, organizational business process outcomes and delightful patient experience of medical travel services.

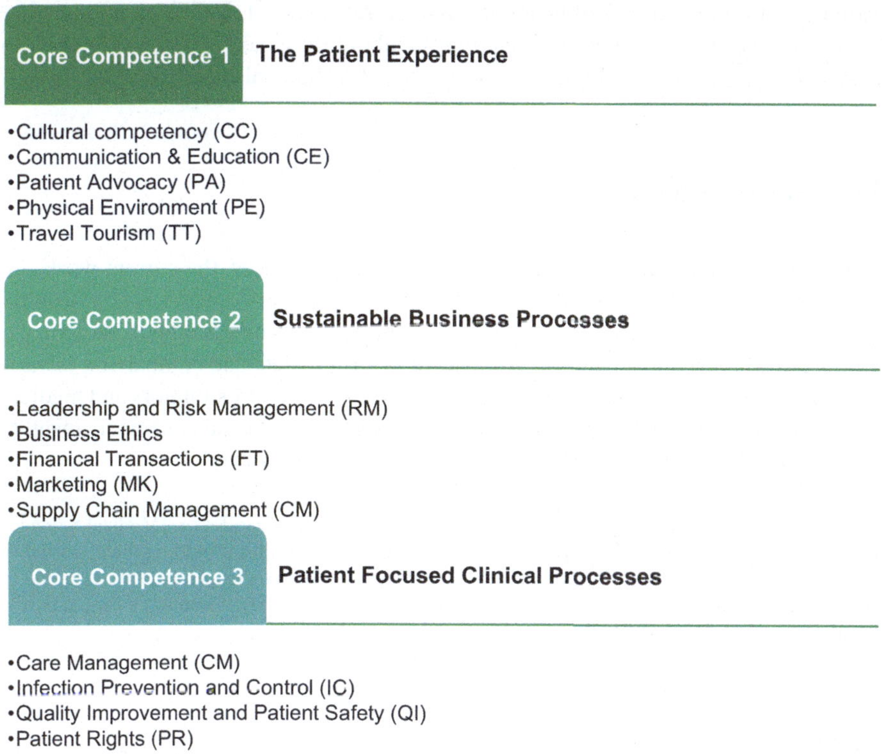

Fig. 5.3 Core competencies of GHA's MTCC program

5.6 Summary and Conclusion

As the medical travel services are gaining its momentum with a huge progressive curve, it becomes imperative to the medical tourism industry players to upgrade their services to 'Quality Assured'. In this context, healthcare quality accreditation plays an important role in terms of good clinical outcomes and best patient experiences. A nationally or internationally certified healthcare facility is known to be the patient choice for selecting the destination services. There are several accreditation agencies such as JCI, ACHS, CBAHI and NABH, which accredit the healthcare facilities of a particular nation or accredit internationally. While few other certification bodies such as ISQua and UKAF accredit the accreditors by certifying the healthcare facilities against the international standards in quality and patient safety services. There are also independent accrediting bodies such as GHA, which provides Medical Tourism Care Continuum Program that mentors the healthcare organizations throughout the process of medical value travel. The accreditation of healthcare facilities is not only about satisfying the international patients with quality services; but on the other hand, it also helps in addressing the needs of the local patients with improved healthcare infrastructure. Thus, it is important that the healthcare organizations become much aware about these accreditation facilities to standardize their services; thereby making place for medical travel services.

5.7 Future Directions

Identifying the importance of healthcare accreditation services, the current work can be further carried out on identifying the healthcare providers' awareness on hospital accreditation services. Few other extensions to the current works include assessing the healthcare organizations' perspective on accreditation system and comparison of various healthcare accreditation bodies across the nations. Role of facilitators and medical tourism agents in assisting the medical travellers and hospitals also gives us insights into operational issues in arranging for medical tourism services.

Acknowledgements The authors would like to acknowledge SDM College of Medical Sciences and JSS Academy of Higher Education & Research and thank them for providing the opportunity and the resources required for drafting this book chapter. Our acknowledgements are also due to The Special Interest Group in Patient Care Management (SIGPCM); Center for Distance and Online Education, JSS AHER.

References

Alkhenizan A, Shaw C (2011) Impact of accreditation on the quality of healthcare services: a systematic review of the literature. Ann Saudi Med 31(4):407–416. https://doi.org/10.4103/0256-4947.83204

Bahadori M, Teymourzadeh E, Ravangard R, Nasiri A, Raadabadi M, Alimohammadzadeh K (2016) Factors contributing towards patient's choice of a hospital clinic from the patients' and managers' perspective. Electron Physician 8(5):2378–2387

CDC (2022) Medical tourism: travel to another country for medical care: U.S. Department of Health & Human Services. Available from https://wwwnc.cdc.gov/travel/page/medical-tourism

Chun J, Bafford AC (2014) History and background of quality measurement. Clin Colon Rectal Surg 27(1):5–9. https://doi.org/10.1055/s-0034-1366912

Frank JR, Taber S, van Zanten M, Scheele F, Blouin D, International Health Professions Accreditation Outcomes Consortium (2020) The role of accreditation in 21st century health professions education: report of an International Consensus Group. BMC Med Educ 20(1):305. https://doi.org/10.1186/s12909-020-02121-5

G20 India Health Track (2023) Azadi Ka Amrit Mahaotsav. Ministry of Health and Family Welfare. Three days 1st Health Working Group Meeting. Medical value travel plays a crucial role in eliminating healthcare disparities across the globe; we aim to provide an impetus to create pathways to bridge this gap. Available from https://pib.gov.in/PressReleasePage.aspx?PRID=1892502

Global Healthcare Accreditation (2020) Raising the standard in medical travel, global health accreditation for medical travel services. Available from https://www.globalhealthcareaccreditation.com

Greenfield D, Pawsey M, Hinchcliff R, Moldovan M, Braithwaite J (2012) The standard of healthcare accreditation standards: a review of empirical research underpinning their development and impact. BMC Health Serv Res 12:329. https://doi.org/10.1186/1472-6963-12-329

Greenfield D, Hinchcliff R, Banks M, Mumford V, Hogden A, Debono D, Pawsey M, Westbrook J, Braithwaite J (2015) Analysing 'big picture' policy reform mechanisms: the Australian health service safety and quality accreditation scheme. Health Expect 18(6):3110–3122. https://doi.org/10.1111/hex.12300

Health and Federation of Indian Chambers of Commerce and Industry (FICCI) (2016) Medical value travel in India enhancing value in MVT

Institute of Medicine (US) and National Academy of Engineering (US) Roundtable on Value and Science-Driven Health Care (2011) Engineering a learning healthcare system: a look at the future: workshop summary. National Academies Press, Washington, p 3. Available from: https://www.ncbi.nlm.nih.gov/books/NBK61963/

International Society for Quality in Health Care (ISQua) (2023). Available at https://isqua.org/membership.html

ISQua (2015) Guidelines and principles for the development of health and social care standards. 4th ed. Available from https://isqua.org/media/attachments/2018/03/20/guidelines_and_principles_for_the_development_of_health_and_social_care_standards__4th_edition_v1.2.pdf

JCI Accredited Organizations (n.d.). Available from https://www.jointcommissioninternational.org/about-jci/accredited-organizations/

Jha AK (2018) Accreditation, quality, and making hospital care better. JAMA 320(23):2410–2411. https://doi.org/10.1001/jama.2018.18810

Johnston R, Crooks VA, Snyder J et al (2010) What is known about the effects of medical tourism in destination and departure countries? A scoping review. Int J Equity Health 9:24. https://doi.org/10.1186/1475-9276-9-24

Joint Commission International (2023). Available from https://www.jointcommissioninternational.org/about-jci/

Joint Commission International (ed) (n.d.) Joint Commission International accreditation standards for hospitals including standards for academic medical center hospitals, 7th edn. Joint Commission International, Singapore

Khan MJ, Chelliah S, Haron MS (2016) International patients' travel decision making process-a conceptual framework. Iran J Public Health 45(2):134–145

Kruk ME, Gage AD, Arsenault C et al (2018) High-quality health systems in the sustainable development goals era: time for a revolution. Lancet Glob Health 6:e1196–e1252. https://doi.org/10.1016/S2214-109X(18)30386-3

Malhotra N, Dave K (2022) An assessment of competitiveness of medical tourism industry in India: a case of Delhi NCR. JGBC 17:215–228. https://doi.org/10.1007/s42943-022-00060-0

Mate KS, Rooney AL, Supachutikul A, Gyani G (2014) Accreditation as a path to achieving universal quality health coverage. Glob Health 10:68. https://doi.org/10.1186/s12992-014-0068-6

Naghipour M, Langarizadeh M, Razzazi M (2019) Identification of the requirements for designing medical tourism information system of Iran. J Educ Health Promot 8:118. https://doi.org/10.4103/jehp.jehp_372_18

National Accreditation Board for Hospital and Healthcare Providers (NABH) International (2023). Quality Council of India. 'What is Accreditation'. Available from https://international.nabh.co/whynabh.aspx

Neil Lunt RS, Exworthy M, Green ST, Horsfall D, Mannion R (2011) Medical tourism: treatments, markets and health system implications: a scoping review. Directorate for Employment, Labour and Social Affairs, London

Sultana S, Haque A, Momen A, Yasmin F (2014) Factors affecting the attractiveness of medical tourism destination: an empirical study on India-review. Iran J Public Health 43(7):867–876

The Australian Council on Healthcare Standards (ACHS) (n.d.). Available from https://www.achs.org.au

The Central Board for Accreditation of Healthcare Institutions (CBAHI) (2022) Hospital Accreditation Program (3rd Version), National Standards for Hospitals. Available from: https://portal.cbahi.gov.sa/english/accreditation-programs/hospital-accreditation-program

The Central Board for Accreditation of Healthcare Institutions (CBAHI) (n.d.). Available from https://portal.cbahi.gov.sa/english/home

Turner LG (2011) Quality in health care and globalization of health services: accreditation and regulatory oversight of medical tourism companies. Int J Qual Health Care 23(1):1–7. https://doi.org/10.1093/intqhc/mzq078

UK Akkreditering Forum Limited (2023). Available from http://www.ukaf.org.uk/about.aspx

Wadhwa R, Huynh AP (2022) The Joint Commission. In: StatPearls. Stat Pearls Publishing, Treasure Island. Available from https://www.ncbi.nlm.nih.gov/books/NBK557846/

Wardhani V, van Dijk JP, Utarini A (2019) Hospitals accreditation status in Indonesia: associated with hospital characteristics, market competition intensity, and hospital performance? BMC Health Serv Res 19(1):372. https://doi.org/10.1186/s12913-019-4187-x

Young M, Smith MA (2022) Standards and evaluation of healthcare quality, safety, and person centered care. In: StatPearls. StatPearls Publishing, Treasure Island. Available from: https://www.ncbi.nlm.nih.gov/books/NBK576432/

Chapter 6
Technology as a Catalyst for Medical Tourism

Kinjal Jani, Bhupinder Chaudhary, and Baljit Saini

Abstract Being a terrain of prosperous and diverse cultural heritage, India is known as one of the renowned destinations for tourism. Besides general tourism, medical tourism has taken off to a new level and gained colossal popularity in India. This act is a massive boon for the entire tourism industry. In India, the grouping of cost-effective treatments, enhanced quality standards, and excellent medical technology attract patients beyond borders. The significant role of technology in medical tourism is undeniable. Technology has added innovation and the best facilities for foreign patients. The upsurge of digital technologies has strengthened communication, sharing of data, and security to explore the streamlined and convenient traveling experience. Major digital technologies ambit have helped medical tourism to be a more credible and feasible option for patients abroad. Cloud computing, data mining, and information technology are pivotal factors in medical tourism. It aids in making Electronic Medical Records available overseas to smoothen the services and helps to avoid second-time diagnoses. External factors (Government Schemes) are strengthening medical tourism related to infrastructure. India's technological advancement from consultation and laboratory tests to surgery and even discharge process adopted technological interventions and it is evident as a catalyst in the healthcare industry. In a nutshell, the role of technology has seeped into the ambit of Indian healthcare, helping India to become a global leader so far as medical tourism and healthcare go hand in hand.

Keywords Medical tourism · Technology · Cost-effective

K. Jani (✉)
Department of Hospital Management, Hemchandracharya North Gujarat University, Patan, Gujarat, India

B. Chaudhary
Department of Hospital Management and Hospice Studies, Jamia Millia Islamia, New Delhi, India

B. Saini
Department of Computer Engineering, K.D. Polytechnic, Patan, Gujarat, India

B. Chaudhary et al. (eds.), *Medical Tourism in Developing Countries*,
https://doi.org/10.1007/978-981-99-8909-6_6

6.1 Medical Tourism

The healthcare sector is known as the robust industry, as is closely associated with other sectors, i.e., travel and tourism, information and wellness, and technology and communication. In the yesteryears, the amalgamation of healthcare and travel segment has witnessed a remarkable movement. It has shaped phenomenal growth in the mobility of individuals around the globe.

Medical Tourism is narrated as an "Occurrence in which healthcare seekers leave their nation of residence to another country with the intention of medical care to the illness that she or he has" (Carrera and Bridges 2006; Puczko and Bachvarov 2015). Predominantly and primarily medical tourism encompasses biomedical procedures united with tourism and travel. Comprehensively, medical tourism is attracting tourists by promoting their well-being services (Goodrich 1987), a popular mass culture, and a business center rather than only a trend (De 2021). Medical tourism is one of the international dimensions for the growth of the healthcare industry. In India, medical tourism has taken off to a new level and gained colossal popularity. A unique basket of services and diversity has been offered by Indian culture for medical tourism, i.e., clinical medicine, yoga, ayurveda, natural herbal treatments, and meditation (Sarngadharam 2009). Primarily medical tourism is agreed upon for the cost benefits in the destination nations. Later on, competitive advantages have been added to medical tourism stem, i.e., low-cost advantages, well-built reputation in the developed healthcare (organ transplant, cardiovascular surgery, eye surgery, etc.), and tourist destination attraction with diversity (Dawn and Pal 2011).

Globalization has shaped medical tourism as one of the agile service industries. This sector is having enough potential to become the utmost foreign exchange earner. Yesteryears have witnessed how the healthcare industry is blooming and patients are cheering the advantages of globalization. The Internet has played a significant role to boost medical tourism widely and to create a new space in the healthcare environment, as a result of this, healthcare is not limited to local territory (Rai 2017). Due to healthcare globalization, governments and hospitals are spending on the utmost quality of healthcare and medical technology to expand their competitive advantages and share in the market in the industry of medical tourism.

Medical tourism in India is attracting visitors from all across the globe. The majority of the influx comes from the SAARC predominantly from Bangladesh, Sri Lanka, Nepal, and the Maldives to whom the main concern is high-quality healthcare services. Traditionally, India has strong accomplices with Middle Eastern countries, i.e., Oman, Saudi Arabia, Qatar, the UAE, and Yemen. East Africa which covers Kenya, Tanzania, Uganda, and Ethiopia approaches India as the best destination for medical tourism. Even ASEAN countries, i.e., Cambodia, Myanmar, Indonesia, and the Philippines along with Cambodia, Myanmar, Indonesia, and the Philippines as well as CIS countries of Kazakhstan, Uzbekistan, and Afghanistan show their preference for healthcare in India. Recently, a new trend has been seen in healthcare seekers from the United Kingdom, the United States, South America, and even Europe they visit India, especially for Proton Therapy. It represents the unprecedented growth of medical tourism in India (Bhardwaj 2022).

6.2 Driving Factors of Indian Medical Tourism

In the modern days, millions of individuals take a trip overseas to obtain medical treatments. For that several motivators play a significant role as pull and push factors. It is evident in the number of studies (Hurley 2004; Kazemi 2008; Singh 2019) that there are important factors that drive the success of medical tourism. It is indeed a fact that several domains of socio-demographic (García-Altés 2005), behavioral (García-Altés 2005), and technological advancement have enhanced the growth of medical tourism (Rai 2017; Singh 2019) (Fig. 6.1).

In the contemporary industrialized globe with the growth of the elderly population in developed nations, the availability of well-being and preventive services are in demand. Even in India, the demand for ethnic treatment, i.e., meditation, yoga, ayurveda, and numerous other treatments along with rehabilitative care, is gradually accelerating, and global acceptance for such kinds of treatment particularly for preventive therapies is also in demand. Globalization, reduced cost of treatment, demand for good health, accreditation and certification, fast-track actions, and technology are the core factors for the growth of medical tourism (Singh 2019).

The excellence in healthcare technology in requisites of cutting-edge procedures and contemporary treatment plays a significant role to attract medical tourists.

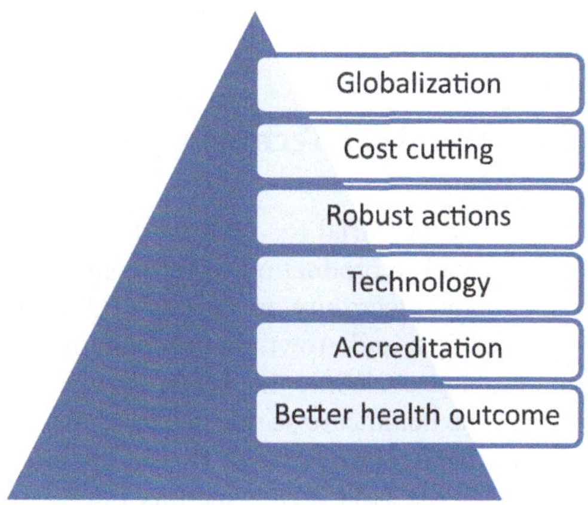

Fig. 6.1 Success factors of medical tourism

6.3 Technology: Driving Shaft to Medical Tourism in India

Other than world-class techno-savvy doctors and hospitals, India has also excelled in the medical technology sector. Technology and medical tourism are interdependent sectors. Technology along with its applications has indeed permeated every living globe and it has created an entry in the scope of medicine. Technology has provided roots to cross the border to gain the best available medical services. Even genetically inherited disorders, therapeutic complications, and abstruse demands for cosmetic and vital surgeries demanded a link up of technology to medical tourism. India ranks as Asia's 4th largest nation to have advanced medical technology equipment (García-Altés 2005). Relate to this, medical technologies in healthcare have always been developing. Nevertheless, a new pattern of disease is constantly demanding a novel course of treatment, and this kind of desirable care is not used to available at an individual's preferred location or area. Therefore, advanced medical technology not only helps to enhance the quality of care and medical precision but also bridges the geographical barrier and makes available services closer and faster. In India, many hospitals have adopted modern technologies in the area of cardiac surgery, organ transplant, well-equipped ICUs, neonatal screening, prenatal diagnostics, advanced imaging technologies, i.e., PET, MRI, CT SCAN, in vitro fertilization options, bone marrow transplant, etc. On the global map, this highly advanced medical technology has positioned India as the preferred destination to get quality medical care.

The technology has proved the concept of healthcare service delivery of "right information" (medical information) to the "right people" (healthcare providers, patients, family, and friends) at the "right time" (during the entire time of treatment and on-demand).

6.4 Trends of Technology Applicable in Medical Tourism

In the first Industrial Revolution, there was a use of mechanics and steam-powered tool to excel in production, whereas the 2.0 industry were known for the mass production and electricity processes. 3.0 has introduced the first sign of technological digitalization, and growth in the economy to reach beyond geographical boundaries at a faster pace. While the 4.0 IR introduced in 2016 took the storm in the progression of the healthcare sector including the medical tourism sector (Wong and Saaid Hazley 2020). In this latest IR digital, physical, and biological spheres are introduced (Bernasconi 2016) such as Internet of Things (IoT), robotics, automation, virtual reality, cloud solutions, artificial intelligence, and big data analytics. This technological advancement has made a tremendous impact like a storm on the medical tourism industry. Major trends of technology that are applicable in medical tourism are stated hereafter.

6.4.1 Cloud

Cloud ranks at the top of this category due to the availability of Electronic Medical Records (EMR) all across the globe accessible to each patient via budgeted solutions. Not only to patients but also real-time access to all medical tourism solutions to doctors and providers is feasible through a cloud. EMR helps to reduce medication errors and unnecessary and repeated diagnoses to stream efficiency in the healthcare industry. It has also profited from system-based data over paper-based data. It is indeed a boon that even EMR can be also accessible via smartphone, escorting to a revolution in the ambit of the healthcare industry.

6.4.2 Data Mining

Data mining is also a significant benefactor of the healthcare sector. Compilation of data in a comprehensive manner in a continuous manner through various sources, i.e., case studies, medical journals, search engines, etc., can help to build an enormous databank of the illness diagnosis system. As medical records can be stored in smartphones that could be encrypted for security even if it requires a password to the way in. To build strong security and access, an OTP protocol is enlisted. A server can store on-demand access to data-intensive information, e.g., CT-scan, and an X-ray at the same time as a phone can store low-bandwidth data.

6.4.3 Telemedicine

Telemedicine is an actual attempt to bridge the gap between healthcare providers and receivers by cutting down the physical distance on travel which encompasses communication and information technologies (Santiago 2020). It is one of the indispensable cogs in the system of medical tourism, due to these facilities; the approach of "know each other" before the actual meeting for treatment can be fulfilled. Case histories of patients, medical visual data, and information in text form are changed to electronic signals and the converted data can easily be accessible via electronic media. It provides on-demand health-related notes starting from the beginning to follow-up sessions irrespective of geographical barriers. Consequently, it has enhanced the efficiency, attractiveness, and productivity of medical tourism (Bhatiya 2015).

Telemedicine is also considered a distance healing (Shen et al. 2021). It is significantly relevant in the field of medical tourism, telemedicine allows the beneficiaries to link between their primary physician and consultant present overseas to elaborate case history and/or to conduct surgery via web conferences, especially in augmenting the course of pre-operative and post-operative care, in the ambit of both patient and medical. Even prior recovery assessment of wounds and healing recovery can be performed by anesthesiologists and surgeons. Thus it helps in the production, transmission, and control of information and data.

6.4.4 The Internet

As medical tourism is rising as a global industry, a wide range of key stakeholders with an interest in commercial output, and website is one stakeholder. A significant driving factor in medical tourism is known as a technological platform that is offered by the Internet to make healthcare information accessible and get advertisements from all over the world (Lunt et al. 2011). Commercialization is the core factor for growth in medical tourism and to achieve it web-based resources offer information, market destination, and advertisement, and generate connections between healthcare providers and agents. Medical Tourism seekers from all around the world use the Internet as a prominent tool to get the answers to their medical tourism-related queries. The Internet also provides a platform for the electronic processing of bookings and E-mail communication. Websites, social media sites, and informational pages are the most trendy mediums of information to know the medical tourism destination (Karimov et al. 2011). The creation and sharing of beneficiary-generated content are enabled by social media sites. Even social networking has created a buzz as it is the finest and most easily accessible platform to be in touch with doctors and consultants from various nations. In the current era, this novel technology has strengthened foreign patients to be in touch with Indian doctors.

6.4.5 Internet of Medical Things

The phrase Internet of Things (IoT) refers to a globe wide network of interrelated things, which are particularly marked by standard communication protocols (Hittinger and Jaramillo 2019). All kinds of physical devices, e.g., autonomous transportation systems, smart appliances, and personal health monitors which are entrenched in digital technologies can be grouped to agree to these devices' interaction with each other through data of communication. IoT has opened a new horizon to monitor patients and beneficiaries from a distance and in a continuous manner ahead of only limited visits, text, and telecommunications (Gatsis and Pappas 2017). There are significant innovations in wearable medical technologies. Smartwatches, Bio patches, and smart hearing aids support the innovations. Even clothes are having the potential to measure the heart rate (Hassan and Bellos 2022). Optical technology such as photoplethysmography (PPG) also tracks the variation in blood composition and volume. The global Medical Internet of Things (MIoT) is expected to accomplish USD 188.2 billion next to 2025 (Evangeline 2022). It shows that doctors can deliver superlative care through remote monitoring in the pre-operative and post-operative phases of treatment by using IoT-enabled devices. It also assists in minimizing the duration and length of stay, in that way IoMT helps significantly to reduce healthcare cost and enhancing treatment outcomes (Bhatia et al. 2020; Tiwari and Tripathi 2019).

6.4.6 Artificial Intelligence

Great healthcare amenities and medical tourism grow hand in hand (Banerjee 2022). AI is developing at an exceptional rate. It is having a bundle of applications. The growth of AI accelerated the efficiencies of machines managing X-rays, MRIs, CT scans, etc. The requirement for such services is mounting as there is a change in the behavior of patients as a customer (Nagar et al. 2021). It also assists to monitor the trend in healthcare tourism that can assist in attracting foreign medical travelers to the nation. It helps to make healthcare more affordable and approachable.

6.4.7 Assistive Technologies

India is one of the preferred nations to have robot-assisted surgeries that help to fetch hefty revenue via medical tourism. It assists to provide minimum invasive surgeries, precision control, and improved ergonomics to surgeons (Bhatia 2021). Moreover, it provides access to a tough-to-access component of the body (Reddy 2022). It provides the best feasible solution to prime problems, inter alia, extended waiting time, for surgeries, delayed recovery, insufficiency of expertise, etc. Along with well-trained robotic surgeons and infrastructure, India is paving to turn into the world leader in the ambit of robotic surgery.

6.4.8 Blockchain Technology

The success of Bitcoin initiated augmented growth of the crypto market mainly focusing on cryptocurrencies. As the financial sector has been the prime focus of blockchain technology, a new range of applications related to other industries and sectors, i.e., governance, tourism, health, etc., have been developing (Davidson et al. 2016). Blockchain is a distributed digital ledger that is made of immutable arranged in chronological order, and decentralized data between allied devices in a system of the blockchain. With blockchain, data from patient's health records are accessible to healthcare providers if only the patient authorizes it (Bhatia et al. 2021; Dinesh Bhatia and Mishra 2022). It allows a hassle-free flow of information beyond borders. Çapar (2020) stated that transactions and cryptocurrencies linked in blockchain affect medical tourism in a positive way that protects the collaborator from monetary risk transactions, also facilitates access to medical care services, and preserves the evidence in case of malpractice. This technology also ensures the quality, origin, and transparency of the data. The core benefits of blockchain in medical tourism are summarized hereafter.

Even blockchain technology assists in issuing medical visa to reduce the waiting time by managing all government documents.

6.4.9 Technology in Biomedical Waste Disposal

In the yesteryears, the prime way out for Biomedical Waste (BMW) was to burn the waste. Numbers of toxins used to produce, inter alia, dioxins, products of incomplete combustion (PIC), and furans during incinerations (Emmanuel et al. 2001). To overcome the environmental and public health challenges various new technologies are introduced for the effective management of BMW. These technologies are grouped into four categories: Thermal, Chemical, Irradiative, and Biological processes.

Thermal-based technology: Low (93–177 °C), medium (177–540 °C), and high (540–8300 °C) heat temperature is used in thermal technologies. Microwaves and autoclaves are used in this technology. A plasma torch is used in plasma pyrolysis (Nema and Ganeshprasad 2002). A wide range of waste is handled in plasma-based technology, i.e., sharp, infectious waste, plastics, hazardous waste, dialysis waste, chemotherapy waste, etc. There is a minimal emission rate, and the inert and sterile residue is the advantage of this technology. Chemical-based technology: Liquid, gas, or dry chemicals are in use to treat BMW. This technology demands a closed system or handled with negative pressure. The exhausted air needs to be passed through HEPA to prevent the aerosol formation at the time of shredding. This technology is categorized into two groups: chlorine and non-chlorine-based technology. Ionizing radiation: the electron beam technology constructs ionizing radiation to strike the object. No toxic emission, no ionizing radiation, and no liquid effluent are produced in the procedure (Emmanuel et al. 2001). Low operational cost and fully automated technologies are the additional advantages of this technology. As healthcare and medical tourism go hand in hand, the same technology is also applicable in the field of medical tourism (Banerjee 2022).

6.5 Medical Value Travel (MVT)

India is estimated to attract 430,000 medical tourists overseas for a market value of 6.4 billion US dollars (Nayar 2017). As the growth forecast of medical tourism in India is brighter, it is necessary to modify and update designs, packages, and post-care services related to the long-term sustainability of services. The term Medical Value Travel (MVT) is being used prominently to refer to medical tourism as

Information and Communication Technology (ICT) and a range of ICT-enabled services and Products. Optimization of patient admission and EMR can be done by ICT utilization. ICT also provides support to integrated service delivery for both tourism and health providers (Ayuningtyas and Ariwibowo 2020). ICT not only provides treatment and care services but also had a significant role in the payment process.

From this perspective, the ambit of technology has a significant role in MVT in India.

Figure 6.2 depicts that communication and information technologies are essential rather than just an option. The largest segment for the attraction of medical tourism is advanced technology and that is 40%.

Along with a quality image and lower cost, advanced technology linked with ICT and ICT-based applications has boosted the sector. India ranked in the top 3 among 184 countries of the globe for the contribution to the travel and tourism sector in the context of the GDP of the country, as of 2016 (Nayar 2020). As of Medical Tourism Index 2020–2021 conducted by Medical Tourism Association, India is lined up at 10th out of 46 nations (Rao 2021). Figure 6.3 narrates the growth of medical tourism in India and as advanced technology is playing a significant role in the growth, it clearly states that advanced technology of medical tourism is contributing to the Indian economy. Regardless of the deliberate impact of the pandemic, by 2022 MVT in India is anticipated to grow to 13 billion USD.

Rising technologies that contribute meaningfully associated with the MVT excel in the cost-effectiveness and efficiency of healthcare (Buhalis 1998) (Fig. 6.4). Improved ICT in India compasses, inter alia, the subsequent:

1. Enterprise Resource Planning (ERP): it assists in the storage, processing, and analyses of information initiated or in use for daily medical operations, concern to all the serviceable areas, i.e., HR, Finance, Accounts, etc. For the success of MVT, an ERP would be a significant player in ICT.

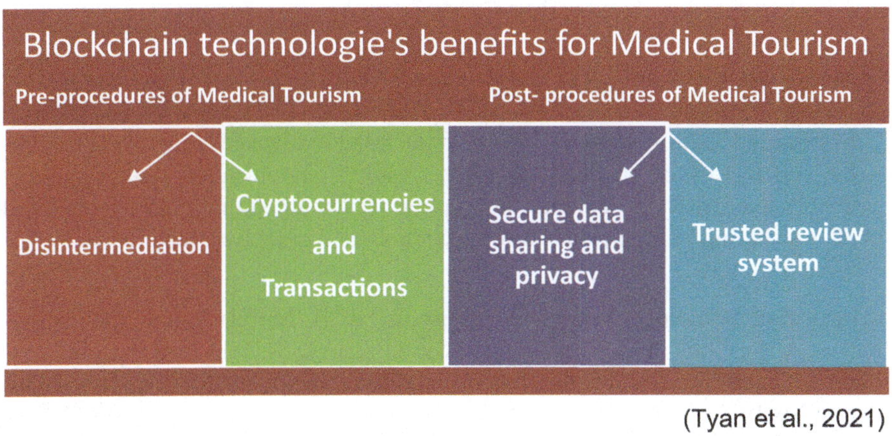

Fig. 6.2 Blockchain benefits in medical tourism (Tyan et al. 2021)

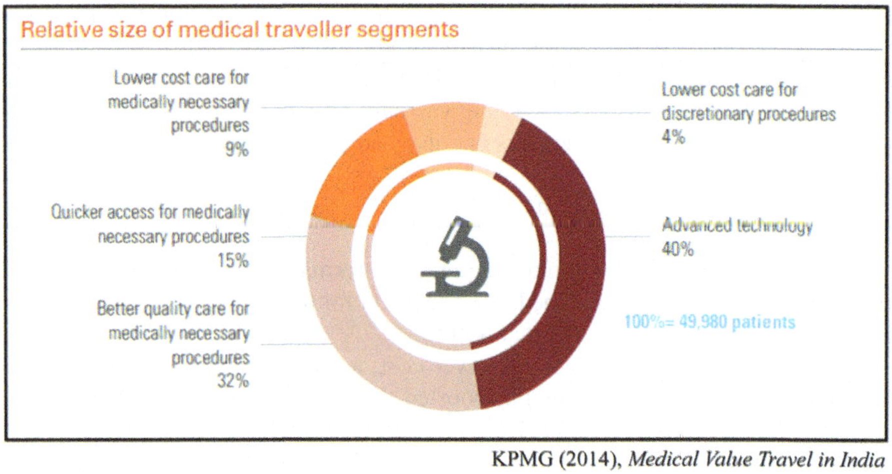

Fig. 6.3 Relative size of the medical travel segment. KPMG (2014), Medical Value Travel in India

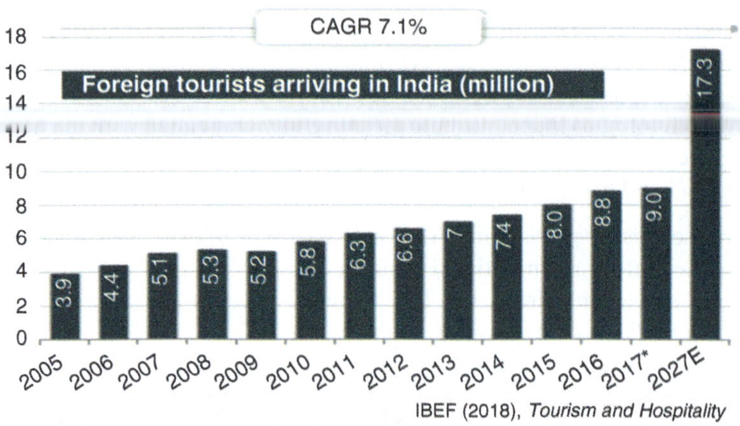

Fig. 6.4 Foreign tourists arriving in India (Million). IBEF (2018), Tourism and Hospitality

2. Electronic Health Records (EHR): it is intended to manage comprehensive profile and history of patients, laboratory results, immunization tests, radiology images, etc. HER also enables the sharing of data among multiple systems and allows sharing of medical histories accurately and quickly to lead real-time services of MVT.

Inter alia, Radiology Information Systems (RIS), Mobile-based Applications (Mobile App), Clinical Decision Support Systems (CDSS), Telemedicine, etc., contribute to macro-level healthcare systems, and the same innovations apply to MVT (Nayar 2020).

6.6 Post-pandemic Era for Medical Tourism and Technology

Although India has been balanced to succeed to achieve the expected growth of medical tourism, inevitably the nation has suffered the collision of the COVID-19 pandemic. As there is a well-known said that "A crisis provides an opportunity", the pandemic has built a winner-high-tech acceptance across the world, and India has led in such upgrades (Times of India 2022). To counter the pandemic, The Government of India and medical industries utilized technology very effectively and eventually assist in the revitalization of medical tourism during and after the pandemic. To get quicker responses and broadcasting of information, operations of healthcare across the nation augmented their reliance on technology. AI, robotics, IoMT, remote diagnosis, and tele-consultancy have helped to understand the pattern and need of service delivery. As per the PwC report, India has used AI with a 45% increased growth during the pandemic compared to other major economies. As initially medical tourism was hit by the pandemic, the same kind of reverse force was observed for sustainable medical tourism assisted with high-tech after the vaccination. Ample of efforts are initiated by the government of India, i.e., chatbots enabled by AI that were in use by MyGov to track the pandemic (Benerjee 2022). "Watson Assistant" has been introduced by the Indian Council of Medical Research (ICMR) that can assist data entry operators and frontline workers. Recently a new initiative, "Heal in India" has been introduced.

6.7 Expected Growth of the Medical Tourism in India

The notable contribution of technologies excels the service delivery and competitiveness of medical tourism to attract the beneficiaries as per World Economic Forum, 2020 summit. Figure 6.5 depicts the expected growth of medical tourism and which is ascending for India as the technology of healthcare is improving with each passing year.

6.8 Future Directions of the Technology

The emergence of IR 4.0 has changed the landscape of healthcare and medical tourism. As technologies are growing day by day, further trends and future shapes will empower medical tourism to relate to the commercialization aspect. Ayurveda, robotic surgeries, surgical camps, and startups will be the core focus area for the future development of medical tourism. Unique combinations of technological devices with skills will lure a larger number of patients to our nation. As the 5G network has paved the industry via satellites, it will strengthen 5 G-enabled robotic surgeries (Ahmed 2022). As demand increases, technologies will create a niche

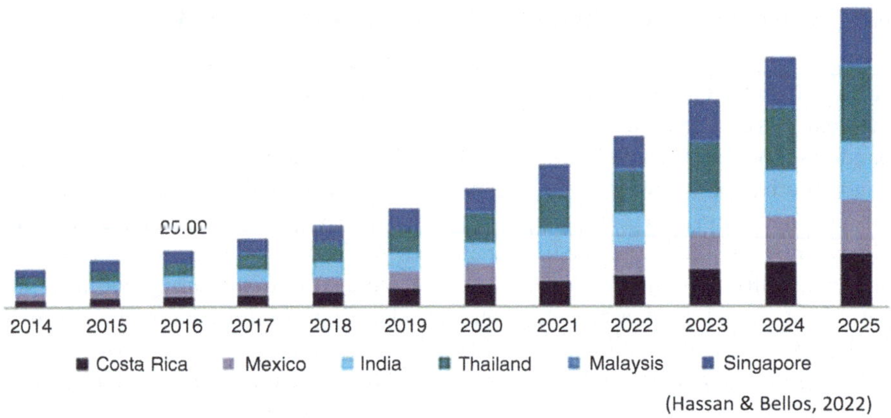

Fig. 6.5 Global medical tourism market size (Hassan and Bellos 2022)

market for medical tourism to lure the patient. It leads ease to conduct complex and lengthy procedures and reduces the waiting period by focusing on cost beneficial to patients. The future of medical tourism assisted by technology seems better and brighter than ever.

6.9 Limitations of Technology

Smart healthcare and advanced medical technology have improved the outcome of medical tourism. There are still many more challenges and untapped areas in the technology that can become the obstacle in medical tourism, i.e., managing Internet-connected technology continuously, handling a colossal amount of healthcare-related data, ambiguity related to ownership of data, the threat of cybercrime, fraudulent insurance claims, to train the manpower to handle the high-tech operations. Intentionally or accidentally by third parties, there may be the possibility of a breach of protected healthcare data. To manage healthcare data, service providers need to be dependent on the external cloud provider, and in that case, cyber security may be at risk.

Cyber risk does not only create a risk to the ransoms or exposure of private data but also altered data can lead to serious health consequences. As medical devices are linked with technology, the device's altered functionality or IoT interruption can even lead to serious health consequences, even death and life circumstances in the worst case. As healthcare professionals and patients are dependent on the data, altered or deleted data can lead to an incorrect diagnosis and treatment. Issues of empathy, miscommunication, the frustration of poor implementation of technology, and too much reliance on technology can weigh limitations over opportunities.

It is indeed a fact that technology can assist the service provider but not replace the manpower, so in that case adaptation of technology in healthcare and medical tourism is still in the infancy phase, as the industry matures, disadvantages are expected to be outweighed by the opportunities.

6.10 Implication of the Chapter

This chapter has mentioned the understanding of advanced technology in healthcare and its applications in medical tourism in India. Readers will be familiar with the advancement in data security, privacy, and assist to promote the modernization and expansion of health facilities in India. As the chapter is descriptive in nature, it will provide the base for situation analysis of medical tourism in India.

6.11 Summary of the Chapter

The adoption of technologies in medical tourism is expected to make looking service delivery overseas more accessible, and affordable. Moreover, health-related data are available in real time. It is worth mentioning that technologies have contributed ample growth to medical tourism that have raised eyebrows in society from the aspect of social, security, and economic development. Medical tourism has progressively incorporated the demand for cultivated and sophisticated medical treatments and equipment above par the customized ones. Pre-operative and post-operative care from customer and medical service perspectives are extremely enhanced by the technology, i.e., IoMT, blockchain technology, mobile healthcare, digital health, etc. To assess the healing and recovery of patients from a distance tele-consultation is in demand. Virtual rehabilitation applications are also adding benefits that integrate wearable sensors along with a recording of a range of motions. Artificial Intelligence and Assistive technologies have upscaled the effectiveness of surgeries. The technology of Biomedical Waste Disposal has helped to relieve public health threats. Thus the growth and application of the technology will surely reshape the healthcare industry in the form of more "understandable, affordable, and accessible". In the end, beneficiaries of medical tourism look forward to getting predictive, integrated, and personalized experiences for health and wellness in India.

References

Ahmed D (2022) Here's how India is shaping the future of medical tourism. Financial Express. Available https://www.financialexpress.com/lifestyle/travel-tourism/heres-how-india-is-shaping-the-future-of-medical-tourism/2707932/

Ayuningtyas D, Ariwibowo DA (2020) The strategic role of information communication technology in succeeding medical tourism. Enfermería Clín 30:170–173. https://doi.org/10.1016/j.enfcli.2020.06.039

Banerjee N (2022) India medical tourism is gearing up for Artificial Intelligence. SME FUTURES

Benerjee N (2022) India's medical tourism is gearing up for AI. SME futures. Available https://smefutures.com/indias-medical-tourism-is-gearing-up-for-ai/

Bernasconi S (2016) The role of medical technology in the 4th Industrial Revolution. MedTec Views. Available https://www.medtechviews.eu/articles/role-medical-technology-4th-industrial-revolution/

Bhardwaj T (2022) Advantage India: the world is coming to India as the country eyes increase in global medical tourism share. Financial Express. [Online]. Available: https://www.financialexpress.com/lifestyle/travel-tourism/advantage-india-india-eyes-increase-in-global-medical-tourism-share-heres-why-the-world-in-coming-to-india/2672596/

Bhatia D (2021) Modern technological intervention advancements for the physically challenged and disabled population. Cambridge Scholars Publishing, Cambridge

Bhatia D, Sanjeevirayar B, Karthick A, Mishra A, Malviya A (2020) Role of the Internet of Things and deep learning for the growth of healthcare technology. In: Trends in deep learning methodologies. Elsevier, Amsterdam, pp 113–127. https://doi.org/10.1016/B978-0-12-822226-3.00005-2

Bhatia D, Mishra A, Mukherjee M (2021) Amalgamation of blockchain technology and internet of things for healthcare applications. In: Blockchain for 5G-enabled IoT. Springer, Cham, pp 571–592. https://doi.org/10.1007/978-3-030-67490-8_22

Bhatiya D (2015) Medical informatics. PHI Learning Pvt. Limited, Delhi

Buhalis D (1998) Strategic use of information technologies in the tourism industry. Tour Manag 19:409–421. https://doi.org/10.1016/S0261-5177(98)00038-7

Çapar H (2020) Using cryptocurrencies and transactions in medical tourism. J Econ Adm Sci 37:677–693. https://doi.org/10.1108/JEAS-07-2019-0080

Carrera PM, Bridges JF (2006) Globalization and healthcare: understanding health and medical tourism. Expert Rev Pharmacoecon Outcomes Res 6(4):447–454. https://doi.org/10.1586/14737167.6.4.447

Davidson S, De Filippi P, Potts J (2016) Disrupting governance: the new institutional economics of distributed ledger technology. SSRN Electron J. https://doi.org/10.2139/ssrn.2811995

Dawn SK, Pal S (2011) Medical tourism in India: issues, opportunities and designing strategies for growth and development. Int J Multidiscip Res 1:3

De M (2021) Rise of medical tourism in Delhi: a case study of AIIMS hospital. Int J Multidiscip Curr Res 3:123–131

Dinesh Bhatia AKP, Mishra A (2022) Blockchain technology for biomedical engineering applications. In: Applications of blockchain and big IoT systems digital solutions for diverse industries. CRC Press, Boca Raton, pp 245–266

Emmanuel J, Puccia C, Spurgin R (2001) Non-incineration medical waste treatment technologies. Heal Care without Harm Washingt, p 61. Available: http://goo.gl/QrK3hB

Evangeline J (2022) Top 3 applications of Internet of Medical Things (IoMT). India Pharma Outlook

García-Altés A (2005) The development of health tourism services. Ann Tour Res 32:262–266. https://doi.org/10.1016/j.annals.2004.05.007

Gatsis GJ, Pappas K (2017) Wireless control for the IoT: power spectrum and security challenges. In: IEEE/ACM second international conference on internet-of-things design and implementation (IoTDI). IEEE, Piscataway, pp 341–342. Available https://www.indiapharmaoutlook.com/news/top-3-applications-of-internet-of-medical-things-iomt-nwid-431.html

Goodrich G (1987) Healthcare tourism-an exploration study. Tour Manag September:217–222

Hassan V, Bellos G (2022) COVID-19: reshaping medical tourism through artificial intelligence (AI) and robotics. Athens J Tour 9(2):77–98. https://doi.org/10.30958/ajt.9-2-2

Hittinger E, Jaramillo P (2019) Internet of things: energy boon or bane? Science 364(6438):326–328. https://doi.org/10.1126/science.aau8825

Hurley T (2004) Managing customer retention in the health and fitness industry: a case of neglect. Ir Mark Rev 17(1):23–28

IBEF (2018) https://www.ibef.org/industry/indian-tourism-and-hospitality-industry-analysis-presentation

Karimov F, Brengman M, Van Hove L (2011) The effect of website design dimensions on initial trust: a synthesis of the empirical literature. J Electron Commer Res 12:272–301
Kazemi Z (2008) Study of the effective factors for attracting medical tourism in Iran
KPMG (2014) https://assets.kpmg.com/content/dam/kpmg/pdf/2014/09/KPMG-FICCI-Heal-Sep2014.pdf
Lunt N, Smith R, Exworthy M, Stephen T, Horsfall D, Mannion R (2011) Medical tourism: treatments, markets and health system implications: scoping review. Dir Employment Labour Soc Aff 2011:1–55, Available http://scholar.google.com/scholar?hl=en&btnG=Search&q=intitle:Medical+Tourism+:+Treatments+,+Markets+and+Health+System+Implications+:+scoping+review#0
Nagar R, Singh Y, Jaglan V, Meenakshi (2021) A review on machine learning applications in medical tourism. In: 2021 fourth international conference on computational intelligence and communication technologies (CCICT). IEEE, Piscataway, pp 208–215. https://doi.org/10.1109/CCICT53244.2021.00048
Nayar R (2017) Medical value travel and Indian economy: a swot analysis. Int J Trade Glob Bus Perspect 6:2319–9067
Nayar R (2020) Role of ICT in promotion of medical value travel in India: a primer role of ICT in promotion of medical value travel in India
Nema SK, Ganeshprasad KS (2002) Plasma pyrolysis of medical waste. Curr Sci 83:271–278
Puczko L, Bachvarov M (2015) Spa, bath, thermae: what's behind the labels? Tour Recreat Res 31:83–91. https://doi.org/10.1080/02508281.2006.11081250
Rai A (2017) Globalization and medical tourism: a spatial study
Rao GKV (2021) Medical value tourism in India: what makes the country a leading medical tourism destination. Financial express. https://www.financialexpress.com/lifestyle/travel-tourism/medical-value-tourism-in-india-what-makes-the-country-a-leading-medical-tourism-destination/2338644/
Reddy S (2022) Robotic surgery to pave the way for medical value tourism. The Times of India. Available https://timesofindia.indiatimes.com/blogs/voices/robotic-surgery-to-pave-the-way-for-medical-value-tourism/
Santiago I (2020) Trends and innovations in biosensors for COVID-19 mass testing. Chembiochem 21(20):2880–2889. https://doi.org/10.1002/cbic.202000250
Sarngadharam VSSM (2009) Health tourism in India. New Century Publications, New Delhi
Shen YT, Chen L, Yue WW, Xu HX (2021) Digital technology-based telemedicine for the COVID-19 pandemic. Front Med 8:1–23. https://doi.org/10.3389/fmed.2021.646506
Singh L (2019) Medical tourism motivations: the driving force. JOMAT 4(2):77–86
Times of India (2022) Pwc India's study finds India leads in AI adoption during Covid-19. [Online]. Available https://www.hindustantimes.com/india-news/pwc-india-s-study-finds-india-leads-in-ai-adoption-during-covid-19/story-2kUMXmBBDbvLnFKOdkFJ1K.html
Tiwari A, Tripathi RP (2019) Advancements in data security and privacy techniques used in IoT-based hospital applications. IGI Global Publications, Hershey
Tyan I, Yagüe MI, Guevara-Plaza A (2021) Blockchain technology's potential for sustainable tourism. In: Wörndl W, Koo C, Stienmetz JL (eds) Information and communication technologies in tourism 2021. Springer, Cham
Wong BKM, Saaid Hazley SA (2020) The future of health tourism in the industrial revolution 4.0 era. J Tour Futur 7(2):267–272. https://doi.org/10.1108/JTF-01-2020-0006

Chapter 7
Impact of Covid-19 on Medical Tourism

N. Shalini, R. Sathish, B. J. Divya Rao, and H. K. Mamatha

Abstract The Covid-19 pandemic has had a significant impact on the global economy, including the medical tourism industry. Medical tourism also known as health tourism refers to the practice of traveling to another country for medical care. The industry has grown in recent years due to the availability of high-quality care at lower costs in other countries. However, the Covid-19 pandemic has caused many countries to close their borders and restrict travel, resulting in a significant decline in medical tourism. Additionally, many hospitals have suspended non-essential medical procedures to focus on treating Covid-19 patients thereby significant decline in revenue generation.

According to the report by the World Tourism Organization, international tourist arrivals fell by 84% in April 2020 compared to the previous year, which affected medical tourism also. A study by the International Medical Travel Journal found that the number of medical tourists visiting Thailand, a popular destination for medical tourism, decreased by 98% in the first quarter of 2020.

Despite the impact of Covid-19 on medical tourism being significant, there is a potential recovery also as many countries begin to ease travel restrictions and more people are vaccinated against Covid-19.

Medical tourism looks promising in the future as individual awareness of health and wellness is increasing in addition to the increasing cost of healthcare in many developed countries.

Keywords Covid-19 · Medical tourism · Pull factors · Push factors · Impact

N. Shalini (✉) · B. J. Divya Rao · H. K. Mamatha
Department of Health System Management Studies, JSS Academy of Higher Education and Research, Mysuru, India
e-mail: shalini.dhsms@jssuni.edu.in

R. Sathish
Department of Oral and Maxillofacial Surgery, JSS Dental College, JSS Academy of Higher Education and Research, Mysuru, India

B. Chaudhary et al. (eds.), *Medical Tourism in Developing Countries*,
https://doi.org/10.1007/978-981-99-8909-6_7

7.1 Introduction

The novel coronavirus is responsible for the outbreak of the current pandemic Covid-19. It originated in Wuhan, China, in December 2019, according to the World Health Organization (WHO), around 216 countries/territories/areas and over 9 million people are affected by Covid globally. The Covid-19 appears to be transmitted through respiratory droplets and close contact in healthcare settings. Healthcare workers (HCWs) are highly vulnerable to both, acquiring and transmission of infection as they are continuously exposed to infected patients and contaminated surfaces. During the pandemic lot of healthcare workers were affected by Covid-19 viruses, leading to loss of life, Covid-19-related complications, thus limiting the healthcare workforce.

The Covid-19 pandemic has affected the human being population in every single possible way. Every sector like Health, Economy, Industry, and Food is jeopardized as of restrictions. The impact is so intense that threatens health as well as the global economy. Medical tourism is a unification of healthcare, and the international travel industry has contributed to the nation's economy and has been adversely affected.

7.2 Health Tourism

In the past few years, health tourism is gaining importance in the health industry. Health tourism also contributes to economic growth globally. Today people are seeking alternatives to healthcare facilities offered in their own country in terms of better quality, lesser waiting time, and affordability.

Health tourism is a wider term for travel that focuses on medical treatments and the use of healthcare services. It covers a wide field of health-oriented tourism ranging from preventive and health-conductive treatment to rehabilitation and curative forms of travel.

The driving force for rapidly growing and developing health tourism in modern times is

- Globalization
- Technological advances
- Travel affordability
- Difference in healthcare costs in developed and developing countries

Health tourism comprises two major sub-categories, which are, wellness and medical tourism (Fig. 7.1).

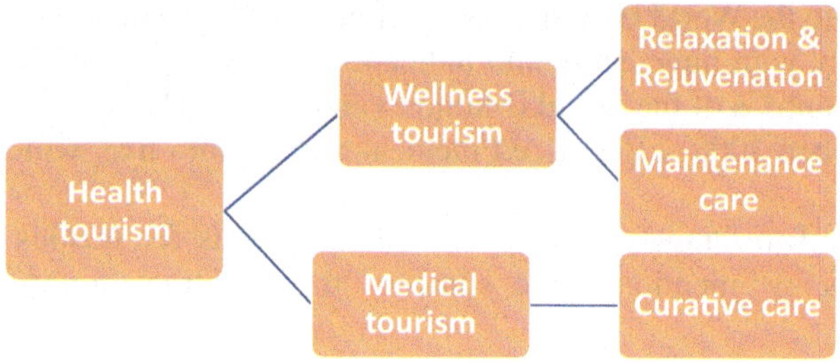

Fig. 7.1 Classification of health tourism

7.3 Wellness Tourism

Wellness is a holistic phrase with an ancient origin that has gained popularity in the modern world. Wellness is most associated with health, which is well-being without any illness. It indicates the positive characteristics of health. Health and wellness are indispensable in the tourism industry. In today's hectic life, we are neglecting our health. A large proportion of people have no time to take care of their health due to stressful work culture. The awareness towards health amongst individuals has raised several folds. Health and wellness as one form a prominent niche tourism market.

Wellness is a broad concept that includes lifestyle, physical, mental, and spiritual health as well as one's relationships with oneself, other people, and the environment.

7.4 Medical Tourism

People were travelling overseas for better health needs in earlier days, but the term MT is getting focused on in recent years and has captured the attention of policymakers, media, and researchers. There is no universally accepted unified definition (https://www.news-medical.net/health/What-is-Medical-Tourism.aspx).

Travelling people from one place/country to other for better health is termed medical tourism. People travel to affordable developing/developed nations thus leading to a change in patient motion both in terms of quality and quantity. The factors contributing to this change are

- Affordable treatment costs in developing countries
- Availability of economic flights
- Intensified marketing
- Online information about the available facilities to the consumer

Medical tourism is an indicator of globalization in the healthcare industry (Malhotra and Dave 2022).

According to the World Health Organization (WHO), Medical tourism is a developing tendency with huge economic indications (Bookman 2007) particularly the developing countries of the world (Malhotra and Dave 2022).

Cohen (Cohen 2008) categorized medical tourists into five, which are given in Table 7.1.

People travel to faraway nations as medical tourists for various health-related procedures, below mentioned are some of the countries preferred for certain procedures.

America, the especially southern and central parts are the preferred destination for cosmetic/plastic/bariatric/dental care treatments.

India, Malaysia, Singapore, and Thailand are preferred for cancer care and cardiac and orthopaedic care.

Keeping in mind patient preferences, services, and satisfaction, sophisticated modern care is being offered under the banner of medical tourism by highly advanced countries like Canada, Belgium, Israel, Italy, and Germany (Horowitz et al. 2007).

Due to the rapid growth of the United States and other developed nations, many employers and insurance providers began to see medical travel to reduce costs. As even more nations throughout the world begin to realize the economic benefits of these emerging markets, they start to offer top-notch medical services at considerably reduced costs. The medical care cost in clinics and hospitals depends on the patient's economic state.

7.5 The Driving Forces for Medical Tourism (Singh 2019)

Travel motivations drive the movement of medical tourists across the world.

Table 7.1 Types of tourists

Type of tourist	Purpose of tour
Mere tourist	Who won't use any medical facility in overseas countries?
Medicated tourist	Who use medical facilities due to some trauma or accident
Medical tourist proper	Who come together with both tourism and medical treatment with intent. This type involves both, those who travel to the host nation with an earlier intention to get treatment during their vacation, as well as those who decide on such treatment only during their stay in the country
Vacationing patient	Who primarily come for therapy, could also have a good time informally or when you are recuperating
Mere patient	Who obtain only treatment but no other vacationing activities

7.5.1 *Major Pull Factors*

In addition to the major pull factors given in Table 7.2, other pull factors include affordable air travel and favourable exchange rates, local transportation associated with escort services, sightseeing, translation, pleasant hotel accommodations, and an array of healthcare procedures with a variety of food and hospitality.

7.5.2 *Push Factors*

Along with the pull factors, some push factors that motivate travellers to travel overseas for health reasons are given in Table 7.3.

These factors have been identified as essential components of medical tourism growth. Medical tourism is a promising and significant segment of the modern tourism industry.

7.6 Impact of Covid-19 on Medical Tourism

Covid-19 outbreak has affected worldwide after Chinese New Year around mid of January. By February western countries commenced the lockdown process after a considerable number of cases were detected (Sharma et al. 2020). The World Health Organisation announced a Public Health Emergency of International Concern on 30 January 2020 and declared Covid-19 as a pandemic on 11 March 2020. Most nations undertook intense measures to control movements and enforce lockdowns to

Table 7.2 Major pull factors for medical tourism

Low cost—medical as well as travel cost
Less waiting time—the patients have to delay their medical treatment for a long time due to overburdened medical delivery systems in developed countries
Availability of treatment—the comprehensive array of health essential services extended at a hospital is of key value for tourists forced to go to other nations to pursue treatment
Quality treatment and care—the quality of services like getting accredited by established authorities like the NABH, and JCAHO (Joint Commission for the Accreditation of Health Care Organisations) is a major pull factor to medical tourism
Availability of tourist attractions—although travelling to a different nation for treatment, it is also likely to visit pleasing places and memorials of that nation
Technology—health tourists are drawn by facilities with supportive staff and tech-savvy medical professionals
Personalization—medical tourists are driven to utilize the medical services of hospitals which have an outstanding repute an important feature luring travellers to choose a medical tourism location is communication efficiency

Table 7.3 Major push factors for medical tourism

Affordability—patients who are unable to pay for expensive medical or surgical procedures in their home country might explore this aspect. This forces them to seek a nation that delivers cheaper treatment without compromising on quality
Adjournment—if the patient is unable to wait, he or she will look for alternative locations to obtain medical treatment or surgery
Unavailability—when some treatments are unavailable or there is a lack of quality care in their home countries, patients are willing to travel across borders
Inferior healthcare services—some nations' healthcare services fall short of international standards due to issues like a lack of follow-up care, poor quality, and a lack of skilled healthcare professionals
Lack of coverage under insurance in home country—medical tourism can be an alternative to the increased costs of healthcare, for those who require procedures without insurance coverage
Privacy and confidentiality—patients travel out of the country for treatment for privacy and confidentiality reasons
Legal liability—in some nations, certain diagnoses, and treatments, such as gender-changing procedures, baby gender determination, egg and sperm donation, abortion, and stem cell treatment, are prohibited by law

minimize the spread of infection. By the time the mere existence and gravity were recognized, it had already crossed national borders (Sharma et al. 2020).

The Covid-19 outbreak is a worldwide emergency since it impacted every nation equally. Especially significant economic disruption has occurred for nations that depend on tourism, travel, hospitality, and entertainment for their growth and well-being. Growing economies and emerging markets are confronting further challenges with unprecedented problems in investment flow as worldwide risk appetite declines, exchange demands as surviving with weaker health systems, and additional limited financial space to support.

Even though Covid-19 is not as contagious and fatal as Ebola, one tends to spread the virus well before suffering the actual symptoms. Moreover, the possibility of asymptomatic transmission rises in various areas with insufficient testing, which is a significant issue. Large-scale travel bans and safety protocols were implemented to combat the pandemic, which caused a loss of around US$2.1 trillion in 2020, according to the WTTC (Dash and Sharma 2021).

Covid-19 spreads by various routes, among which predominant modes are aerosol, other body fluids, and secretions, fomites, or surfaces like furniture and fixtures existing within the immediate atmosphere of a contaminated patient and items used like stethoscope or thermometer on the affected person (Karia et al. 2020).

Covid-19 has become a global pandemic. The reason for Covid-19 to become a global pandemic is mainly by travelling from one geographic location to another with the help of carriers. The main carrier for this virus is humans. People usually travel from one place to another, either for business, tourism, or healthcare purposes. Once the Covid-19 pandemic was announced, a lot of tourists cut short their travel and returned to their respective places, thus creating a mad rush in travel places, and facilitating transmission of the virus from pandemic areas to non-pandemic areas.

Governments were necessitated to take drastic measures in response to the Covid-19 pandemic, which had a significant impact on all economic sectors, although some were more severely impacted than others. The adoption and application of technology have contributed to addressing some of these difficulties, which include the intense demand in the health sector to provide patients with lifesaving care (Chhabra et al. 2021). The pandemic has had a significant impact on medical tourism, raising concerns about what steps could be taken to aid in both short- and long-term growth (Chhabra et al. 2021).

The travel agencies and tourism sector had a major business setback as the government health regulatory bodies directed for the closure of borders between the cities/countries, barring people from travelling from one place to other. All the tourist destinations which are potential places of people congregation were shut down, thus controlling the fast Covid-19 virus spread (Chhabra et al. 2021).

Cost is one of the key determinants that influence medical tourism, but there are also risks. Traveling to nations in addition to fewer stringent surgical specifications and post-operative restoration facilities may put themselves at more risk because of the varying ethical and legal protections, quality standards for hospitals and patients, and other factors. Hospitals are the key source of infection, and hygiene standards differ from nation to nation (Chhabra et al. 2021). There may also be ethical concerns regarding some processes in the destination country for medical tourism, such as the illegal buying of organs or tissue for transplantation. The patients' legal rights may not be effectively covered if problems occur during or after the procedure, which could lead to significant physical and psychological issues (Chhabra et al. 2021).

The business sectors and a lot of people faced an economic/financial crisis during the Covid-19 pandemic. People became very cautious in financial management, spending only for very important needs like groceries, medicines, and personal protective equipment. The plans of travel either for vacation or health or wellness reasons were cancelled or the reasons being Covid-19 transmission or financial problems.

7.7 The Impact of the Pandemic and Challenges

Global job losses were significant because of lockdowns that halted manufacturing, construction, and service activity completely in most nations. In addition, the pandemic has caused a significant number of deaths and the closing of numerous businesses, equally large and small. Healthcare and the digital services sector, on the other hand, are among those that have been to a smaller extent impacted but have faced pressure because of the situations. However, hospitality and tourism are among the industries that have been impacted the most severely (Chhabra et al. 2021).

The greater impact of the Covid-19 pandemic is likely to persist until 2025 and beyond, and the IMF predicted that world GDP would shrink by more than $22 trillion (Chhabra et al. 2021).

Medical tourism has been impacted by the pandemic's cancellation of elective surgeries and postponement of various treatments, as well as travel restrictions. The pandemic has impacted all sectors of the hospitality and tourism industry. People travelling for medical reasons have had much fewer options for treatment options owing to the unpredictability of whether border crossings would be open or closed and the varying requirements for quarantine. However, the extent of preparedness for medical tourists has been a secondary factor because of the significant burden placed on intensive care units and other healthcare facilities (Chhabra et al. 2021).

On a medical visa, 234,000 people entered India in 2015. That number increased to 495,056 in 2017 and 697,000 in 2019, or 6.9% of all foreign tourist arrivals. However, the insurmountable challenges posed by the pandemic have led to a rapid decline in this sector for India and other leading nations in medical tourism (Chhabra et al. 2021).

During the pandemic, all the hospital/health sectors were having Covid-19 management as the prime priority. To prevent the Covid-19 transmission and reduce its burden on healthcare providers, the treatments for other non-Covid-19 ailments were limited only to emergency conditions. Hospital visits were very limited, telemedicine facility was utilized for health-related consultations. All the elective/cosmetic procedures were deferred, and people made them a secondary priority due to Covid-19, which in turn affected the health tourism industry directly.

To curb unnecessary travel during Covid-19, restrictions were put on a travel visas, vaccination status was an important criterion because travelling was a problematic procedure, which discouraged travelling and thus vacations.

7.8 The Positive Impact of the Pandemic

Though Covid-19 has caused a lot of problems in terms of health and business, there are some positive outcomes in the form of

- Increased awareness among people worldwide regarding personal hygiene
- Implementation of hygiene protocols at hospitality, and tourist places
- Compliance with hand hygiene protocols
- Cough etiquettes
- Importance of social distancing
- Consciousness about a general health condition
- Improved standards of sterilization at healthcare centres
- Adaptation to scientific methods of biomedical waste disposal
- Improved protocols in patient appointment schedules

7.9 The Impact of the Pandemic and Opportunities

Given Covid-19 spreading rapidly, most nations have established new rules for international visitors. Importance was given to updating protocols in terms of hygiene and safety, just like in the hospitality and tourism industry. For medical tourism, these changes may bring innovations that might transform healthcare delivery in the future (Chhabra et al. 2021).

In the time following the pandemic, the widespread use of technology-driven consultations will make affordable medical tourism more accessible. Medical tourism is at a crossroads right now, and practices used during the pandemic may continue and make it easier for more people to get health services after the pandemic is over.

However, many people will return to medical tourism as vaccines become more widely available. As a result, this is a good time for stakeholders of medical tourism to form associations to ensure that testing and sanitization processes are followed consistently. Medical tourism canters should align their existing facilities to meet the shifting demand patterns. Medical tourism's future is also heavily dependent on government involvement.

7.10 Conclusion

Covid-19 is the pandemic that has caused a significant catastrophe to people in terms of health and the economy. It has made it even more important for nations to work together to share real-time information about disease outbreaks and be transparent about how to respond to and contain them. Healthcare professionals and health facilities have been able to provide patients with remote medical care and counselling because of incorporating technology as a response to the pandemic. Priority had to be given to updating standard operating procedures (SOPs) regarding hygiene practices for medical tourist-associated facilities and hospital premises. Implementation of the Covid protocols as well as training support has allowed essential services to continue during the pandemic, this may start significant shifts in medical tourism and healthcare. Government agencies should play an important role in implementing appropriate policies to ensure medical tourists' safety and protect service providers' rights.

References

Bookman M (2007) Medical tourism in developing countries. Springer, Cham

Chhabra A, Munjal M, Mishra PC, Singh K, Das D, Kuhar N, Vats M (2021) Medical tourism in the Covid-19 era: opportunities, challenges, and the way ahead. Worldwide Hosp Tour Themes 13:5

Cohen EC (2008) Medical tourism in Thailand. AU-GSB e-Journal 1:1

Dash SB, Sharma P (2021) Reviving Indian Tourism amid the Covid-19 pandemic: challenges and workable solutions. J Destination Mark Manage 22:100648

Horowitz MD, Rosensweig JA, Jones CA (2007) Medical tourism: globalization of the healthcare marketplace. MedGenMed 9(4):33. PMID: 18311383; PMCID: PMC2234298.

Karia R, Gupta I, Khandait H, Yadav A, Yadav A (2020) COVID-19 and its modes of transmission. SN Compr Clin Med 2(10):1798–1801. https://doi.org/10.1007/s42399-020-00498-4. Epub 2020 Sep 1. PMID: 32904860; PMCID: PMC7461745

Malhotra N, Dave K (2022) Int J Glob Business Competitive 17:215–228

Sharma A, Vishraj B, Ahlawat J, Mittal T, Mittal M (2020) Impact of COVID-19 outbreak over medical tourism. IOSR J Dent Med Sci 19(5):56–58

Singh L (2019) Medical tourism motivations: the driving force. J Multidiscip Acad Tour 4(2):77–86

Chapter 8
Dental Tourism in India: An Emerging Market

Pooja Sharma and Vineet Golchha

Abstract **Background and context:** The concept of having to travel to another country to pursue medical service has been in practice for generations. As technology and medical facilities advanced, it witnessed a flow of people from developed to developing countries. The 21st century has observed a boom in oral infections due to dietary habit changes; also the awareness towards dental health is also increasing at an equal rate with individuals aspiring to seek appropriate unraveling of their dental problems. Many multi-chain dental players having centers throughout India are focusing to cater the patients and are advertising abroad in newspapers and popular Web sites. Along with Delhi and Mumbai, many other states like Kerala, Goa and Jaipur are now becoming a hub of dental tourism.

Significance and conclusion: Dental tourism is an emerging new tool for marketing dental health, and promoting dentistry together with tourism. With an expected projection in the costs of oral healthcare, the scope for dental tourism is expanding and is predicted to widen at a greater pace in the coming times.With times to come dental tourism will facilitate international patients to considerably reduce on their dental expenses and at the same time explore the Indian heritage. This will in turn facilitate contribution to the growth of health economies.

Keywords Dental tourism · Dental market · Oral health · Dental industry

P. Sharma (✉)
Department of Hospital Management and Hospice Studies, Jamia Millia Islamia, New Delhi, India
e-mail: psharma@jmi.ac.in

V. Golchha
Department of Orthodontics and Dentofacial Orthopedics, Inderprastha Dental College and Hospital, Ghaziabad, UP, India

B. Chaudhary et al. (eds.), *Medical Tourism in Developing Countries*,
https://doi.org/10.1007/978-981-99-8909-6_8

8.1 Health Tourism

Tourism is an important indicator of economic growth in the modern world. It is an important area that can provide tremendous opportunities for the development of the society. Travelling is not just a journey anymore, it has transformed into lifelong cherished memories and experiences for an individual. This phenomenon has evolved over time and augments the economic development of that region (Cohen 1974). Tourism requires constant adaptability to the changing demands and aspirations of the customers. The prime focus of this dynamic and competitive industry is on the entertainment, safety and satisfaction of their travellers. Countries all over the world have realized the economic power of tourists and are now busy developing infrastructure to showcase their places as tourist hubs.

Medical tourism is currently a means of movement of people in search of physical and mental well-being combined with recreation and vacations is very prevalent nowadays. As per the medical tourism index 2020–2021 India ranks 10th among the leading countries in the world (https://www.medicaltourism.com/destinations/india). Among the top countries generating tourists for India during 2021, USA (28.1%) was the highest, followed by Bangladesh (15.8%), UK (10.7%), Canada (5.3%), Nepal (3.4%), Afghanistan (2.4%), Australia (2.2%), Germany (2.2%), Portugal (2.1%), France (2.0%), Maldives (1.7%), Sri Lanka (1.7%), Russia Federation (1.2%), Iraq (1.1%) and Netherlands (1.0%). As per the Ministry of Tourism, FEEs from tourism (2021) were US $8.7970 billion as compared to US $6.9580 billion in 2020 with a growth rate of 26.4% (https://health.economictimes.indiatimes.com/news/industry/challenges-and-opportunities-in-the-dental-tourism-market-in-india/95671471). Many travellers are now exploring probabilities for better healthcare services in India, and it has emerged as a potential growth stimulus for the tourism industry.

8.2 History of Medical and Dental Tourism

The concept of having to travel to another country to pursue medical service has been in practice for generations. Medical practitioners in England, Norway, and similarly other colder regions had always advised their clients diagnosed with vitamin D deficiency to travel to warmer places. Since the 1990s with the advancement of technology and communication the concept of medical tourism started spreading to Asian and African countries. For years, medical tourism in Asia was not a planned business but due to the currency crisis in Thailand in 1998, private group of hospitals started addressing international travellers.

Due to advancement in the field of medical technology, there is a flow of patients from developed to developing countries. The population which was without insurance or underinsured moved swiftly to developing countries to get the same quality of treatment probably at one-tenth of the cost. This "medical outsourcing" phenomenon has become common in countries like India, Thailand, and Turkey as these countries have emerged as the hub of medical tourism. The Medical Tourism market in India will grow at a CAGR of 21.1% between 2021–2028 and reach $53.51 billion in 2028 (Fortune Business Insights n.d.) (a report by Fortune Business Insights).

Similarly, people from the USA migrated to Mexico for cost-effective dental treatment. Mexico being a border state to America has over the years evolved as a dental treatment hub due to its lower cost of treatment; almost 25% of tourists coming here do seek dental treatment (Adams et al. 2018). Hungary owing to its geographical location and low-cost dental treatment charges is the hot spot for European tourists. The key factors involved are the availability of the latest medical technologies at reduced cost and compliance with international quality standards. The big corporate hubs as a new trend to reduce disbursement bills are encouraging their employees to avail low-cost dental treatment through dental tourism. Introduction of measures like removal of visa restrictions and the visa-on-arrival scheme for those seeking medical or dental treatments has also facilitated the concept of medical tourism.

8.3 Dental Tourism

Dental tourism provides dental care services outside one's native healthcare systems in combination with leisure or vacation (Turner 2008). American Dental Association in 2009 defined dental tourism as "act of travelling to other country for purpose of obtaining dental treatment". In European countries, it is being called as "dental vacations or vacation for ones teeth". Dental tourism amounts to about 10% of the total medical tourism industry in India (Frost & Sullivan). The global dental tourism market will reach to a valuation of US$ 6.7 billion in 2022. The demand in the market is predicted to grow at an astounding 13.6% CAGR, elevating the market valuation to US$ 24.3 billion by 2032 (Dent Care Publications 2015).

As per the Indian Dental Association, the market for dental equipment and material is estimated to increase by 25–30% annually. Currently, there are around 5000 Dental Laboratories, 125,000 dental professionals and 292 Dental Institutes in India providing graduation to about 20,000 dental students per year. The Indian healthcare market is among the world's top ten markets and the potential of dental care service market is approximated at about US$ 600 million. Additionally, dental equipment and appliances market is growing at a rate of 10% per annum, dental implants segment account for 25.6% of the total market share in 2022. The total sales in the dental tourism market are expected to represent nearly 4.0% of the overall US$ 152.3 Billion worth medical tourism market in 2022 (Dent Care Publications 2015) (Future Market Insights)

A report to Congress (2012) stated that about 130 million Americans live without dental insurance which is called as "Dental Crisis in America". A very few per cent of the Americans are acquainted with the concept of dental insurance. This is one of the prime reason that makes them travel to countries where the cost of the treatment is much less. Countries that benefited from this phenomenon included India, Hungary, Chile and Southeast Asian countries like Thailand. As per estimate, an American could save around 50% on dental procedures such as crowns, root canals and implants, if they visit another country and this cost also includes the cost of travelling and stay. In the UK, the National Health Service covers only a fraction cost of the dental treatment whereas in Australia dental care can get quite expensive even for people with insurance. For example, a single implant in the UK will cost you around 3000–3500 USD while the same internationally brand implants cost you only 800 USD. Similarly, a root canal and teeth whitening procedure costs around 2200 pounds (around Rs. 1.56 lakh), which is quite high as compared to India where it costs only around 280 pounds (Rs. 20,000) (Kamath et al. 2015) (Table 8.1).

As per the case report of Ms. Natalie who came on a 45-day holiday trip exploring the magnanimous palaces of Jaipur and other cities in Rajasthan in India, managed to save about 1920 pounds (Rs. 1.36 lakh) during this trip. The savings were a clear joy that was the result of her decision to get her dental treatment done in Jaipur. In London, where she belongs to, the procedure for a root canal and teeth whitening would have made her shell around 2200 pounds (around Rs. 1.56 lakh). She after the advice of her insurance company, planned to undergo her treatment in a dental hospital in Jaipur, India. Where the treatment costed her only around 280 pounds (Rs. 20,000). She stated that "That's when I decided to come to India. For the money that I would pay my dentist in London, I could afford air tickets as well as a holiday package," says the advertising executive, whose entire holiday, along

Table 8.1 Comparison of dental treatment costs between Western countries and India (adapted) (https://www.researchgate.net/publication/352642068_Dental_Tourism_in_India_The_Fast_Growing_Opportunity_For_The_Budding_Dentists)

Dental Procedure	Cost in US & UK ($)		Cost in India ($)
	General Dentist	Top End Dentist	Top End Dentist
Smile Designing	-	8,000	800-1000
Metal Free Bridge	-	5,500	500-800
Dental Implants	-	3,500	800-1000
Porcelain Metal Bridge	1,800	3,000	300-400
Porcelain Metal Crown	600	1,000	90-130
Tooth Impactions	500	2,000	90-130
Root Canal Treatment	600	1,000	80-100
Tooth Whitening	350	800	100-130
Tooth Colored Composite Fillings	200	500	20-40
Tooth Cleaning	100	300	60-80

with the dental treatment, cost her Rs. 1.45 lakh (about 2000 pounds) still saving a few hundred pounds and gaining a memorable trip to remarkable India (Ortiz 2011).

The twenty-first century has observed a boom in the number of cases related to oral infections whose prime reason being changes in dietary habits. At the same time, there is an increase in the awareness towards dental health with individuals aspiring to seek appropriate treatment for their dental problems. Together with dental treatment services, nowadays there is an increasing demand for cosmetic dentistry like whitening, tooth reshaping, etc. suggesting that there is an increase in the awareness of individuals related to self-appearance. The key here is to balance the high work-pressure life and minimum time with nominal expenditures. The solution can be in Dental tourism. Tourists can easily undergo dental treatment during their vacations due to the mostly non-emergency nature of dental treatment. India is considered a holiday destination for many foreign nationalities; dentists can easily render their services to them with affordable margins.

The giant hospital groups like Apollo and Fortis have their tie-ups with local tour operators and insurers abroad. Many multi-chain dental services providers are also following the same footsteps. They are also involved in spreading awareness in the other countries among the public for their services through advertisement in the newspapers and popular websites in India Delhi, Kerala, Goa, Jaipur and Mumbai have become a major hub of dental tourism. New Delhi has emerged as a prime destination for cardiac care, Chennai for eye care, and Kerala and Karnataka for state-of-the-art ayurvedic healing and meditation centres. India is becoming an attractive place for travellers due to the availability of experienced health practitioners, good medical staff with efficient communication abilities, a combination of allopathic with alternative systems of medicine, advanced diagnostic equipment, the availability of super speciality centres and these premium services at a comfortable cost (Youngman 2014).

There is a structured flow of the process to be followed that includes patients contacting the tour operators or the dentist directly, following which the tour operators arrange all the documents for them and facilitate the trip to the tourist country where they undergo the treatment. Post treatment the tour operators facilitate the trip taking care of all the facilities and finally the traveller may visit the dentist again as per treatment requirement (Fig. 8.1).

8.4 Factors that Contribute to Make India a Global Hub for Dental Tourism

8.4.1 Affordable Dental Treatment at Low Cost

India having the highest workforce of dental graduates and specialists offers quality dental care at very reasonable costs. The wide population base with ever-growing dental treatment needs has already attracted all major dental companies to set up

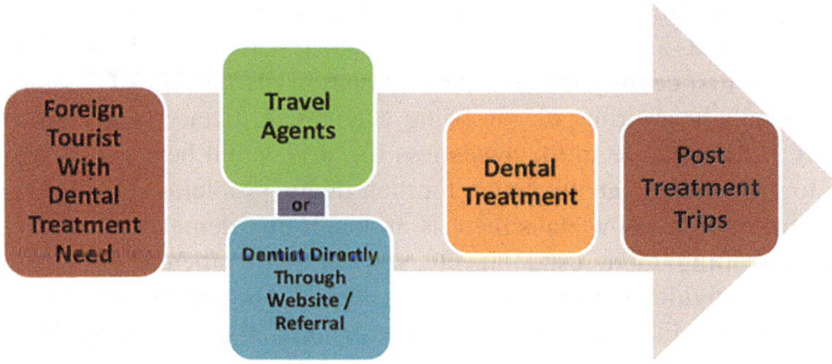

Fig. 8.1 Flow chart of dental tourism (self-drawn)

their base in India hence quality product availability is no issue at all. For example in Implants international brands like Nobel Biocare, Straumann, Dentsply Sirona, and Biohorizons are well established in India. Indian Dental Association and Dental Council of India, the governing body of dental education, have setup guidelines to ensure the highest level of competence and skills amongst its members. Availing international standards at fractional cost makes India a lucrative option for travellers with dental needs (Ortiz 2011).

8.4.2 Psychological Benefits to Foreign Patients

In India, the medium of higher education especially medical and dental is mostly in English. Almost all the dental practitioners working in India are well-versed in English and all dental documentation is prepared in English. English also being most commonly spoken language across the globe, travellers tend to have more confidence and less fear as communication can be direct, no translators, and any miscommunication due to translation is avoided.

8.4.3 Immediate Treatment

Most of the dental treatments being non-emergency and elective can be well planned in advance. The dentist here are well aware of the patient's needs, the equipments needed, the travel schedule of the patients and hence if carefully planned patient gets immediate treatment. Less or no waiting time ensures maximum utilization of travel schedule for leisure and site seeing.

8.4.4 *Quality Treatment*

The government and dental bodies monitor the standard norms for establishment of the hospital and clinic pan India. National Accreditation Board for Hospitals & Healthcare Providers (NABH) and Bureau of Indian Standards (BIS) keep a quality check on the standards of equipment, following strict sterilization methodology and proper Biowaste management. All ensuring only quality treatment is delivered to the patients whether Indian or overseas.

8.4.5 *Less Medication Cost*

India has evolved as the third-largest drug manufacturer in the world. It is also a major exporter of Pharmaceuticals, with more than 200 countries served by Indian exports. India supplies over 50% of Africa's requirement for generics, 40% for the US and 25% for the UK. India is a leading supplier of DPT, BCG and Measles vaccines which account for around 60% of global vaccine demand and 70% of WHO's vaccines (as per the essential Immunization schedule) are sourced from India (https://www.investindia.gov.in/sector/pharmaceuticals). The availability of drugs and their cost price have never been an issue for India.

8.4.6 *Low Labour Cost*

Mostly dental treatments do not require a lot of post-surgical care or the need for paramedics but still if required most of the Hospitals have surplus staff for post-operative care. Also availability of over 5000 dental labs with trained technicians ensures work is done in a limited time. Overall trained and un-trained labour cost is quite less in India as compared to the world making treatment less expensive.

8.4.7 *Geographic Location*

India with his rich heritage is one of the oldest civilizations in the world and one among the most popular tourist destinations in the world. It Extend from the Himalayan heights in the north to the tropical rain forests of the south, from the exclusive beauty of North East to the deserts and palaces of Rajasthan. With the beaches of Bay of Bengal on the east and the Arabian Sea on the west it's just Incredible to explore India. India stands apart with its diverse cuisines, faiths, arts, crafts, music, nature, lands, history and adventure. As the 7th largest country in the world, India is well connected by air, land and water to the rest of the world. It is accessible from every corner of the world through its 35 international airports and 14 ports and the Government is investing majorly in infrastructure and roads to keep the travel hassle-free.

8.4.8 Alternative Medical Proposition

Alternative medicine encompasses any treatment or therapy that departs from mainstream medical practice. India has always been the world leader in these remedies that have been utilized all across the world, Ayurveda, homeopathy, naturopathy, acupuncture, massage, yoga, meditation, herbal medicine, and other forms of traditional alternative medicine are examples. Foreign tourists can also get benefits from these systems and spend time in international centres of naturopathy and yoga for complete mental and physical wellness. The Government of India through its Ministry of AYUSH in 2014 has successfully tried to integrate and streamline the five traditional systems of medicine, namely Ayurveda, Yoga & Naturopathy, Unani, Siddha and Homoeopathy.

8.4.9 Political Stability

Being the largest democracy in the world, India always has strong political stability, secular nature of the country with robust law mechanism all for safe and convenient vacations is also a major factor in its tourism growth.

8.4.10 NRI Citizens

With a large proportion of Indians working abroad, Non-Resident Indians (NRIs) also contribute to facilitating medical and dental treatment growth (32 million NRIs and OCIs residing outside India, Ministry of External Affairs report). When travelling to India they also make a point to get their dental treatment done here well aware of the economic benefits of these.

8.5 Need of the Hour

There is a need for a collaborative effort to explore and take advantage of the tourism sector. There is a huge possibility of collaboration with national and international tour agencies and insurance service providers. The Indian government has spent over 2% of the country's GDP on healthcare (2022). It is predicted to reach about 2.5% by the financial year 2025. Measures are being taken to have quality services and infrastructure to encourage dental tourism. Campaigns like "Swach Bharat, Athithi Devo Bhava and Incredible India", the government is trying its level best to install a positive attitude among overseas patients making India a hub for tourism (Delta Dental of Arizona 2008).

The call of this hour is to have a harmony among policymakers and private players to reap maximum benefits from tourism. Despite having an infinite opportunity in this sector due to our strengths of dental knowledge and skills, geographical location advantage, and cultural richness to attract tourists, it is still only marginally utilized. We can also learn and implement policies like Singapore and Malaysia, create a medical hub, promote medical and dental tourism, extend the medical visa from 1 to 6 months and may be even plan a yearly event to advertise its potential.

8.6 Dental Tourism Myths

The most common myth among the patients is that cross-border dental care being inexpensive may be substandard (Delta Dental of Arizona 2008). An important threat is that dental procedures carried out in foreign countries do not bear any guarantee and patients have to pay huge amount of money in their native countries to get rid of any complications that may arise later. The international companies have an important role to play at this point where they can provide an international warranty to their inhabitants.

An another concern may be related to the agencies which regulate sterilization and infection control standards, as these may vary from country to country and can have an impact on the patient's state of oral health (Turner 2009).

8.7 Conclusion

The main opportunity presented by dental tourism is its contribution to the growth of health economies. Although there are limitations existing currently as lack of coordination among different players in the industry, the negative perceptions about India in relation to hygiene standards, misconceptions related to accreditation and regulation system of the hospitals, yet there is a huge potential and great scope in the domain of dental tourism.

The central and the state governments have been initiating great efforts to promote medical tourism in India like government's big budget market campaign, declaring medical tourism as services export, expanding airports in the country, introduction of medical visa for medical tourists, there still exist a need to formulate more effective and structured processes to facilitate dental tourism at large.

To conclude, this chapter highlighted the significance of Dental tourism as an emerging new tool for marketing dental health, and promoting dentistry together with tourism. With an expected rise in the costs of oral healthcare, the scope for dental tourism is expanding and is predicted to widen at a greater pace in the coming times. Dental treatment in India is being favoured by foreign travellers due to reasons like cost-effectiveness and affordability, diversity of tourist destinations and increasing strength in information technology which is making the process easy. With times to come dental tourism will facilitate international patients to considerably reduce their dental expenses and at the same time explore the Indian heritage.

References

Adams K, Snyder J, Berry NS, Crooks VA (2018) A critical examination of empowerment in medical tourism: the case of dental tourism industry in Los Algodones, Mexico. Glob Health 14(1):1–10

Cohen E (1974) Who is a tourist? A conceptual clarification. Sociol Rev 22(4):527–554

Delta Dental of Arizona (2008) Trouble in paradise, the untold story of dental tourism: dangers and risks of cross- border dentistry; facts & issues. Delta Dental of Arizona, Glendale

Dent Care Publications (2015) Dental tourism: reasons for smile

Fortune Business Insights (n.d.) Medical tourism market size, growth|research report [2028]

Kamath K, Hugar S, Kumar V, Gokhale N, Uppin C, Hugar SS (2015) The business and plea-sure of teeth: dental tourism. Int J Contemp Dent Med Rev 2015:1–4

Ortiz M (2011) Is the risk of 'foreign' dental treatment worth the savings? J Am Dent Assoc [illegible]

Turner L (2008) Cross-border dental care: 'dental tourism' and patient mobility. Br Dent J 204(10):553–554

Turner L (2009) Dental tourism: issue surrounding cross-border travel for dental care. J Can Dent Assoc 75(2):117–119

Youngman I (2014) Trends in the dental tourism market

Chapter 9
Medical Tourism: Exigency for Economy

Sushman Sharma, Nishi Gandhi, B. S. Dhillon, Kesha Bhadiyadra, and Monika

Abstract Medical tourism is the across-border travel for healthcare services by patients from various European and Asian countries. India is one of the preferred choices for medical treatments being the low-cost healthcare service provider along with the holistic quality care. Globalization and Liberalization are two important factors leading to the potential growth of the medical tourism market all over the globe.

The current study undertakes the evaluation of potential factors for the growth of the medical tourism market in the country like cost benefits, qualified and expertise pool of medical staff, certification and accreditation and role of government in it. Based on these opportunities evaluation the strategy necessary for the exponential growth of the market is recommended. The medical tourism market is growing at a high pace of 30% yearly. The study aims to focus on the strategy to boost the economy of the country through the growing medical tourism market.

Indian medical tourism market has been valued at US$ 2.89 billion in the year 2020 and the country has been ranked 10th out of world's top 46 counties for medical tourism by the Medical Tourism Index 2020–2021. Thus, the paper highlights the in-depth analysis of growth drivers to boost the economy of the country through the exponential growth of medical tourism market.

Keywords Strategy · Exponential growth · Cost benefits · Medical tourism market · Low-cost healthcare facilities · Economy

S. Sharma (✉)
HNG University, Patan, Gujarat, India

N. Gandhi
Sterling Hospital, Vadodara, India

B. S. Dhillon
Department of Hospital Administration, PGIMS, Rohtak, Haryana, India

K. Bhadiyadra
Department of Hospital Management, HNGU, Patan, Gujarat, India

Monika
Department of Tourism and Hotel Management, NEHU, Shillong, Meghalaya, India

B. Chaudhary et al. (eds.), *Medical Tourism in Developing Countries*,
https://doi.org/10.1007/978-981-99-8909-6_9

9.1 Introduction

India is one of the countries' leading regional healthcare hub for the different Asian and European countries as it provides low-cost quality medical and surgical treatments along with the promising and preventable treatments of Indian medicines called Ayurveda and yoga. Globalization and the highly emerging liberalization is leading to the progression of the medical trade in the world. In the upcoming era, tourism is looking forward for medical and health tourism which was limited with student tourism, religious tourism and other festive tourism.

Medical tourism is often as similar to health tourism. Medical tourism predominantly encloses the treatment procedures like biomedical procedures, consultation, high-tech surgeries etc. Well-developed technologies and medical advancements have supported the medical travels from varied countries to India. Boost in the potential market of the medical tourism is due to emergence of the low-cost advantages with travel package to the country. Infrastructural facilities provided by the private players in the country make India a preferred destination for treatment from all over the world. Even the Indian market has been successful in making its space in the international healthcare market.

9.2 Emergence of Medical Tourism in India

India is a country with a rich and diverse culture along with the core of hospitality nurtured with the "ATITHI DEVO BHAVA". India has always been a remarkable destination in the hospitality sector all over the world. Since the Vedic times, India has been rich with the knowledge of the medicines witnessed by the writings of the Charak Samhita and Sushruta Samhita in 800 BCE. The roots of today's modern surgeries like rhinoplasty and various other medical procedures and treatments are found in these writings. India has also grown exponentially in accepting and providing modern medicine in the post-independence era. The amalgamation of these modern medicine practices with holistic Indian medicine and wellness has made India the preferred destination for the treatment.

9.3 Current State of Medical Tourism in the Country

Month-wise Foreign Tourist Arrivals India, Jan 2018-June 2020 (Provisional)

Month	Foreign Tourist Arrivals (FTAs) in India				
	2018	2019	2020 (P)	Percentage (%) Change	
				2019/18	2020/19
January	10,45,027	11,11,040	11,18,150	6.3	0.6
February	10,49,259	10,90,516	10,15,632	3.9	–6.9
March	10,21,539	9,78,236	3,28,462	–4.2	–66.4
April	7,45,033	7,74,651	0	4	–100.0
May	6,06,513	6,15,136	0	1.4	–100.0
June	6,83,935	7,26,446	0	6.2	–100.0
July	8,06,493	8,18,125		1.4	
August	7,85,993	8,00,837		1.9	
September	7,19,894	7,51,513		4.4	
October	8,90,223	9,45,017		6.2	
November	10,12,569	10,92,440		7.9	
December	11,91,498	12,26,398		2.9	
Total (Jan-June)	51,51,306	52,96,025	24,62,244	2.8@	–53.5@
Total (Jan-Dec)	1,05,57,976	1,09,30,335		3.5	

Source: https://tourism.gov.in/sites/default/files/2020-09/ITS%20at%20a%20glance_Book%20%282%29.pdf

India is ranked 10th in medical tourism as per the Medical Tourism Index 2020–2021 by Medical Tourism Association. India has experienced 3.5% of annual growth rate in the foreign tourist arrival as per the data shown in the tourist Statistics. From the total tourist arrival 6.4% of share is of the medical tourism in India. The top countries showing the foreign tourist travel are Bangladesh, the United States, the United Kingdom, Australia, Canada, Malaysia and Sri Lanka.

9.4 India as a Leading Medical Tourism Destination

1. Cost benefits and contribution:

   India is the preferred choice for the medical treatments as the patient has to pay only a fraction of the amount for the similar treatment which they pay for in their home country. The quality healthcare with the cheaper price is provided at the best and leading hospitals of the country. Indian hospitals provide excellent treatment with the latest technological advancements in healthcare, experienced staff, good food and accommodation services, and the world-class infrastructure. Thus, under medical tourism the country ensures the safety, excellence and quality of healthcare service to the medical tourists.

Medical tourism in India has the 22–25% of growth yearly. It has a contribution of over 2 bn in the healthcare market of the country.

Indian medical tourism market has been valued at US$ 2.89 billion in the year 2020.

Treatment cost comparison

Procedures	US ($)	Costa Rica ($)	India ($)	Korea ($)	Mexico ($)	Thailand ($)	Malaysia ($)
Heart bypass	$144,000	$25,000	$5200	$28,900	$27,000	$15,121	$11,430
Angioplasty	$57,000	$13,000	$3300	$15,200	$12,500	$3788	$5430
Heart valve replacement	$170,000	$30,000	$5500	$43,500	$18,000	$21,212	$10,580
Hip replacement	$50,000	$12,500	$7000	$14,120	$13,000	$7879	$7500
Knee replacement	$50,000	$11,500	$6200	$19,800	$12,000	$12,297	$7000
Dental implant	$2800	$900	$1000	$4200	$1800	$3636	$345
Breast implants	$10,000	$3800	$3500	$12,500	$3500	$2727	N/A
Rhinoplasty	$8000	$4300	$4000	$6000	$2500	$3901	$1293
Retina	N/A	$4500	$850	$10,200	$3500	$4242	$3000
IVF treatment	N/A	$2,800	$3250	$2180	$3950	$9091	$3819

Source: https://www.medicalindiatourism.com/treatment-cost.html

2. Qualified pool of doctors:

   There is the availability of a large pool of qualified and experienced staff in the country. The number of registered allopathic doctors under the IMC Act (National/State Medical Council) has increased from 0.83 million in 2010 to 1.27 million in 2021. As per the data, the medical colleges in India are 558, also 221 homoeopathy and 339 Ayurveda government-registered colleges. With the unbound support of qualified doctors and experienced medical staff the country is able to cater the need of medical tourists in a varied range of medical services.

3. Certification and accreditation of hospitals:

   Most of the corporate and private hospitals of the country have been certified/accredited under various agencies like the JCI, NABH, CRISIL etc. It helps to raise confidence and provides quality of care to medical tourists. Through this, the standards of the facilities for healthcare as well as healthcare infrastructure are well maintained in the country. The uniformity and the standardized care attract medical tourists to the country.

4. Government contribution:

For the organized and institutional management for the promotion of medical and wellness tourism in the country, the Government has constituted the National Medical and Wellness Board. The board examines the demand regarding the liberalization of the medical visa, facilitation of the healthcare service and enhancing strategy for the same. One of the major key hurdles was the availability of the medical visa, the process of which is now eased with the multiple entries and longer stay which contributes to exponential growth of medical tourist visits to the country. Even the Ministry of Tourism provides financial support and assistance to medical tourists by facilitating hospitals like JCI-accredited and NABH-accredited hospitals of the country under the extended scheme of the ministry called Medical Development Assistance. Thus, the Ministry of Health and Family Welfare along with the Ministry of Tourism contributes to streamlining the process of medical tourism in India. The easy and simplified process of the medical visa attracts more cross-borders travel for the healthcare service. India also has a dedicated four-entry medical visa system for this purpose.

5. Process streamlining:

   Individuals seeking medical treatment contact the facilitator in the country wherein all the reports, doctor's opinion letter, history and all other required additional information are provided. Registered and certified doctors or healthcare providers are recommended and if required specialists are consulted. Also, the individual is intimated about the choice of hospital, doctors, cost of treatment, length of stay and other information regarding transport, accommodation, etc. Recommendation for the application of medical visa is also provided to the relevant embassy so that the process is eased. Medical assistance is also provided with the help of the portal which provides all the necessary information. After the patient undergoes the surgery, the individual is counselled for the additional post-operative care, follow-up checks and lastly provided the certificate for the fit to fly.

6. Other contributing factors:

   (a) No waiting period for the major surgeries in the country unlike the US and UK.
   (b) No language barrier in the developed states and major cities of the country offering medical services to foreign tourists.
   (c) Holistic treatment packages with modern and preventive Indian medicines.
   (d) Growing Pharmaceutical Sector and Medical Device Sector of the country.

9.5 Strategy for Promoting Medical Tourism in the Country

1. To leverage the leadership in medical tourism, India should have the:

   (a) Short-term focus: Specifically in the leading expertise services like cardiology, orthopaedics and many other high-tech services like neurology, oncology and cosmetic surgeries. They should focus on the development of the

AYUSH Health market for the amalgamation of holistic care to medical tourists.
(b) Long-term focus: Should focus on building the credibility of the services in fertility, weight loss surgeries and dentistry.

2. Develop India as a brand for the medical treatment destination:

   (a) India offers the best of both modern medical treatment along with traditional medical treatments for the holistic care of patients, there is an urgent need to focus on the branding and highlighting of the combined wellness treatment for the patient. "Heal in India" campaign is one of such branding campaigns for medical and wellness tourism. Tourist-friendly and the patient-centric branding of medical tourism is desirable as a successful strategy to promote medical tourism.

3. Digitalization of the service:

   (a) Under the current situation, the country needs to develop a medical tourism portal for catering the informational needs of the patients. It can facilitate the knowledge about the facilitators, appointments availability, immigration, insurance companies and all information for the journey throughout the treatment in the country. It will ease and streamline the process of treatment, increase transparency and visibility of the service providers and enhance the users' experience throughout the journey.
   (b) It will facilitate in providing the information for better decision-making and strategy development within the country.

4. Robust ecosystem:

   (a) To bring together and create strong linkage between all the stakeholders for the medical tourism development like Government, hospitals/service providers, airlines, insurance companies, hotels and other regulatory bodies. Strengthening of this ecosystem can lead to the improvised and encouraging medical service in the country.

5. Other strategies:

   (a) Standard pricing policy for all health service providers throughout the country.
   (b) International linkages of the hospital to increase the visibility of the healthcare service provided in the country.
   (c) Develop value-added service for the patient with the contribution of all the stakeholders in the medical travel to the country.
   (d) Legal support in the country for the fastest grievance handling of the patients.
   (e) Development of the wellness hubs at various destinations of the country other than the metro cities.
   (f) Quality revolution by the accreditation agencies to signify the provision of the healthcare by the providers.

9.6 Path Ahead

The medical tourism sector can provide the potential contribution in the GDP, economy of the country, improvement of infrastructure of the facilities and employment opportunities. India has the quality and cost-effective advantage which can help to leverage the Indian medical tourism market as the world leader. Thus, by the addition of the foreign exchange revenue the overall economy can be boosted. In growing competition in the medical tourism sector, we need to adapt the pace with certain tax relaxation on various duties for the medical equipment, tax incentives and cooperation among all the stakeholders like public and private. Department of health, tourism and information and communication can together create, build and promote a high-quality patient care destination.

9.7 Conclusion

Based on the data, we can conclude that India has shown immense growth in the medical tourism sector. The potential to boost the country's economy by threefold lies in the strategy building for the development of medical tourism in the country. More of accredited hospitals with safe and quality, standardized cost and pricing mechanism, value-generating and effective utilization of available human resources (Medical and Paramedical practitioners) can cater the maximum needs of the medical tourists visiting the country. The country has been moving towards the own startups which can meet the requirement of the assets (medical equipment, instruments) for providing the best treatment in the most cost-effective manner. Also, the pharmaceutical industry should incline more towards R & D, which can add value. Accessible, affordable and quality holistic healthcare is the boon to attract maximum medical tourists which in turn boosts the economy of the country. Summing up the initiatives and efforts in the right direction can help India to lead in the medical tourism sector post-pandemic era.

9.8 Limitation of Study

Study is limited to the Indian market only. The further scope of the study is to understand the contribution of medical tourism to nation's economy in other Asian countries also. The comparative analysis of the Asian market for medical tourism can add value to the study. The gap analysis and the level of the interventions required to build strategy with thorough understanding of Indian Market are incorporated in the study. Although understanding of the perspective of local residents needs to be closely monitored. Feedback analysis on the prior and current experience of medical tourists will provide new insights and will help in decision-making for path ahead. Thus, the future research study has the opportunity to study the customer experience which is significantly important to propose better and improvised revenue generation model for the country.

Further Reading

https://www.financialexpress.com/lifestyle/travel-tourism/medical-value-tourism-in-india-what-makes-the-country-a-leading-medical-tourism-destination/2338644/

https://globalresearchonline.net/journalcontents/v34-1/46.pdf#:~:text=Medical%20tourism%20is%20a%20new%20form%20of%20niche,study%20was%20conducted

https://tourism.gov.in/sites/default/files/2020-09/ITS%20at%20a%20glance_Book%20%282%29.pdf

https://www.medicaltourism.com/mti/home

https://www.medicalindiatourism.com/treatment-cost.html

https://www.ibef.org/industry/healthcare-presentation

https://tourism.gov.in/sites/default/files/2021-03/Annual%20Report%202021%2021%20English.pdf

https://tourism.gov.in/sites/default/files/2021-06/Draft%20Strategy%20for%20Medical%20and%20Wellness%20Tourism%20June%2012.pdf

Chapter 10
Sustainability Through Community-Based Tourism Development (CBTD): Planning Initiatives, Concerns, and Strategies in the Growth of Medical Tourism

Monika, Punit Gautam, and Dinesh Bhatia

Abstract The Community-Based Tourism Development (CBTD) approach encompasses sustainable tourism practices through a community approach. It promotes a feeling of belongingness among residents of a community in whose vicinity the tourism resource lies. It helps in the development of tourism activities by residents with conservation of natural resources thereby protecting their natural heritages and traditional customs. The success of CBTD-based management practices influences the livelihood and survival of communities by employing best business practices. If such practices are ignored then it may cause environmental degradation, loss of natural resources, displacement from natural surroundings, loss of foreign exchange, and reduced revenues which affects the overall economic scenario of the region and the country at large as per the report of the World's Summit on Sustainable Development, 2002. The growth and success of CBTD could be replicated in the development of sustainable and best CBTD practices in medical tourism.

Keywords Resources · Community · Medical Tourism · Healthcare · Environment · Sustainable

10.1 Introduction

The tourism industry has been considered a strong engine of growth which has provided livelihood, tremendous revenues, employment, and means of sustenance to the masses of the country. It has strong socioeconomic, cultural, and

Monika · P. Gautam
Department of Tourism and Hotel Management, North Eastern Hill University, Shillong, Meghalaya, India

D. Bhatia (✉)
Department of Biomedical Engineering, North Eastern Hill University, Shillong, Meghalaya, India

B. Chaudhary et al. (eds.), *Medical Tourism in Developing Countries*,
https://doi.org/10.1007/978-981-99-8909-6_10

environment-related dimensions that have grown through civilizations and progressed with time. It is considered one of the fastest growing industries that is an effective source of foreign exchange and revenues with protection and conservation of natural resources and cultural aspects. It encourages innovation, start-ups, and entrepreneurship along with the holistic development of destinations (Agrawal and Gibson 1999; Trejos and Chiang 2009). The success of medical tourism and widespread acceptability of low-cost best practices could be developed as an economically viable and self-sustaining practice in the long run with the involvement of a community-based approach wherein other available resources could be utilized to help in improving the existing healthcare infrastructure and improved customer experience of visiting the facility.

Throughout history, culture has consistently held sway over travelers' decisions, beckoning them to embark on journeys of exploration. Cultural attractions serve as pivotal players in the global tourism stage, with Europe and Asia taking center stage in their significance. These attractions embody the very essence of worldwide cultural undercurrents, ultimately resulting in the prestigious designation of World Heritage sites, annually attracting countless tourists. At the grassroots of society, culture molds personal identities and fosters a profound sense of belonging. Recent times have witnessed a burgeoning interest in heritage tourism, particularly in developing nations, as culture assumes a central role in defining personal identities. This trend, fueled by a blend of nostalgia and the innate human desire to reaffirm one's roots, leaves an indelible mark on the realm of cultural tourism. It is undeniably clear that cultural attractions stand as indispensable cornerstones of the global tourism landscape (Blackstock 2005; Chuenpagdee et al. 2002).

Cultural tourism, situated within the broader context of culture, encompasses two interrelated perspectives: the psychological aspect, involving people's thoughts (attitudes, beliefs, ideas, and values), and their behaviors (ways of life, artworks, artifacts, and cultural products). From a psychological viewpoint, culture represents organized systems of knowledge and beliefs that shape individuals' experiences, perceptions, actions, and choices (Subhajit and Priyom 2012). Therefore, culture can be regarded as both a psychological and physical phenomenon. As Reid articulates in this context, culture arises from human psychology and finds expression in the physical realm, often purposefully crafted as technology to enhance life, including the beautification of technological objects or art. Traditionally, cultural tourism has largely emphasized the physical aspects of culture, such as visiting cultural sites and monuments. However, an ideal approach to cultural tourism should encompass both the psychological and physical expressions of people within a particular setting. As noted by Dekadt in 1979, cultural tourism extends beyond the consumption of historical cultural artifacts to include contemporary culture and the "way of life" of a people or region (De Kadt 1979). Hence, cultural tourism can be understood to encompass both "heritage tourism" (related to historical artifacts) and "art tourism" (related to contemporary cultural creations).

To effectively promote culture as a tourist attraction, two dimensions warrant attention: the Cultural Richness of destinations and the Cultural Psychographics of both the destination community and tourists. The former is pivotal in providing the necessary resource base and directly impacting the tourism appeal of the destination region. The latter is vital for the welcoming nature of the indigenous community, socio-cultural sensitivity, and responsible behavior of guests. Thoughtful management and development of these aspects can yield substantial benefits, including increased employment opportunities, cultural heritage preservation, rejuvenation of fading art/craft forms, improved living standards, enhanced global understanding, and more. This concern prompted many tourism-dependent countries, particularly in the 1980s with the advent of mass tourism, to explore innovative strategies to transform their cultural resources into alluring yet gentle tourist attractions. This shift gave rise to new forms of tourism activities distinct from earlier phases. Today, the focus is on delivering unique and exotic cultural experiences that serve as primary attractions (Dogan 1989; Aref et al. 2010). Consequently, sustainable practices in Cultural-Based Tourism Development (CBTD) have the potential to bolster medical tourism by offering alternative solutions for disease prevention, diagnosis, and treatment. Satisfied clients could become regular customers in need of ongoing treatment for chronic health conditions, contributing to optimized advertising, publicity, branding, and the overall reputation of the facility.

10.2 Sustainability and Cultural Tourism

An essential aspect of Cultural-Based Tourism Development (CBTD) is its utilization of local knowledge within broader frameworks of cultural tourism business models. This approach enables the active participation of local communities at the management level and often results in a more profound understanding of the business landscape. Leveraging inherited knowledge also facilitates an easier entry point into the tourism industry for locals whose livelihoods are impacted by their regions being used as tourism destinations. The involvement of local communities restores ownership of these businesses to the community itself and provides an alternative sustainable pathway for development in regions and environments that may struggle to support other forms of development. The pursuit of cultural sustainability through CBTD (Felstead 2000) is guided by the following principles:

- *These endeavors play an active role in preserving both natural and cultural heritage.*
- *The planning, development, and operation of these initiatives involve local and indigenous communities, enhancing their overall welfare.*
- *Stakeholders possess the capacity to explain the destination's natural and cultural heritage to visitors.*
- *The products and services provided result in greater satisfaction for independent travelers and participants in small-group organized tours.*

Tourism serves as a significant indicator of development, reflecting mobility and social interaction. It not only demands but also provides opportunities for income redistribution from the privileged to the less fortunate, promotes knowledge access, fosters partnerships, encourages diverse engagement and participation, and facilitates the exchange of cultures. Moreover, it signifies the level of achievements across borders (Getz and Jamal 1994; Giampiccoli and Kalis 2012). Cultural heritage, as previously discussed, holds a strong appeal for tourists and encompasses a broad concept that extends well beyond historical artifacts, architecture, and history. It includes elements such as language, folklore, ethnographic items, the traditional natural environment, and intangible cultural aspects like group legacies. Tangible cultural heritage assets encompass historical structures like monuments, forts, palaces, cemeteries, archaeological sites, rock art, sculptures, ancient settlements, museums, and historical sites, among others (Guzmán et al. 2011).

Intangible cultural heritage comprises languages, stories, myths, music, songs, dances, traditions, handicrafts, literature, rituals, customs, ways of life, and more, offering valuable insights into the past. It embodies the softer facets of culture, representing the people, their traditions, and their accumulated wisdom (Haywood 1988). Folklore, in particular, encompasses the rich tapestry of tradition-based creations within a cultural community, expressed by both groups and individuals, and recognized as reflections of the community's cultural and social identity (Kamarudin 2013) (Fig. 10.1).

Moreover, this approach adheres to tangible steps, including:

- Ensuring that all stakeholders are equally, effectively, and actively engaged, with access to complete information.
- Recognizing the rights of indigenous communities to decline tourism development and to be thoroughly informed to actively participate in the planning of tourism activities within their communities, lands, and territories.
- Facilitating procedures for indigenous groups and local communities to have authority over and sustain their resources (Kibicho 2008).

As a result of the points/principles mentioned above, strategic community planning for tourism can result in:

- *Enhanced comprehension of the interrelationship between attractions and service providers.*
- *Greater communal harmony by avoiding friction and related problems.*
- *Reduction in business failures by assuring sound growth.*
- *Fostering community acceptance of tourism on a large scale.*
- *Assisting in obtaining the much-desired human and financial resources (*L"Allier 2005*).*

If not properly planned, tourism can have a detrimental impact on the environment, particularly heritage sites. Conversely, well-planned tourism can support and promote conservation efforts. Therefore, tourism presents a dual-edged sword and, unless managed effectively, can become a potential negative force. Many cultural resources, particularly tangible ones, are non-renewable, meaning that once lost, they cannot be recovered at any cost. Consequently, sustainable tourism necessitates the prudent use of such vulnerable resources and requires the effective management of tourists to ensure the proper conservation, protection, and utilization of land and

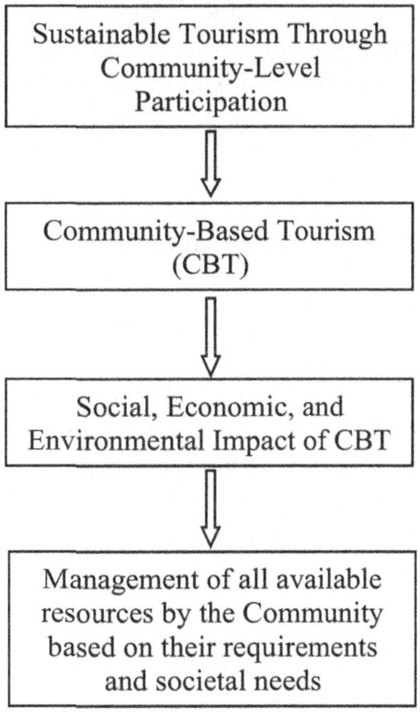

Fig. 10.1 Community-based tourism approach

the environment. Sustainable tourism is defined as a form of development that satisfies the needs of present-day tourists and host regions while safeguarding and enhancing opportunities for the future (WTO 1997). Although Agenda 21, adopted at the Rio Summit, highlights the potential of sustainable tourism as a tool for poverty alleviation, the practical aspect is that sustainable tourism has the capacity to contribute to a region's comprehensive growth, encompassing cultural, economic, and social aspects, not to mention aesthetic values. Below are some of the key characteristics of sustainable tourism:

- Sustainable tourism prioritizes the preservation of *local culture and traditions.*
- Sustainable tourism is educational, serving not only to inform tourists about destinations but also to enlighten locals *about the culture and civilization of tourists.*
- This form of tourism is geared toward *conserving the resources of the destinations* being visited.
- Sustainable tourism encourages *greater engagement of local communities*, offering opportunities for local residents to earn a livelihood. Above all, Sustainable Tourism emphatically emphasizes the integrity of tourist destinations.

Sustainable tourism typically involves the preservation of resources used for tourism purposes. Sustainable tourism practices often revolve around the management of tourist sites by local communities. This approach is grounded in the belief that those living near a resource are best equipped to protect it when they recognize the potential benefits of adhering to specific practices. Consequently, tourism activities and businesses are developed and run by local community members, with their consent and support, aligning with the philosophy of Community-Based Tourism Development (CBTD) (Lepp 2008; Liepins 2000). Consistently following such practices in the field of medical tourism could prove beneficial, aiding in the long-term prevention, detection, and diagnosis of diseases.

10.3 Consequences

- A better understanding of the interdependence between attractors and service providers.
- Greater communal harmony by avoiding friction and related problems.
- Reduction in business failures by assuring sound growth.
- Fostering community acceptance of tourism on a large scale.
- Assisting in obtaining the much-desired human and financial resources (MacDonald and Jolliffe 2003).

10.3.1 Planning Initiatives

Tourism is just one of the many activities that require careful planning and coordination within a community or region. This bulletin offers a simple framework and basic guidelines for comprehensive tourism planning at the community or regional level. Planning involves defining objectives and assessing the methods to achieve them. When we talk about comprehensive planning, we mean considering all aspects of tourism within a region, including its resources, organizations, markets, and programs. Such planning also takes into account the economic, environmental, social, and institutional dimensions of tourism development.

Tourism planning has evolved from two interrelated but distinct sets of planning philosophies and methods. On one hand, tourism is among the activities in an area that should be considered as part of physical, environmental, social, and economic planning. As a result, it's common to find tourism addressed, at least partially, in regional plans covering land use, transportation, recreation, economic development, or comprehensive planning. The extent to which tourism is integrated into such plans depends on its significance to the community or region and the planning authority's awareness of tourism activities (Manyara and Jones 2007).

Alternatively, tourism can be viewed as a business in which a community or region decides to participate. Individual tourism businesses engage in various planning activities, including feasibility assessments, marketing strategies, product development, promotion efforts, forecasting, and strategic planning. If tourism plays a significant role in an area's economy or development plans, there's a need for regional or community-wide marketing plans to coordinate the development and marketing activities of different tourism stakeholders within the community (Okazaki 2008; Scheyvens and Scheyvens 2015).

A comprehensive approach combines strategic marketing planning with traditional public planning activities, ensuring a balance between meeting the needs and desires of tourists and those of local residents. A formal tourism plan serves as a platform for various community interests to collaborate and pursue shared objectives. It also serves as a means of aligning tourism with other community activities.

Like any other product or service, tourism planning is goal-driven, aiming to achieve specific objectives by aligning available resources and programs with people's needs and desires. Comprehensive planning requires a systematic approach, typically involving a series of steps. The process should be viewed as iterative and ongoing, with each step open to modification and refinement at any stage of the planning process. Generally, the core steps in the planning process should be considered when involving the community in tourism development, including defining goals and objectives, conducting a thorough analysis of the tourism system (including resources, organizations, and markets), exploring alternative options, evaluating those alternatives, selecting the most suitable development approach, and implementing it. Periodic monitoring, evaluation, and adjustments are also crucial.

In the case of community-based tourism development, with a focus on cultural sustainability, planners, governmental bodies, NGOs, and social activists should take proactive steps to lay the foundation for holistic tourism development that can ensure long-term success. These initiatives may encompass the following (Simpson 2008):

1. ***Awareness Campaigns***: In countries like India general public is least informed and bothered about, tourism-related activities. And, as a result, are not aware of the role they can play in the growth and development of this economic booster. The concerned parties and organizations must aggressively plan awareness campaigns. We must not forget that *knowledge is the key to innovative openings.*
2. ***Stimulation Drives***: After making people aware of the opportunities where they can get involved, the next step is to motivate them to actively participate in the related ventures. This can be done by conducting micro-level studies to discover destination-specific possibilities with the help of the residents. Career counseling can do miracles in this regard. Some fiscal or non-fiscal incentives can be planned to motivate the destination community to participate in the developmental process.
3. ***Capacity Building Programmes***: The Ministry of Tourism, Government of India has already initiated *Capacity Building Programmes* for the non-skilled and semi-skilled persons directly or indirectly involved with the business of tourism. These are aimed at developing a tourist-friendly attitude and enhancement skills related to various spheres of the trade. Somehow the State level organizations have not been able to implement the scheme to the optimum use. At present, it is essential to train a group of individuals at all well-visited and promising tourist destinations to professionally attend to the needs of tourists.
4. ***Conduction of Workshops on Benefits and Costs of Tourism Development***: Every business or trade has both faces, i.e., positive and negative. It solely depends upon how the business is conducted as to which of these dimensions

emerge as a consequence. The community should be informed of the benefits and costs of tourist pursuits from time to time. It becomes even more crucial to consider the ever-evolving nature of the tourism and travel industry, marked by continuous changes in typology and forms, each resulting in a diverse range of operational outcomes.

5. ***Regular Inputs About the Market Trends*:** The tourism industry features one of the most unpredictable market segments. Their motivations, perceptions, expectations, and activities keep on changing. We need to keep the practitioners aware of the present and future trends so that they can understand the needs and wants of the target market(s) and can plan efficiently in advance to enhance their chances of getting a better share.

10.3.2 Concerns and Strategies—Tabular Form

Many challenges arise from various factors when aiming for cultural sustainability through the engagement of indigenous communities in the development process. However, it is evident that these challenges, while not entirely eliminable, can be significantly managed through the effective implementation of strategic planning. This section of the paper endeavors to emphasize key concerns and corresponding improvement strategies (Stettner 1993; Taylor 1995)

10.4 Modernization and Globalization

Modernization and globalization serve as indicators of a region's development quotient. They represent both affluence and drivers of economic growth. Undoubtedly, they create opportunities for accessing knowledge, expanding partnerships, fostering diverse involvement and participation, and promoting cultural exchange. However, the impact of globalization on intangible cultural heritage is significant because the priority spectrum of individuals with modern and global perspectives differs markedly. This apathetic approach has adverse effects on customs, traditions, handicrafts, and folklore. The pace of change in cultures has accelerated over the years, surpassing previous rates. Consequently, this has a profound impact on the thinking and attitudes of people, especially the younger generation, toward preserving both tangible and intangible heritage, which are essential for sustaining cultural tourism (Kamamba, 2003). Therefore, the challenge lies in preserving tangible and intangible heritage within this modernized global society.

- ***The culture needs to be promoted as an antidote to the escalating stress and strain caused by the typical mechanical lifestyle in the modernized global world. Our cultural "roots" are an inherent part of everyone, and with effective efforts, they can become a "pull" factor in the context of tourism. Such a***

strategy, on the one hand, will keep the youth awakened about their culture and, at the same time, will prove to be a rejuvenating exercise to conserve the traditional heritage.

10.4.1 Cultural Osmosis

Whenever persons from different cultural backgrounds interact, for quite an extended period, there is bound to be some mutual exchanges of thoughts, ideas, traditions, ethics, and values. This effect is termed ***cultural osmosis***. Past experiences have shown that such a transition cannot be avoided and somehow *demonstration effect* has also caused cultural transformations. This phenomenon is quite applicable to both tourists and hosts. Many times this is argued upon as cultural dilution.

- ***Mutual exchange, due to prolonged interactions, is bound to affect the cultural ethics of any society. This may be an enriching situation as well. The strategy should focus on slowing down the rate of transition so that the costs and benefits can be clearly understood by the societies concerned and the transition/ osmosis is healthy (*****Taylor** 1995***).***

10.5 Negative Impacts of Tourism

While we discuss tourism as a potential boon for developing countries, it's crucial to acknowledge that tourism can also lead to exploitation and degradation in the social, cultural, economic, and environmental aspects of an area if mechanisms to control and mitigate its negative impacts are not in place. One significant concern is the cases where a majority of profits leave local communities, often due to vertical integration. It's essential to examine power dynamics and the uneven development relationships in the context of globalization.

Effective and responsible tourism management is paramount to prevent excessive exploitation and the erosion of land and cultural norms and traditions. Thus, it's imperative to identify and eliminate illegal medical practices to ensure that vulnerable patient populations are not subjected to exploitation or victimization, which could result in more harm than good.

10.6 Participation of Communities

Efficiently engaging the local community in the planning processes emerges as a pivotal concern within this context. Local neighborhoods contend with a spectrum of challenges, encompassing the steady surge of tourists, amplified noise levels, potential escalations in goods and services pricing, and the surge in traffic. Consequently, it becomes imperative to factor in their welfare across all phases of planning, development, execution, and management. In addition, garnering insights from local inhabitants concerning environmental dynamics, the unfolding narrative of tourism, communal aspirations, and even the perspectives of the visitors themselves holds immense importance. Rather than adhering strictly to conventional reactive planning methodologies, we should venture into innovative avenues of management, guided by the feedback derived from local residents and stakeholders. This proactive planning strategy strives to anticipate issues before they arise, contrasting sharply with the traditional approach of merely reacting to challenges. The active involvement of local communities and other stakeholders in the planning process offers the potential to preemptively address conflicts that may surface between tourists, residents, and the surrounding environment (Telfer and Sharpley 2008).

10.7 Effects of Authorities

Just as cultural systems encompass both tangible and intangible elements that cannot be separated, development itself possesses a significant intangible dimension that requires recognition and nurturing for true sustainable development (UNESCO 2002). Sustainable diversity plays a crucial role in fostering intangible development, and without this intangible aspect, achieving sustainable development is impossible. Despite numerous attempts to view development comprehensively, acknowledging the integral role of people, values, and social capital, there persists a strong inclination to define and measure development primarily through material indicators, such as schools, hospitals, infrastructure, and more. However, the challenges of development underscore that these material objectives cannot be sustained through material means alone. They demand knowledge, vision, commitment, and training to ensure they are driven democratically, culturally legitimate, and socially sustainable. Unfortunately, these intangible dimensions of development have not been adequately linked to cultural capacities and cultural diversity. This mindset represents a particular perspective, and unless it is transformed through various means, including education, training, and active engagement of the youth in local traditions, customs, and overall culture, the very essence of cultural heritage, which is a significant tourist attraction, could be at risk of fading away.

10.8 Combining Cultural Heritage and Tourism

Cultural tourism is inherently connected to people's curiosity and their desire to explore the history and heritage of different cultures. The growth of cultural tourism is intertwined with the development of a "tourism culture" itself. It is acknowledged as a valuable resource with the potential to address issues of poverty. Cultural resources, in this context, refer to elements that can be made accessible for various purposes, including visual enjoyment, recreational activities, satisfying historical curiosity, facilitating academic and scientific research, providing opportunities for camping and picnicking, and even as souvenirs for purchase. The primary challenge is to establish effective and practical strategies that can transform these cultural resources into marketable commodities. Once cultural resources become tangible commodities, it becomes crucial to implement suitable strategies to improve the economic conditions of the nearby communities. Achieving this transformation from cultural heritage to marketable commodities requires the development of promotional strategies for tourism at sites like museums, cultural centers, monuments, and historical locations. Key considerations in the promotion of cultural tourism encompass the effective management of resource marketing and the assessment of cultural tourism's impact on the local economy, all while preserving the integrity of cultural heritage.

10.9 Cultural Heritage Quality

The quality of cultural heritage and its presentation play a pivotal role in reaping the benefits of tourism. For instance, Tanzania boasts a rich cultural heritage, including evidence of human evolution in Olduvai, 2000 years of history along the coast with world heritage sites like Kilwa Kisiwani and Songo Mnara, and renowned Makonde carvings. Africa's cultural heritage is among the best, but for it to truly shine, it must be easily accessible, well-presented, effectively interpreted, and supported by appropriate facilities and amenities. Society bears the responsibility of ensuring the enhancement and support of cultural heritage quality. Challenges such as a lack of qualified experts, funding, marketing efforts, and adequate facilities persist in many developing African regions, especially in sub-Saharan Africa (Telfer and Sharpley 2008; Tosun 2000).

10.10 Cultural Heritage and Financial Support

An investigation into tourism in Africa highlights that "Tourism has the potential to significantly boost their economies, but for sustainable development, it must be seamlessly integrated into the country's overarching policies and economic planning strategies." According to a World Bank report titled "Tourism in Africa 1999," the growing optimism regarding tourism's future growth is prompting several countries to explore ways in which tourism can catalyze economic expansion and diversification. However, many governments face challenges in knowing where and how to initiate such efforts and whom to seek assistance from to kickstart these initiatives. The funding of cultural heritage endeavors remains a particular concern, given that cultural activities in developing countries often receive insufficient backing due to their perceived lack of economic viability.

10.11 Tourism Delicate Business

African nations, especially those in sub-Saharan Africa, hold great potential to attract tourists globally due to factors such as prevailing peace, political stability, ethnic diversity, and rich cultural heritage. However, it's crucial to recognize the tourism industry's delicate nature, as it can swiftly respond to political, social, economic, cultural, and religious events, along with issues like hygiene and disease outbreaks. A significant concern lies in substantial investments made in the tourism sector that often remain underutilized due to a lack of demand, attributable to the aforementioned factors. There have been instances of hotels and restaurants established to cater to this industry, only to sit empty due to a single event, be it political, religious, or cultural, that jeopardized the safety of anticipated tourists or customers. Such situations present challenges not only for business owners but also for the communities relying on the sector's success (Tosun 2000; Zorn and Farthing 2007).

Table 10.1 shows how the different C-factors could contribute toward community-based tourism, which would allow optimum resource utilization thereby improving customer satisfaction and building a long-term relationship. If the perceived notions or misperceptions could be removed, then judicious usage of all resources would enhance outcomes by showing improved customer caring and involvement of all factors toward the achievement of desired targets for developing a sustainable community-based model approach to revive the tourism sector and also aid in developing customer trust and satisfaction. This is even more required in the healthcare setup where a lot of uncertainty and variations in the provision of desired healthcare outcomes may be seen. Further, with improved outcomes, it has the potential to convert temporary clients to permanent ones who may require routine treatment for their chronic ailments. With the availability of socio-cultural resources and economic viability, the same could be utilized continuously by prospective customers to satisfy their needs and those of their known contacts. With enhanced satisfaction, it could be possible to have better word-of-mouth publicity and/or referrals which may be beneficial for the sector in the long run. Thus, it holds the capacity to rejuvenate the medical tourism sector and make a long-term contribution to the economy.

Table 10.1 The C-Factors

Tourism components	Concerns of society	Planning requirements	Expected outcomes
C-1: CUSTOMERS (Target segment/Patients)	• Changing Perceptions • Uncaring Attitude	• Correctly Informed • Properly Directed	Potential interested customers
C-2:CATALYSTS (Intermediaries/Agents/Medical Support Staff)	• Out-dated Information • Misleading	• Socio-Cultural Compatibility • Eco-Conscious • Effective Information Upgrade and Dissemination	Influence customers to clients
C-3:CHARISMA (tourist attractions with resources/ healthcare set-up with modernized facilities)	• Mis-perceptions • Notions Consumption • Carrying Capacity	• Judicious Interpretation • Resources Optimization • Monitoring of resources	Optimum utilization of resources for the community
C-4:CARE-TAKERS (service providers/healthcare service providers)	• Lack of Professionalism • Simulated by Monetary benefits	• Adequate Literacy • Caring Attitude	Customer satisfaction and building relationship
C-5:INDIGENOUS COMMUNITY	• Passiveness • Perceived opposition to changes	• Active Involvement • Costs & Benefits Analysis	Improved benefits and resource utilization

10.12 Conclusion

Heritage tourism in developing countries has the potential to significantly contribute to heritage conservation by channeling tourism-generated revenue into conservation efforts. This form of tourism also addresses seasonality and the tourism sector's vulnerability to external factors. It plays a pivotal role in transforming traditional sun-and-sea resort destinations into sophisticated, multidimensional locations that offer high-quality experiences. Such a shift benefits not only local communities but also the broader regional and national economies. Building strong partnerships with heritage-conscious hotel guides and tour operators is key to fostering economically and environmentally sustainable tourism development.

Additionally, there's a compelling argument for creating opportunities in regions across the global South where tourism has significant potential, which could greatly improve the lives of impoverished communities. Recently, the World Bank renewed its commitment to the role of culture and tourism in poverty reduction. President J. Wolfensohn emphasized that culture is an often-overlooked resource in many developing countries, capable of generating income through tourism, crafts, and other cultural enterprises. Therefore, it's vital for all stakeholders to comprehend the intricate relationship between tourism and cultural heritage conservation to nurture a mutually beneficial synergy. Heritage acts as a magnet, drawing visitors, empowering local hosts, and promoting sustainable practices (FICCI 2001).

To ensure that tourism development in the sub-region is community benefit-orientated, the strategy seeks to:

- Expand opportunities by bringing tourists to villages and towns in provinces with high incidences of poverty, or linking poor communities to the tourism industry through the supply of handicrafts, agricultural, and other products.
- Ensure that tourism is recognized as a major actor in the poverty reduction policies, plans, and programs of the GMS countries.
- Provide a framework for local populations to engage in businesses and indirect employment in the tourism area.
- Create indirect employment opportunities from the production of tourism-related inputs.

Ecotourism offers many opportunities to reflect on the importance of sustainability and the possibilities of implementing approaches that move us in a new direction. But it also suggests that there are significant obstacles. A new correlation of social forces, a move toward broad-based democratic participation in all aspects of life, within each country and in the concert of nations is required to overcome these obstacles. Strategies to face these challenges must respond to the dual challenges of insulating these communities from further encroachment and assuring their viability (Zorn and Farthing 2007).

In the healthcare sector, with improved outcomes, it has the potential to convert temporary clients to permanent ones who may require routine treatment for their chronic ailments. With the availability of socio-cultural resources and economic viability, the same could be utilized continuously by prospective customers to satisfy their needs and those of their known contacts. With enhanced satisfaction, it could be possible to have better word-of-mouth publicity and/or referrals which may be beneficial for the sector in the long run. Hence, it has the potential to revive the medical tourism industry and contribute to the economy in the long run (Telfer and Sharpley 2008; Zorn and Farthing 2007).

References

Agrawal A, Gibson CC (1999) Enchantment and disenchantment: the role of community in natural resource conservation. World Dev 27:629–649

Aref F, Redzuan M, Gill SS (2010) Assessing level of community capacity building in tourism development in local communities. J Sustain Dev 3:1

Blackstock J (2005) A critical look at community based tourism. Community Dev J 40(1):39–49

Chuenpagdee R, Fraga J, Euan-Avila JI (2002) Community perspectives toward a marine reserve: a case study of San Felipe, Yucatan. Mexico Coastal Management 30(2):183–191. https://doi.org/10.1080/08920750253504706

De Kadt E (1979) Tourism: passport to development? Perspectives on the social and cultural effects of tourism in developing countries. Oxford University Press, New York

Dogan HZ (1989) Forms of adjustment: socio-cultural impacts of tourism. Ann Tour Res 16(2):216–236

Felstead ML (2000) Master plan for community-based eco-tourism inUlgan Bay, Palawan, Republic of the Philippines. Puerto Princesa City (PPC), Philippines: UNESCO-UNDP- PPC

FICCI (2001) International Conference and Exhibition on Rural Tourism in India, Sept., 8,-12

Getz D, Jamal TB (1994) The environment–community symbiosis: a case of collaborative tourism planning. J Sustain Tour 2(3):152–173

Giampiccoli A, Kalis JH (2012) Community-based tourism and local culture: the case of the ama-Mpondo. Revista de Turismo y Patrimonio Cultural 10:173–188

Guzmán TZ, Osvaldo B, Ana MC (2011) Community-based tourism in Cape Verde—a case study. Tour Hosp Manag 17(1):35–44

Haywood KM (1988) Responsible and responsive tourism planning in the community. Tour Manag 9(2):105–118. https://doi.org/10.1016/0261-5177(88)90020-9

Kamarudin KH (2013) Local Stakeholder's Participation in Developing Sustainable Community-Based Rural Tourism (CBRT): The case of three villages on the East Coast of Malaysia. International Conference on Tourism Development 2013

Kibicho W (2008) Community-based tourism: a factor-cluster segmentation approach. J Sustain Tour 16(2):211–231

L"Allier. (2005) Built environment for sustainable tourism, Conference, Sultanate of Oman

Lepp A (2008) Attitudes towards initial tourism development in a community with no prior tourism experience: the case of Bigodi, Uganda. J Sustain Tour 16(1):5–21

Liepins R (2000) New energies for an old idea: reworking approaches to 'community' in contemporary rural studies. J Rural Stud 16(1):23–35

MacDonald R, Jolliffe L (2003) Cultural rural tourism: evidence from Canada. Ann Tour Res 30(2):307–322. https://doi.org/10.1016/S0160-7383(02)00061-0

Manyara G, Jones E (2007) Community-based tourism enterprises in Kenya: an exploration of their potential as avenues of poverty reduction. J Sustain Tour 15(6):628–645. https://doi.org/10.2167/jost723.0

Okazaki E (2008) A community-based tourism model: its conception and use. J Sustain Tour 16(5):511. https://doi.org/10.2167/jost782.0

Scheyvens R, Scheyvens R (2015) Ecotourism and the empowerment of local communities ecotourism and the empowerment of local communities. Tour Manag 20(APRIL 1999):245–249. https://doi.org/10.1016/S0261-5177(98)00069-7

Simpson MC (2008) Community benefit tourism initiatives conceptual oxymoron? Tour Manag 29(1):1–18. https://doi.org/10.1016/j.tourman.2007.06.005

Stettner AC (1993) Commodity or community? Sustainable development in mountain resorts. Tour Recreat Res 18(1):3–10

Subhajit D, Priyom RK (2012) Village tourism in Sikkim, India; a pre-colonial approach for sustainability. Int J Soc Sci Tomorrow 1:4

Taylor G (1995) The community approach: does it work? Tour Manag 16(7):487–489. https://doi.org/10.1016/0261-5177(95)00078-3

Telfer DJ, Sharpley R (2008) Tourism and development in the developing world. Routledge, London

Tosun C (2000) Limits to community participation in the tourism development process in developing countries. Tour Manag 21:613–633

Trejos B, Chiang L-HN (2009) Local economic linkages to community-based tourism in rural Costa Rica. Singap J Trop Geogr 30

Zorn E, Farthing LE (2007) Communitarian tourism. Hosts and mediators in Peru. Ann Tour Res 34(3):673–689

Chapter 11
Healthcare Sector, Medical Tourism and Employment Relations in India: Emerging Paradigms, New Directions and Future Trajectory

Abhishek Mishra, Ajay Wagh, and Hanee Sunil Vinchu

Abstract Healthcare professionals have often been acclimatised as one of the most challenging (and promising as well) when it comes to the management of people at workplaces. Strange but true, the aspects of employment relations at workplaces have received little research consideration in healthcare sector even in the developed countries. India, becoming one of the most attractive destinations for medical tourism, has given substantial impetus to the healthcare sector which gave birth to new forms of employment relations practices in the sector. Adopting a qualitative approach where literature research along with the use of search engine using selected key words, the authors in this chapter intend to identify the emerging paradigms and new directions of employment relations in the sector. The objectives in this chapter will also centre on mapping the future trajectory of employment relations in the healthcare sector with specific considerations for medical tourism in India.

Keywords Employment Relations · Healthcare sector · Medical Tourism · Paradigms · Trajectory

---

A. Mishra
Department of Business Administration (Human Resource), The University of Burdwan, Bardhaman, West Bengal, India
e-mail: amishra@mbahr.buruniv.ac.in

A. Wagh (✉)
Department of Business Management, Indira Gandhi National Tribal University, Amarkantak, Madhya Pradesh, India
e-mail: ajay.wagh@igntu.ac.in

H. S. Vinchu
Department of Commerce, Indira Gandhi National Tribal University, Amarkantak, Madhya Pradesh, India
e-mail: hanee.vinchu@igntu.ac.in

B. Chaudhary et al. (eds.), *Medical Tourism in Developing Countries*,
https://doi.org/10.1007/978-981-99-8909-6_11

11.1 Introduction

India in recent years has become one of the preferred destinations for patients suffering from different diseases and ailments from all across the globe. The well-timed interventions by the government and the private players in the healthcare sector gave the much required impetus to the growth, development and promotion of the very idea of 'medical tourism' which in recent years has received much attention from avid researchers and scholars. However, it needs to be clarified that medical tourism remains as one of the components of healthcare industry or sector, including other components like hospitals, pharmaceuticals, diagnostic centres, health and medical insurance, medical instruments and devices and telemedicine (Sarwal et al. 2021). The lessons learnt during the global pandemic had facilitated our understanding towards focussing more on improving the increasing healthcare infrastructure of the country. Also, increasing healthcare consciousness, better life-styles due to spurt in household incomes, penetration of medical insurance along with several other factors had given the sector an immense boost. These factors have also pushed the demand for qualified workforce in the sector. The sector still is undergoing issues related to not only the quality of manpower but also the quantity of the manpower to meet the current as well as the future requirements (Mistry et al. 2022). Currently, the sector employs around 4.7 million people[1] which is expected reach 12 million by the year 2030 (Sharma 2022). This is an obvious indication towards the yawning gap between demand and supply of manpower in the sector. Along with this, the management of employment relations in the sector also remains an underrated issue since the sector still is emerging and evolving giving enough scope for employment relations to take shape of its own when faced with issues and challenges related to management of relationship in the sector. The exponential growth of the small diagnostic centres across the nooks and corners of the country, the penetration of multi-chain hospitals in semi-urban and rural areas, the mobility of manpower with relevant experience and academic qualifications to different regions of the country in search of better employment along with several other concerns are gradually giving shape to employment relations in the sector. There are enough linkages to establish that employment relations are directly linked to the quality of healthcare facilities provided by any organisation, either large or small (Kabene et al. 2006). Efficiency has been directly linked with human resource management practices in the healthcare sector in different parts of the globe (Kabene et al. 2006). While most of the studies have been and are still being conducted in the developed countries owing to their advanced infrastructural healthcare system, there is paucity of literature available on employment relations and human resource management in the healthcare sector in India due to the still evolving nature of the sector. Thus, the healthcare sector in India largely remains unexplored when it comes to exploring the aspects related to human resource management by the practitioners and academicians. The authors in this chapter intend to bridge this gap by

[1] https://www.ibef.org/industry/healthcare-india

drawing the existing framework of employment relations in the sector. The chapter will also explore and highlight how the evolving employment relations is affecting medical tourism in the country. The chapter shares policy considerations for HR fraternity to get prepared in advance to fulfil the expectations of the world through offering best medical experiences by adopting appropriate employment relations strategies and practices paving multiple ways to promote medical tourism in the country.

11.2 Contextualising the Agenda

Healthcare sector remains as one of the fundamental pillars for economy and society along with other critical parameters for achieving the goals for sustainable development (WHO, 2023). The significance becomes all the more significant in developing countries like India where majority of the population remains deprived of quality healthcare amenities and attention. Health remains one of the most valued possessions for any individual since it enables him or her to pursue things which he or she believes to be of some value to their lives (Sen 1999). Thus, health can be considered as human capital which promotes productive power of the workforce along with the development of the economy (Bloom and Canning 2003). The healthcare sector mainly comprises different organisations, institutions and actors who offer healthcare facilities to the people with a common objective of promoting, restoring and maintaining health of the public at large (Burns 2014). The Indian healthcare sector has different sub-sectors including hospitals, nursing homes, wellness centres, health centres, diagnostic centres, pharmaceuticals, biomedical chemical manufacturing, health insurance, telemedicine, medical and surgical equipment production and several other ancillary services. With such an exhaustive scale of operations, the sector undoubtedly provides employment to a large chunk of working population in the country. The cheap and pocket-friendly medical treatment in India has also made it one of the most preferred countries when it comes to better medical treatments among the Asian countries. Medical care recipients from different countries like Bangladesh, Nepal, Bhutan, Nigeria, Afghanistan, Kenya, Fiji and several other countries prefer to visit India for their treatments which makes the country turn into a hub of medical tourism (Das 2022). Considering all these, the healthcare sector in India not only has immense potential to grow in terms of fiscal advantages, but it can also cater to the need of employment generation for an employment-hungry country like India. There were around 69,000 public and private hospitals in the year 2019 in India (Kanwal 2022). The total number of health diagnostic centres was estimated to be more than 100 million (Sahay 2020). Since the sector is highly fragmented in nature and several unregistered enterprises remain operational in the sector, specifically in the semi-urban and rural areas, it is difficult to project the exact number of these entities in the country. Post COVID, there has been immense surge in the number of these healthcare-providing centres. Respective governments have also taken serious note of the infrastructural discrepancies existing in the healthcare sector and had started paying attention to address the same. With the rise in the existing number of these healthcare-related facilities, there is also an outburst in the demand for employment in the sector. It is estimated that every year the sector needs around 500 million people to meet the manpower requirements in the country (Bajaj 2021). Interestingly, the healthcare sector along with the hospitality industry did not receive much attention in previous years. Medical tourism, as one of the aspects of healthcare sector, has largely remained affected by the policy deficits. Still at its nascent stage, medical tourism not only can serve the need for employment generation at a large scale, but it can also provide lucrative avenues for foreign revenue generation. However, the type of manpower required in the sector is quite different as compared to other sectors. The manpower in the sector is expected to be highly sensitive to the needs of the patients, along with other qualities like self-managed, social awareness, human relation skills, expertise in handling stressful situations and many more (Sisodia and Agarwal 2017). The list is endless, and it clearly indicates that possession of 'soft skills' and 'human skills' is the prerequisite for successful performance of jobs in the healthcare sector and promotes medical tourism in the country. Adopting the best human resource management practices leads to best performance outcomes. For the sector which is highly dependent on qualified employees, following best employment relations practices becomes a must for the organisation. Positive employment relations, which are manifested in the form of showing care and concern for their co-workers by the managers' help establish positive relationship with the healthcare recipients as well (Dickson-Swiftet et al., 2014). There are enough empirical evidences in the forms of reports what are available which unfortunately highlight the poor working conditions, heavy workloads with unequal and insufficient payment structure and inadequate training opportunities which highlight the existing aspects of employment relations in the sector (Weber and Nevala 2011). While the practices related to workers' unionisation and collective bargaining are strongly felt in countries like the United States, Britain and some other developed European countries, 'collectivism' does receive a setback in the healthcare sector, particularly in the private sector in India which was mainly due to the failure on the part of the trade unions (Krinsky and Miller 2007). There are also issues related to 'trust' in the sector (Kim and Kim 2012). The upcoming section explores the emerging aspects of employment relations in the healthcare sector in India.

11.3 Employment Relations in Healthcare Sector: Emerging Paradigms and New Direction

Employment relations in the healthcare sector can still be considered to be in an embryonic stage as the sector has started gaining prominence in recent years. The inherent diversification in the sector makes it more challenging for the researchers to come up with any model of employment relations in the sector. Small hospitals may have different set of employment relations practices as compared to large chain hospitals. Similarly, small diagnostic centres and wellness centres are assumed to be significantly different from the pharmaceutical industry and rest of the others. Thus, divergences in terms of employment relations form one of the most significant characteristics of employment relations in the healthcare sector. With different staffing needs and organisational structure, management of employment relations in the sector itself has become challenging (Buchan 2000). And it will continue to change dramatically with the unveiling of the future and examination of the different workplaces issues (Townsend and Richards 2011). With the sector getting highly competitive in recent years, the healthcare organisations have realised the significance of employment relations in order to improve quality and efficiency and safety to the services extended to the healthcare recipients (Greenfield et al. 2014). To understand the emerging paradigms of employment relations in the healthcare sector, the authors underwent a review of existing literature which was not exhaustive in nature, but relied more on the literature which threw significant light on the theme of the research. Database of JSTOR has been accessed using the institutional login by the authors. Using the Advance Search option on JSTOR, a search was carried out 'employment relations' as the primary word and 'healthcare sector' as the secondary word. For further filtration, only the articles, reports and reviews were selected for the search purpose, and dates for filtration were selected between 2010 and 2022. To add more filtration, only the academic materials published in the journals related to business, law, sociology, social work, industrial relations, employment relations and organisational behaviour were selected for the search purpose. It was found that 1204 academic publications were available on the related subject. On examination it was observed that majority of the literature could not any way be related to the present theme of the study. Therefore, selective reading based on suitability and convenience was performed to explore the emerging paradigms of employment relations in the healthcare sector in India. Interestingly, very little amount of literature exists on the aspects of human resource management in the healthcare industry in India which itself is the indicative of the fact towards the dire need for qualitative study in the domain. Institutional publications such as reports from International Labour Organization and World Health Organization throw considerable light on the existing patterns of employment relations in the sector. ILO (2019) points out how patterns of employment like the non-standard forms of employment including agency work, temporary, fixed-term contract, etc., are making the relationship more fragmented in nature. This fragmentation of relationship has resulted in making the sector overpowered by feelings of job insecurity, inadequate payment system, denied rights to unionisation and collectivism, little or no access to social security provisions apart from other regulatory violations. This has made employment relations in the sector characterised by authoritarianism and Unitarianism with little left to the discretion of the employees at workplaces. The ultimate decision-making happens from the top of the organisational hierarchy. Intensity of work has been strategically used by the managers to exercise control on the employees in the sector (Bach 2004). Thus, mobility of employees remains one of the main challenges in the healthcare sector. This also makes difficult for the healthcare organisations to retain quality employees which pose more difficulty in sustaining of the organisations in the long run.

Interestingly, few organisations have started to accept the strategic importance of employment relations in the sector. With the orientation of the sector shifting from public to private sector, organisations have slowly started to realise the vital role employment relations play in the long-run survival of the business. To attract more and more healthcare recipients and promote medical tourism, the organisations have adopted employment relations policies which are more customer-centric in nature (Lethbridge 2015). All the actors in the employment relations model in the healthcare sector have become more oriented towards marketisation where focus is more on efficiency, effectiveness and better experience. With the increase in technology-enabled medical services like telemedicine, mobile clinics, better coordination, teamwork and supervision with the employees and among the employees including the doctors, nurses, suppliers, etc., have become essential. To provide better services and as a sign of relief to the employees, shift arrangements have been implemented. However, these shifts are full of workload and sometimes become highly stressful. This has given encouragement to the practice of sick days leave among the employees resulting in reduced number of employees during peak hours (Böhlke 2008). Since the payment structure including the supplemental pay is not very competitive in the sector, voluntary exits and high mobility of the employees remain an issue in the sector. The issue of supplemental pay is yet to be introduced in the healthcare sector in India. The aspect related to sufficient pay along with the supplemental pay is a cause of grave concern for the healthcare employees employed as Accredited Social Health Activist or the ASHA workers who extend their services as local medical trainers and promoters in the rural areas of the country. This 'scheme-based' employment of employees in the sector is turning out employment relations to be a troubled one. In recent years, ASHA workers have frequently resorted to strikes in order to draw attention of the policy-makers towards regularisation of their services, payment of minimum wages and pension scheme. Similarly, nurses of some of the premier government hospitals also wage strike and protest against their contractual appointments, pay disparity and other related issues. Interestingly, majority of the protests are waged in the government sector where employees do have the right (or the privilege) of organising collectively against their employing authority. However, collectivism does receive a setback in the private sector where employees resorting to collective against are terminated without any reason. Thus, while employment relations in the public sector are still oriented towards 'collectivism', the same witnesses 'individualism' in the private sector. While the collective actions on the part of the healthcare professionals and practitioners can be justified from different perspectives, it creates a trust deficit between the patient community and the healthcare service provider. With frequent strikes and refraining to perform their duties, the image of the healthcare organisation gets tarnished which in long run may fail India to achieve the status of preferred destinations for 'medical tourists'. Employment relations can only flourish when all the stakeholders in an enterprise look at each other with mutual respect, trust and confidence. While employment relations in the healthcare sector have become more collaborative in nature, there still remain certain sticking points which need to be given a clarion call to make employment relations more conducive and productive. The healthcare sector has rightly been recognised as one of the sectors which employ largest number of knowledge workers (Halpern et al. 2001; Matney et al. 2013). This is one of the main reasons why collective actions and existence of trade unions as one of the institutional mechanisms in employment relations framework have received a setback in the sector. But at the same time, this has also resulted in making the working environment, specifically in the private sector, one of the best in the country. With the advent of latest technological advancements, the healthcare sector employees feel engaged and often feel to be justifying with their roles and responsibilities. Thus, technological environment along with the market orientation is shifting the employment relations in the sector. Technology offers the strategic advantage to the organisations in the highly competitive world of healthcare sector. Use of technology not only improves the efficiency and accuracy of the job, but at the same time, it also facilitates the identification of impending risks and challenges. Thus, the work becomes engaging, enriching and error-free at the same time. This is indicative towards the fact that employment relations in the healthcare sector are also determined by the work itself. Interesting is the fact that in spite of the rise of automation, artificial intelligence and robotics in the sector, it is very unlikely that the sector will replace skilled human hands in the upcoming future. This makes the sector highly stable in terms of employment relations.

Healthcare sector, in recent years, remains witness to one of the changing paradigms of employment relations in terms of its increased orientation and focus towards High-Performance Work Systems (HPWS). Key findings of the limited literature being conducted on this aspect of employment relations glorified 'high involvement', 'high commitment', 'employee empowerment' as being significantly important to business performance of enterprises (Lewin 2011). Considering the nature of high risk and complexities the sector involves in, the organisations have been right in their approach in implementing the High-Performance Work Systems in the healthcare sector, more specifically, the hospitals and critical care centres. Specialisation, interdependence and high workflow make the work performance more based on team work and inculcation of safety culture (Mielke et al. 2019). However, research studies are indicative of the fact that high-performance work systems often lead to high stress and exhaustion on part of the employees which can only be managed on focussing on the perceived nature of employment relations between the different stakeholders in the organisational set-up (Mihail and Panagiotis 2016). As an outcome, the value system of both the employers and employees falls in line with each other in order to offer the best services to the clients. However, the downside of this 'compliance to value system' often ignores the hidden grievances and complaints of the employees which very explicitly reflect the unitary perspective of employment relations in the healthcare sector.

One of the significant factors affecting employment relations in the healthcare sector is the rise of franchising enterprises in recent times. Franchising enterprises, regarded as one of the most sought-after business models, have considerable implications on the course and practices of employment relations in the healthcare sector

(Kellner et al. 2011). While the franchising model is still at its nascent stage in India, the trend is one the rise considering the profitability that this business model has to offer. Big hospitals and diagnostic centres are the main players in the franchising model of business in India. There also remains a big research deficit on exploring employment relations in the franchising enterprises in the healthcare sector in India. One of the biggest drawbacks of the model bearing significance on employment relations practices is the limited freedom to implement enterprise-specific employment practices as the policy making and decision-making are mostly finalised by the dominant employer (Kinnie et al. 2005). It has been observed that regulatory violations have become a general trend in the franchising sector where there still remains little legislative monitoring due to the lacunas in the regulatory framework of India. Mainly adopted as a business strategy for expansion in the 1800 century in the United States of America, this model has been observed to highly advocate the violation of labour and employment rights (Easton et al. 2021). For a country like India which aims to achieve the goal of becoming one of the most favoured medical tourist hubs, it is important that employment relations in the franchising enterprises do adopt to 'tailor-made' employment relations practices to suit the needs of the manpower employed in that particular enterprise. The services offered by the franchising enterprises often shape the customer perception of the parent organisation. The customers are rarely aware of the fact that they are availing the services of franchising enterprise and not the actual organisation. As a result, poor and inefficient services which mostly happen due to ill-managed human resource policies and practices affect the image of the parent organisation. Unfortunately, more empirical research studies are required to fill this research deficit and come up with substantive findings on the emerging practices on employment relations. Recent literature highlights informal recruitment practices, no unionisation, absence of training initiatives and employment standards to be existent in the sector (Kellner et al. 2011). The inconsistent employment relations practices are attributed mainly to the size and operation of the franchise enterprises. While small franchising enterprises are yet to come up with substantive employment relations policies and practices, the big enterprises have adopted a more suitable and concrete policies.

Since the eruption of the global pandemic, the diagnostic and wellness centres have taken a huge surge considering our awareness towards health and maintaining healthy lifestyles. Increased customer demand has given the sector huge push which endorsed the opening of health diagnostic centres across the nooks and corners of the country. Diagnostic market has immense potential in India and as per estimates, the subsector is estimated to reach 20 billion dollars by the end of 2026 (De 2022). The employees engaged in the sector face heavy workload which is facilitated by use of technology. Most of the recruitments are made through job portals in big cities while in small towns and cities, recruitment through referrals is a common practice. Jobs exist in good numbers in the sector. But the diagnostic centres mainly rely on affordability, quality and punctuality of the services. And there is huge competition in the sector as new ventures are coming up on daily basis due to its immense profit potential. But things take an ugly turn in the form of layoffs when these diagnostic centres fail to deliver in the highly competitive market. Big players in the sector have started giving serious consideration over aspects related to employment relations to attract and retain best professionals in the segment. Daily meetings with employees, lab technicians and other staff members, open to suggestions and ideas, organising regular conferences, incentivising employee efforts, mentoring under eminent experts, etc., are some of the emerging trends which are standardising employment relations practices in the segment. However, the segment is still immune from collective organisation by the employees. The diagnostic centres still lack any well-established HRM mechanism. This can again be attributed to the size of the enterprise. Since most of the diagnostic centres are small in nature, establishment of full-fledged HRM mechanism appears an expensive initiative for the employer. The employer himself takes the role of human resource manager and facilitates the functioning of the diagnostic centres.

11.4 Implications for Medical Tourism

The inclination of the travellers to visit India to avail treatment in the country can be seen as one of the most remarkable phenomena in recent times. In other words, the country has rightly earned the reputation of medical tourism considering the large number of patients visiting in search of better treatments for different chronic and non- chronic ailments. India ranks tenth in the Global Medical Tourism Index which is much above of the rank of the developed countries like Germany, Japan, South Korea, France and United Kingdom (Agnihotri 2022). Realising the immense potential of medical tourism in the country, the Government of India also launched scheme called 'Heal in India' to position the country as a global leader in the healthcare sector and offer best medical care services to the travellers on their medical journey to the country. Crooks et al. (2011) identified the highly trained medical staff members as one of the main drivers for this spurt growth in medical tourism, specifically the language skills. Sadly, there is very little literature available to highlight the correlation between employment relations and medical tourism in management literature. Authors like Ebrahim and Ganguli (2019) and Beladi et al. (2017) have to some extent underlined the strategic role of human capital on the growth of medical tourism in the country. Drawing cue from discussion in the previous sections, it can rightly be inferred that performance is very much dependent on employment relations practices existing at the organisational or firm level. Management of foreign travellers seeking medical services and facilities is a very sensitive affair. A very minute flaw or negligence in the process may give a severe blow to the reputation and image of the country. Addressing the issues and concerns at the level of employment relations can address this problem to a larger extent. It has been well accepted that extending training to the staff members facilities in building more productive, conflict-free and coordinative workplaces (Guile and Unwin, 2019). Since employees in the healthcare are expected to be highly skilled, skill acquirement shall remain one of the prioritised aspects not only for the employees in the sector but also for the employers. Skill acquirement facilitates employees to make adjustments with the changing nature of employment requirements in the sector. Employers shall also include investment in training as part of policy consideration as skill up-gradation, reskilling, etc. facilitate building up competencies and bring economic prosperity to the organisation (ILO 2005). The fact that India still lacks competencies to address healthcare needs shall be given enough consideration. The review of some major research works related to the theme identified patient management, public health knowledge, relationship management, cultural competency, international healthcare legislative knowledge, communication, etc., as some of the emerging competency requirements in the healthcare sector. Therefore, equipping employees with these competencies (technical, behavioural and motivational) for delivering successful performance becomes an imperative for the human resource management systems in the healthcare sector (Fattahi et al. 2020). Employees in the sector, through equipping with latest and required competencies, must be offered appropriate avenues to 'involve', 'participate' and 'commit' to meet the goal of offering best services to the treatment recipient. This will directly add value to the organisational performance and profitability and will create a sustainable image of the country as conducive for medical tourism (Lewin 2011). Healthcare sector, predominantly representing service sector, is characterised by 'indeterminacy of labour' which means since labour is not a commodity, it can only be realised once it is executed only (Warhurst et al. 2011). Thus, 'aesthetic labour' and 'emotional labour' become one of the primary requisites for the employees working in the sector. The healthcare sector is mainly dependent on face-to-face or voice-to voice interaction with the patients which requires control and regulation of feelings for expected service outcome. The bodily and face dispositions during patient interactions also are crucial to make the treatment seekers feel good which is one of the most essential criteria to attract foreign travellers seeking treatment in India (Warhurst et al. 2011). The trajectory of employment relations in the healthcare sector is changing very fast considering its interactive nature and tech-driven approach. As previously discussed, there is ample scope for employment for growing medical destination like India. Therefore, investing on improving the quality of manpower, specifically in soft and emotional skills in the sector, shall become an utmost concern for the public as well as private players in the sector.

As India takes a swift turn towards becoming an attractive destination for medical tourists, the possible implications can be manifested in the form of high stress at workplaces to cater to the needs and demands of the foreign treatment seekers. Under these considerations, 'trust' in employment relations becomes an essential and critical ingredient. For the employees to perform to their best, it is important that they must believe in the management that the employees will be provided with supportive working environment, suitable and attractive remuneration, rewards along with fair treatment and avenues for employee voice and representation (Davis et al. 2000). This not only encourages employees to perform even during times of extreme stress but also mitigates unnecessary monitoring and control which in turn fosters employment relations in sectors like healthcare where expectations and obligations run hand in hand (Dietz et al. 2011). As stakeholders in employment relations, there is equal onus on the employers and employees to nurture this aspect of trust in relations at workplaces to make the different forms of organisations functional in the sector highly adaptable to the changing needs and requirements of the sector. It is important that HRM shall get appropriate place in every aspect of organisational strategies to make the Indian healthcare sector more attractive for medical tourists. And this can only happen when organisations and its different stakeholders accept the strategic role human resource can play in delivering the best to the medical tourists from a holistic perspective.

11.5 The Conclusion

With the increasing number of healthcare recipients in India and from different other countries, the nation has good reasons to establish its brand image as a medical tourist destination. Metropolitan cities like Bangalore, Hyderabad, Chennai, Gurugram, New Delhi and Noida extend some of the best medical treatments when it comes to extending healthcare facilities in India. To boost medical tourism in the coming years, there is an emergent need to address the demand-supply deficit in terms of the number of healthcare centres in India. With this, there is also the dire need to prepare the existent manpower in the sector to meet the demands of the patients and other recipients who in majority are likely to visit the country for medical treatments. Under these considerations, it becomes imperative to focus on employment relations along with infrastructural and technology needs of the organisations operational in different segments under the healthcare sector. Due to lack in appropriate employment relations policies, employment relations remain one of the most neglected aspects in organisations in the healthcare sector. Uniform monetary policies are found to be absent with little focus on training needs. The aspect of collective voices, union representation and grievance handling mechanism are the areas that need urgent attention. The disparities prevalent in the public and private entities make the issues more complex. However, the future trajectory of employment relations appears to be shifting to a positive note where the government has started to give suitable considerations over the policy issues in the healthcare sector. Specialised professional courses are being run by the institutes of national importance to impart learning and training to the prospective employees to meet the future needs of manpower in the sector. Institutions like Employees' State Insurance Corporation which are crucial parts in regulating employment relations are becoming more vocal in favour of uniform monetary compensation to the employees in the sector. Employers' organisations like the Association of Healthcare Providers in India (AHPI) have also realised that without sound employment relations, the dream of India becoming a hub of medical tourism will remain unfulfilled. Therefore, they have come up with policies to take necessary and corrective actions to bridge the demand and supply of the manpower in the sector, extending training to the manpower and making healthcare sector more safe and secure. Unfortunately, no clear-cut policies regarding employment relations are suggested by the employers' side.

Since the employees and the workers employed in the sector are poorly organised and highly fragmented and they do not have any mechanism to express their voices at workplace which in future can hinder the workplace process in some way or the other, it is important that the employers and the government, as 'actors' in the employment relations framework, take cautious attempts to address employment relations issues in the sector. Employment relations in no case can remain the neglected side of healthcare sector in the sector. The very edifice of the healthcare sector is based on sentiments, emotions and experiences, and it is the feeling and emotion of an employee that can make or mar the experiences of healthcare recipient. Therefore, employment relations must be given due and high importance to make the country one of the most preferred destinations for medical tourists.

References

Agnihotri A (2022) *Medical tourism in India: top destinations, scenarios and all you need to know*. Retrieved from https://www.hindustantimes.com: https://www.hindustantimes.com/lifestyle/travel/medical-tourism-in-india-top-destinations-scenarios-and-all-you-need-to-know-101668163467932.html

Bach S (2004) Employment relations in the health service: the management of reforms. Routledge, Oxfordshire

Bajaj [illegible] (2021) *Healthcare industry in 2021: developments and expectations for 2022*. Retrieved from https://health.economictimes.indiatimes.com: https://health.economictimes.indiatimes.com/news/industry/healthcare-industry-in-2021-developments-and-expectations-for-2022/88578958

Beladi H, Chao C-C, Ee MS, Hollas D (2017) Does medical tourism promote economic growth? A cross-country analysis. J Travel Res 58(1):121–135

Bloom D, Canning D (2003) Health as human capital and its impact on economic performance. Geneva Pap Risk Insur 28(2):304–315

Böhlke N (2008) The impact of hospital privatisation on industrial relations and employees: the case of the Hamburg hospitals. Work Organ Labour Glob 2(2):119–130

Buchan J (2000) Health sector reform and human resources: lessons from the United Kingdom. Health Policy Plan 15(3):319–325

Burns LR (2014) India's healthcare industry: a system perspective. In: Burns LR (ed) India's healthcare industry: innovation in delivery, financing, and manufacturing. Cambridge University Press, Cambridge, pp 3–37

Crooks VA, Turner L, Snyder J, Johnston R, Kingsbury P (2011) Promoting medical tourism to India: messages, images, and the marketing of international patient travel. Soc Sci Med 72(5):726–732

Das T (2022) *Hospitals taking initiative to boost medical tourism*. Retrieved from https://www.sundayguardianlive.com: https://www.sundayguardianlive.com/news/hospitals-taking-initiative-boost-medical-tourism

Davis JH, Schoorman FD, Mayer RC, Ton HH (2000) The trusted general manager and business unit performance: empirical evidence of a competitive advantage. Strateg Manag J 21(5):563–576

De A (2022) *More preventive check-ups, lower test pricing: how covid has transformed the diagnostics sector*. Retrieved from https://news.abplive.com: https://news.abplive.com/india-at-2047/how-covid-has-transformed-the-diagnostics-sector-preventive-check-ups-lower-test-pricing-1566253

Dickson-Swift V, Fox C, Marshall K, Welch N, Willis J (2014) What really improves employee health and wellbeing: findings from regional Australian workplaces. Int J Workplace Health Manag 7(3):138–155

Dietz G, Martins A, Searle R (2011) Trust, HRM, and the employment relationship. In: Wilkinson A, Townsend K (eds) The future of employment relations: new paradigms, new developments. Palgrave Macmillan, Hampshire, pp 141–162

Easton MD, Noack AM, Vosco LF (2021) Are franchisees more prone to employment standards violations than other businesses? Evidence from Ontario, Canada. Econ Labour Relat Rev 32(1):39–64

Ebrahim AH, Ganguli S (2019) A comparative analysis of medical tourism competitiveness of India, Thailand and Singapore. Tourism: An International Interdisciplinary Journal 67(2):102–115

Fattahi H, Gorji HA, Bayat M (2020) Core competencies for health headquarters: a systematic review and meta-synthesis. BMC Public Health 891. https://doi.org/10.1186/s12889-020-08884-2

Greenfield D, Kellner A, Townsend A, Wilkinson A, Lawrence SA (2014) Health service accreditation reinforces a mindset of high-performance human resource management: lessons from an Australian study. Int J Qual Health Care 26(4):372–377

Guile, D., & Unwin, L. (2019). VET, expertise, and work: situating the challenge for the twenty-first century. In D. Guile, & L. Unwin, The Wiley handbook of vocational education and training (pp. 17–40). New York: John Wiley & Sons, Inc.

Halpern RS, Perry SC, Narayan S (2001) Developing clinical practice environments supporting the knowledge work of nurses. Comput Nurs 19(1):17–23

ILO (2005) Skills, knowledge and employability: skills working paper no. 21. International Labour Organization, Geneva

ILO (2019) The future of work in the health sector. International Labour Office, Sectoral Policies Department, Geneva

Kabene SM, Orchard C, Howard JM, Soriano MA, Leduc R (2006) The importance of human resources management in health care: a global context. Hum Resour Health 4:20. https://doi.org/10.1186/1478-4491-4-20

Kanwal S (2022) *Estimated number of public and private hospitals across India in 2019*. Retrieved from https://www.statista.com: https://www.statista.com/statistics/1128425/india-number-of-public-and-private-hospitals-estimated/

Kellner A, Townsend K, Wilkinson A (2011) Franchise firms: changing employment relations. In: Wilkinson A, Townsend K (eds) The future of employment relations: new paradigms, new developments. Palgrave Macmillan, Hampshire, pp 67–82

Kim YH, Kim D-O (2012) Trust and employment relations: a workplace-level analysis. *16th ILERA World Congress*. ILERA, Philadephia. Retrieved from ilera2012.wharton.upenn.edu/RefereedPapers/KimYoonHo%20DongOneKim.pdf

Kinnie N, Swart J, Purcell J (2005) Influences on the choice of HR system: the network organization perspective. Int J Hum Resour Manag 16(6):1004–1028

Krinsky EB, Miller RU (2007) Patterns and issues in health care collective bargaining. Int J Public Adm 5(4):401–418

Lethbridge J (2015) Health care reforms and the rise of global multinational health care companies. Public Services International Research Unit, University of Greenwich, London

Lewin D (2011) High performance human resources (HPHR). In: Wilkinson A, Townsend K (eds) The future of employment relations: new paradigms, new developments. Palgrave Macmillan, Hampshire, pp 11–29

Matney SA, Maddox LJ, Staggers N (2013) Nurses as knowledge workers: is there evidence of knowledge in patient handoffs? West J Nurs Res 36(2):171–190

Mielke J, Geest SD, Beckmann S, Leppla L, Luta X, Guerbaai R-A et al (2019) The German version of the high-performance work systems questionnaire (HPWS-G) in the context of patient safety: a validation study in a Swiss university hospital. BMC Health Serv Res 19(356):356. https://doi.org/10.1186/s12913-019-4189-8

Mihail DM, Panagiotis KV (2016) The effects of high-performance work systems on hospital employees' work-related Well-being: evidence from Greece. Eur Manag J 34(4):424–438

Mistry L, Singh A, Bhattacharya S, Sharma H, Sarker B, Narula A (2022) Strengthening healthcare workforce in India: the 2047 agenda-top 20 priorities. FICCI & KPMG, New Delhi

Sahay P (2020) Diagnsotic sector. Edelweiss Professional Investor Research, Mumbai

Sarwal R, Prasad U, Madangopal K, Kalal SA, Kaur D, Kumar A et al (2021) Investment opportunities in India's healthcare sector. NITI Ayog, New Delhi

Sen A (1999) Development as freedom. Knopf Doubleday Publishing Group, New York

Sharma NC (2022) *India can create 12 million jobs by 2030 by investing in healthcare sector: Report*. Retrieved from https://www.businesstoday.in: https://www.businesstoday.in/latest/in-focus/story/india-can-create-12-million-jobs-by-2030-by-investing-in-healthcare-sector-report-323703-2022-02-23

Sisodia S, Agarwal N (2017) Employability skills essential for healthcare industry. Inf Technol Quant Manag 122:431–438

Townsend K, Richards J (2011) Developing a contemporary approach to conceptualizing employee actions. In: Wilkinson A, Townsend K (eds) The future of employment relations: new paradigms, new developments. Palgrave Macmillan, Hampshire, pp 101–121

Warhurst C, Broek DV, Nickson D, Hall R (2011) Heads, hearts, and now bodies: employee looks and lookism at work. In: Wilkinson A, Townsend K (eds) The future of employment relations: new paradigms, new development. Palgrave Macmillan, Hampshire, pp 122–140

Weber T, Nevala A-MN (2011) Employment and industrial relations in the health care sector. European Foundation for the Improvement of Living and Working Conditions, Dublin

World Health Organization: WHO. (2023, October 5). Universal health coverage (UHC). https://www.who.int/news-room/factsheets/detail/universal-health-coverage-(uhc)

Chapter 12
A Bird's-Eye-View on Technological Advancements in Medical Tourism

Kanakavalli K. Kundury, Shyam Prasad Shetty, and G. B. Kuldeep

Abstract Technology has significant impact on the medical tourism industry, enabling patients to access information about healthcare providers and facilities, schedule appointments and receive care even remotely. Advancements such as virtual reality, blockchain technology, artificial intelligence, medical devices and wearables, medical mobile applications and cloud computing have played key roles in the development and expansion of medical tourism. But, the integration of these technologies also poses challenges such as lack of coordination and communication, limited information, quality assurance, legal and regulatory compliance, technical compatibility, limited follow-up care and lack of training. Additionally, it is important to be cautious when taking decisions based on the information available with these applications, as advancements in technology don't always mean correct and reliable. Thus, this chapter focuses on providing an overview on the healthcare technologies in supporting medical tourism services.

Keywords Medical Tourism · Healthcare · Technologies · Telemedicine · Artificial Intelligence

K. K. Kundury (✉)
Department of Health System Management Studies, JSS Academy of Higher Education and Research, Mysuru, Karnataka, India

Special Interest Group in Patient Care Management, JSS Academy of Higher Education and Research, Mysuru, Karnataka, India
e-mail: kanakavalli.dhsms@jssuni.edu.in

S. P. Shetty
Department of Cardiothoracic and Vascular Surgery (CTVS), JSS Medical College & Hospital, JSS Academy of Higher Education and Research, Mysuru, Karnataka, India

G. B. Kuldeep
Department of Hospital Administration, JSS Medical College & Hospital, JSS Academy of Higher Education and Research, Mysuru, Karnataka, India

B. Chaudhary et al. (eds.), *Medical Tourism in Developing Countries*,
https://doi.org/10.1007/978-981-99-8909-6_12

Abbreviations

3D	3-Dimensional
AI	Artificial Intelligence
EHR	Electronic Health Records
EMR	Electronic Medical Records
VR	Virtual Reality

12.1 Medical Tourism and Healthcare Technologies

Medical tourism and healthcare technologies are closely related as advancements in healthcare technology have made it possible for patients to access a wider range of medical treatments and providers around the world (Neil Lunt et al. 2011).

Technology plays a significant role in the growth of medical tourism by making it easier for patients to find and compare medical treatments and providers around the world (Gu et al. 2021). The internet and social media platforms have made it easier for patients to research medical treatments and providers, as well as to find reviews and testimonials from other patients who have undergone similar treatments (Ventola 2014a). Additionally, telemedicine and virtual consultations have made it possible for patients to consult with doctors remotely, which can save them time and money on travel costs (Gu et al. 2021). Additionally, the developments in medical technology have made it possible for more complex treatments to be performed, which has led to an increase in the number of medical tourists seeking these treatments (Neil Lunt et al. 2011).

12.2 Outcomes of Technological Advancements in Medical Tourism

Technological advancements in medical tourism have led to a number of positive outcomes for both patients and healthcare providers (Hwang et al. 2018). One of the major benefits is improved access to specialized medical care for patients. With the use of telemedicine and remote consultations, patients are now able to receive treatment from doctors and specialists in other countries, even if they are unable to travel (Gu et al. 2021). This has increased access to high-quality medical care for people living in remote or underserved areas and has also made it easier for patients to receive second opinions from top medical experts around the world.

Another benefit of technological advancements in medical tourism is the increased efficiency and cost-effectiveness of the healthcare system (Neil Lunt et al. 2011). The use of electronic medical records, cloud computing and other technologies has made it easier to share patient information between healthcare providers,

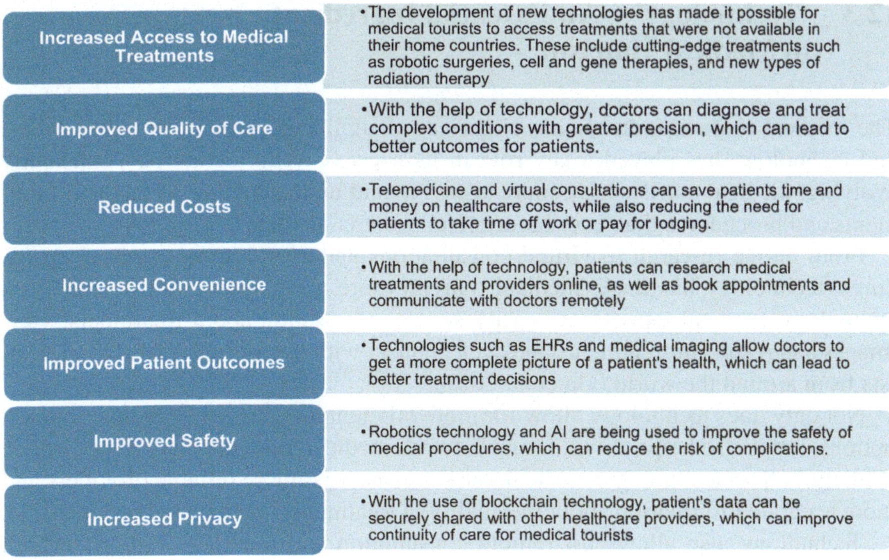

Fig. 12.1 Outcomes of technological advancements in medical tourism

which has helped to improve the coordination of care and reduce the risk of medical errors (Ozair et al. 2015). Additionally, the use of telemedicine and remote consultations has reduced the need for patients to travel for medical treatment, which can save time and money for both patients and healthcare providers.

The use of technology in medical tourism has led to improved access to specialized medical care, improved coordination and continuity of care and cost savings for both patients and healthcare providers (Gu et al. 2021). New technologies can help to reduce the cost of medical treatments by making them more efficient and less invasive. For example, remote surgery can help to reduce the cost of travel and accommodation, and 3D printing can help to create customized medical devices and implants at a lower cost than traditional manufacturing methods (Ventola 2014b). These technological advancements can also enhance the capacity of service providers in medical tourism and healthcare industries, thus meeting the needs of several patients. Outcomes of technological advancements in medical tourism also include (Wong and Hazley 2021) the following (Fig. 12.1).

Overall, technological advancements in medical tourism have the potential to improve the quality, accessibility and affordability of medical care for patients around the world (Wong and Hazley 2021).

12.3 'Technology'—An Essential Ingredient in Medical Tourism

The medical tourism industry has experienced significant growth in recent years, and technology has played a key role in its success. With technology constantly evolving, medical tourists have more access to and understanding of medical treatments and procedures than ever before (Neil Lunt et al. 2011).

From online research to virtual consultations and even remote medical procedures, technology has made medical tourism more accessible and efficient. With technology, medical tourists can easily access information about treatments, view images and results of treatments and even connect with doctors and medical specialists from around the world (Gu et al. 2021).

Not only does technology allow for more efficient and effective medical tourism options, but it also helps to build trust between medical tourists and their providers. With the help of technology, medical tourists can access more reliable providers and more accurate information about the quality of treatments (Wong and Hazley 2021).

Technology also allows for remote consultation and treatment options, which makes it easier for medical tourists to receive the treatments they need without having to travel for them. This is especially beneficial for those who have physical or financial limitations that make travelling difficult (Gu et al. 2021).

12.3.1 Knowledge Advancement

Technology has been a major driving force for the growth of medical tourism. With the availability of high-speed internet, medical tourists can now research and gain access to the latest medical information at their figure tips. In addition, technological advances have allowed for more efficient communication between medical tourists and their providers, allowing for more streamlined processes (Wong and Hazley 2021).

The use of electronic medical records (EMRs) has also made it easier for medical tourists to transfer vital patient information between countries with ease. This has been a huge boon for medical tourists, as it eliminates the need to carry hard copies of their medical records (Hwang et al. 2018).

The internet has made it possible for patients to access a wealth of medical information, including information on medical treatments, providers and costs (Tonsaker et al. 2014). This can help patients make more informed decisions about their healthcare.

Telemedicine and virtual consultations have made it possible for patients to consult with doctors remotely and access specialists who may not be available in their home country (Gu et al. 2021). This has increased the range of treatments and providers available to medical tourists.

Technology such as big data analytics, machine learning and artificial intelligence have been used to analyse large amounts of medical data, allowing researchers to identify patterns, trends and new insights in medical treatments and outcomes (Khan and Alotaibi 2020). Cloud computing, blockchain technology and other technologies are being used to securely store and share medical data, which can improve continuity of care for medical tourists for post treatment follow-up (Shen et al. 2019).

Technology has made it easier for medical tourists to access personalized services. Using online platforms, medical tourists can now easily find the right medical facility and treatments that are tailored to their individual needs. By utilizing sophisticated algorithms, medical tourists can find the most suitable and affordable healthcare option for their needs.

All in all, technology has been a major contributor towards the growth of medical tourism. It has allowed medical tourists to access a higher quality of medical services and to easily transfer vital patient information across borders (Wong and Hazley 2021). In addition, technology has enabled medical tourists to access personalized services that are tailored to their individual needs.

12.3.2 Better Customer Service

Technology has revolutionized customer service for medical tourism, making it easier and more efficient than ever before. With the advancement of the internet and mobile applications, medical tourists have access to a premium information, such as medical procedure packages, medical facilities and medical tourism specialists within minutes (Tonsaker et al. 2014). In addition, the use of sophisticated data management systems and artificial intelligence (AI) has further improved customer service, making it easier to find the right medical tourism package and get the best quality services (Khan and Alotaibi 2020).

AI-driven chatbots have made it simpler for medical tourism companies to manage customer interactions and provide quick responses to queries. Such bots can also help medical tourism customers identify the right medical provider with ease, ensuring that they get the best treatment at the lowest cost (Khan and Alotaibi 2020). Video conferencing has been another major technology advancement for medical tourism (Gu et al. 2021). This technology has provided a smooth channel of communication between customers and medical tourism providers, reducing physical visits, paperwork and delays.

The advancements in payment systems have made it easier for patients to pay for medical tourism packages, as well as receive refunds in the event of any issues (Institute of Medicine (US) 1991). This ensures a seamless and secure payment experience for patients; also, easier claims management with insurance service providers.

Overall, technology has revolutionized patient service for medical tourism, allowing for improved communication, access to information and secure payments, ultimately leading to a better experience.

12.3.3 Cost Reduction and Revenue Generation

With the help of the internet, healthcare providers can now connect with clients in different countries and provide them with reliable and cost-effective medical services (Institute of Medicine (US) 1991). Furthermore, with the development of sophisticated technologies, medical tourism businesses can provide their services at low costs, still not compromising on the quality (Hwang et al. 2018).

For example, telemedicine technology enables doctors to consult with patients remotely, eliminating the need for patients to travel (Gu et al. 2021). Additionally, medical tourism businesses can benefit from automated appointment scheduling systems and remote patient monitoring, which can significantly reduce operational and labour costs associated with managing appointments (Snoswell et al. 2020).

Overall, technology has made medical tourism more accessible and cost-effective for businesses, helping them to reach more patients and generate more revenue.

12.3.4 Creation of Medical Tourism Portals

In the past, traveling to a foreign country for medical treatment was not so comfortable as now, and it would have taken a great deal of time and effort to find providers and compare prices (CDC 2022). Now, however, medical tourism portals allow people to quickly and easily compare medical costs, treatment options and more (Tonsaker et al. 2014). By leveraging technology, medical tourism portals allow potential travellers to quickly and easily find the best medical care at the lowest possible cost (Tonsaker et al. 2014).

The use of such portals has made it easier and more affordable for people to seek the best care for their medical needs. In addition, the use of technology has made it easier for providers to market their services to potential customers, increasing the number of clients that they can serve (Tonsaker et al. 2014). As such, technology has been a major driver in the growth of medical tourism, making it easier and more affordable for people to travel for medical care. With the use of these portals, medical treatment is not only more affordable but also more accessible to a wider range of people.

12.3.5 Securing Medical Data Transfer

Technology has revolutionized medical care, making medical data transfer secure and more efficient, providing a reliable platform for the growth of medical tourism. Long-distance medical care is now a reality, making it possible for patients to travel for medical treatment without having to worry about their data being compromised.

Data encryption and other security measures have been implemented to ensure that patient information access is available to the privileged medical professionals involved in the patient's care (Kruse et al. 2017). This has enabled a safe and secure transfer of medical information, making it as an essential factor for medical tourism to thrive (Kruse et al. 2017).

Moreover, medical tourism has been greatly aided by the advent of telemedicine and remote medical services. Telemedicine can bridge the gap between medical professionals and patients, providing medical care even when the patient is in a different country or time zone (Gu et al. 2021).

In conclusion, technology has been a great contributor to the growth of medical tourism, providing secure and reliable data transfer; telemedicine and remote monitoring services (Gu et al. 2021; Ozair et al. 2015; Kruse et al. 2017). This has allowed patients to receive the medical care they need without having to worry about data theft, making medical tourism a viable option for many.

12.3.6 Mobile Medical Technology

The development of mobile medical technology has revolutionized the medical tourism industry, allowing people to receive medical care using the latest technologies and treatments regardless of their physical location. With the advancement of the Internet, people have the capability to access medical care from any corner of the world, even if they are not physically present in the region (Tonsaker et al. 2014). This has opened doors to hundreds of different medical treatments and services, from cosmetic procedures to complex treatments that require a high level of expertise.

Thanks to mobile medical technology, medical tourists can now access medical services quickly and conveniently (Chang 2022). For example, if a patient is looking for a specific type of surgery or doctor in another country, they can find the best professional for their needs and get the necessary treatment with the help of mobile apps or websites. Additionally, medical tourists can access medical information such as patient reviews, doctor ratings and even read up on their chosen treatment before scheduling an appointment.

The introduction of mobile medical technology has also resulted in the growth of telemedicine, which allows a doctor and a patient to communicate and share information without the limitations of physical distances (Gu et al. 2021). Telemedicine not only makes it easier for medical tourists to access medical care but also makes the process more efficient, as doctors can review records and analyse data remotely (Gu et al. 2021).

Over the years, mobile medical technology has drastically improved the medical tourism industry by providing medical tourists with the opportunity to access medical services from anywhere in the world. With the help of this technology, doctors and patients can communicate and collaborate more effectively, and medical tourists can get the help they need from the comfort of their own homes.

12.4 Technological Breakthroughs in Medical Tourism

There have been several technological breakthroughs in medical tourism that have had a significant impact on the industry. Some of these include the following:

12.4.1 Telemedicine

Telemedicine is also playing an increasingly important role in the field of medical tourism. This allows patients to consult with doctors and specialists in other countries before travelling for treatment (Hong 2016). This can help ensure that the patient is receiving the best possible care and that the treatment is appropriate for their condition. This tele consultation also creates the necessary confidence to the patient on the service providers, giving them the comfort required for care continuum (Hong 2016).

With telemedicine, patients can also continue to receive follow-up care once they return to their home country (Reed et al. 2021). This can be especially important for medical tourists who have undergone major surgeries or treatments, as it allows them to receive the care, they need without having to travel back to the country where they received treatment (Reed et al. 2021). Telemedicine can also be used to facilitate communication between the patient's local doctor and the medical team in the destination country (Muschol et al. 2022). As a result, telemedicine has made it easier for people to receive medical treatment in other countries and still receive the same level of care they would receive at home.

12.4.2 Electronic Health Records (EHRs)

Electronic Health Records (EHRs) are digital versions of patients' medical history, which can be accessed and shared by healthcare providers (Ehrenstein et al. 2019). In Medical Tourism, EHRs can play a critical role in ensuring continuity of care and reducing errors. With EHRs, patient's medical information can be easily shared between healthcare providers in different countries, allowing doctors and specialists to have a complete understanding of the patient's medical history before providing treatment (Ehrenstein et al. 2019).

EHRs can also help to reduce errors by providing accurate and up-to-date information about patient's medical history, allergies, medications and other relevant information (Nguyen et al. 2022). This can be especially important in medical tourism, as patients may be receiving care from healthcare providers who do not have access to their complete medical history. EHRs can also be accessed remotely, which means that patients can have their vital medical information portable and easily accessible after returning home (Evans 2016). Additionally, EHRs can be used to track the progress of the patient, which can help in ensuring that the patient is receiving the best possible care (Bouri and Ravi 2014). Thus, EHRs can play a key role in ensuring continuity of care and reducing medical errors for patients who travel for medical treatment.

12.4.3 Medical Imaging

Medical imaging is an important aspect of healthcare and is used to diagnose and treat a wide range of conditions. In the context of medical tourism, medical imaging can play a crucial role in ensuring that patients receive the right treatment in a timely manner (European Society of Radiology (ESR) and European Federation of Radiographer Societies (EFRS) 2019). With the help of medical imaging, healthcare providers can get a detailed view of the patient's internal organs and tissues, which can help in identifying the underlying cause of the problem and determining the best course of treatment (European Society of Radiology (ESR) and European Federation of Radiographer Societies (EFRS) 2019).

Medical imaging can also be used to monitor the progress of treatment and determine if any modifications in the current therapies to be made. For example, imaging can be used to track the healing process after surgery or to monitor the growth of a tumour (Kessler and Bhatt 2018). Additionally, medical imaging can be used to plan and execute complex surgeries, which can help to reduce the risk of complications and improve the outcomes for patients (Kessler and Bhatt 2018). Telemedicine has also made it possible for patients to receive medical imaging remotely, which can be particularly useful for medical tourists who need to receive follow-up care (Haleem et al. 2021a). Overall, medical imaging plays a vital role in ensuring that patients receive the best possible care, especially when travelling for medical treatment.

12.4.4 Medical Robotics

Robotics technology has made it possible for surgeries to be performed with greater precision, which has led to an increase in medical tourism for procedures such as joint replacements and other orthopaedic surgeries (Kolessar et al. 2022). Medical robotics is a rapidly growing field that uses advanced technology to assist healthcare professionals in the diagnosis, treatment and monitoring of patients (Lanfranco et al. 2004). In medical tourism, medical robotics can play a significant role in improving the quality of care and outcomes for patients (Lanfranco et al. 2004). Medical robots can be used to perform complex procedures, such as surgery, with greater precision and accuracy, which can result in faster recovery times and fewer complications (Lanfranco et al. 2004).

Medical robotics can also be used to assist with remote monitoring and telemedicine facilities, allowing patients to receive care from healthcare professionals remotely (Lima et al. 2021). For example, robots can be used to perform remote consultations, allowing patients to receive medical advice and treatment from specialists located in other countries. Additionally, medical robots can be used to perform remote diagnostic procedures, such as imaging and lab tests, which can help to reduce the need for travel and make healthcare more accessible for patients (Lima et al. 2021). Medical robotics can also be used to assist with rehabilitation and physical therapy, helping patients to regain their strength and mobility after an injury or surgery (Zhang et al. 2013).

12.4.5 3D Printing

3D printing is a rapidly evolving technology that allows for the creation of physical objects by laying down successive layers of material. In the medical field, 3D printing can be used to create prosthetic limbs, surgical guides and even replacement body parts (Ventola 2014b). 3D printing can be used to create customized medical devices and implants that are tailored to the specific needs of individual patients (Ventola 2014b).

3D printing can also be used to create models of patients' internal organs, which can be used for surgical planning and training (Bozkurt and Karayel 2021). This can help to reduce the risk of complications and improve the outcomes for patients. Additionally, 3D printing can be used to create patient-specific surgical guides, which can help to ensure that the surgery is performed accurately and with minimal invasiveness (Bozkurt and Karayel 2021). 3D printing can also facilitate the production of customized medical devices and implants, which can be particularly useful for patients who have unique medical needs or who have difficulty finding the right fit with off-the-shelf products (Bozkurt and Karayel 2021). Overall, 3D printing is a rapidly growing technology that has the potential to significantly improve the quality of care and outcomes for patients who travel for medical treatment.

These technological breakthroughs have significantly improved the accessibility, affordability and quality of medical treatments for patients around the world and have also driven innovation in the healthcare industry.

12.5 Challenges in Integrating Technological Advancements in Medical Tourism

Though the integration of healthcare technologies with medical tourisms has yielded immense benefits, the challenges associated with this integration are still a major concern for both patients and healthcare providers (Neil Lunt et al. 2011).

One of the major challenges of integrating technology in medical tourism is ensuring the security and privacy of patient information (Kruse et al. 2017). As medical information is shared and stored electronically, it is important to have proper security measures in place to protect against data breaches and unauthorized access (Kruse et al. 2017). This includes implementing encryption, secure login protocols and regular security audits. Another challenge is the lack of standardization in the technology used in medical tourism (National Research Council (US) 1997). Different healthcare providers and countries may use different electronic medical record systems, which can make it difficult to share patient information and coordinate care (National Research Council (US) 1997). This can also lead to issues with compatibility and data interoperability.

Additionally, technological integration in medical tourism requires significant investment in infrastructure and training, which can be a barrier for some healthcare providers, especially those in developing countries (Neil Lunt et al. 2011). It also requires a good internet connection, which is not always available or reliable in some places. Another challenge is the need to ensure that medical tourism providers are properly trained in the newest medical technologies (Tonsaker et al. 2014). This includes not only providing training to medical staff but also ensuring that they understand how to use the technology to its full potential. Without adequate training, healthcare teams in medical tourism services may not be able to provide the highest quality of care and may not be able to provide the best experience for their patients (Neil Lunt et al. 2011).

There are several other challenges associated with technology integration in medical tourism, including (Ventola 2014a; Cesario 2018) (Fig. 12.2):

12.6 Technological Trends in Medical Tourism

Along with the technological advancements, there are several technological trends that are currently impacting the medical tourism industry, which include the following:

12.6.1 Virtual Reality

Virtual reality (VR) technology is increasingly being used in the field of medical tourism as a way to enhance the patient experience. VR can be used for a variety of purposes, such as providing patients with virtual tours of medical facilities before they arrive, allowing patients to visualize and prepare for their procedures and even providing virtual post-operative recovery support (Rogers 2020). Using VR technology, medical providers can help patients understand and prepare for the medical procedures they are going to undergo. This includes the procedure itself, the recovery process and the overall medical experience, which can help reduce anxiety and fear in the patient (Rogers 2020).

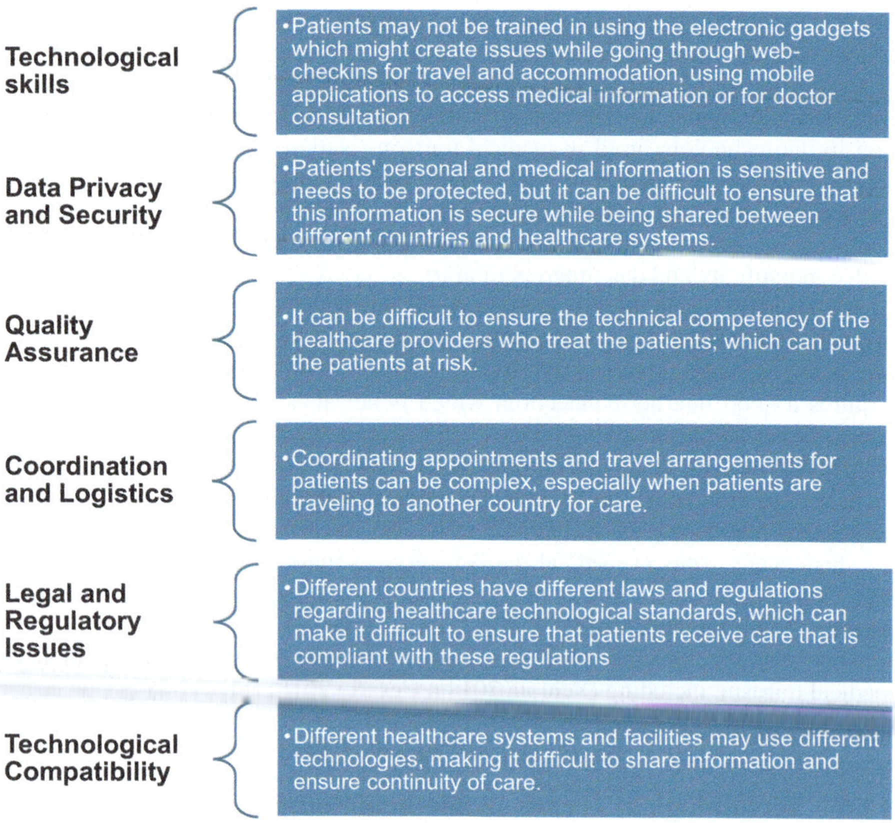

Fig. 12.2 Technological challenges in medical tourism

In addition to its benefits for patients, VR technology can also support medical providers by allowing them to more effectively communicate with patients and provide accurate information about procedures and recovery (Palanica et al. 2019). Additionally, VR can be used to train medical professionals, allowing them to practice procedures in a safe, virtual environment before performing them on real patients (Palanica et al. 2019). This can lead to improved outcomes and increased patient satisfaction. The use of VR technology allows the medical provider to simulate a wide range of procedures, from routine surgeries to complex procedures, which can help medical professionals gain confidence and improve their skills (Javaid and Haleem 2020).

Another advantage of VR technology in medical tourism is cost reduction. With VR technology, patients can undergo virtual consultations with specialists from all over the world and also can save cost on travel expenses (Rogers 2020). Additionally, the use of VR technology can also reduce the cost of medical procedures themselves, by allowing medical professionals to practice procedures in a virtual environment before performing them really on patients (Rogers 2020). Overall, VR has the potential to revolutionize the way medical tourism is conducted, making the process more efficient, effective and cost-effective.

However, VR technology also has some challenges and limitations. VR technology can be complex and difficult to use, and it requires specialized equipment and software (Terashima 2002). VR can only provide limited information about the facilities, staff and services, and it can't replace a physical visit. VR can raise privacy and security concerns, as it involves the transmission of sensitive patient information (Terashima 2002).

Virtual reality technology is being increasingly adopted in the medical tourism industry, and it is expected to continue to grow as technology improves and more patients and healthcare providers adopt it.

12.6.2 Blockchain Technology

Blockchain technology has the potential to revolutionize the field of medical tourism by providing secure and transparent ways to manage patient data and financial transactions (Shen et al. 2019). One of the key advantages of blockchain technology is its ability to create tamper-proof records, which can help ensure the security and privacy of patient data. This can be especially important in the context of medical tourism, where patient data may need to be shared across borders and between different medical providers.

Another advantage of blockchain technology in medical tourism is the ability to streamline financial transactions (Tyan et al. 2021). Blockchain technology can be used to create smart contracts, which are self-executing contracts with the terms of the agreement between buyer and seller being directly written into lines of code (Tyan et al. 2021). This can facilitate the payment process for medical procedures and other related expenses, reducing the need for intermediaries and increasing transparency (Tyan et al. 2021).

Moreover, blockchain technology can also enable the creation of a decentralized healthcare system, where patients have more control over their medical records and can share them with different medical providers as needed (Haleem et al. 2021b). This can help to improve the coordination of care and reduce the risk of errors. With the ability to provide patients with a unique medical history that is verifiable by multiple parties, it could also be used to validate medical certifications and qualifications of medical professionals, helping to ensure that patients receive the highest quality care (Haleem et al. 2021b).

On the flip side, blockchain technology also has some challenges and limitations, such as it can be complex and difficult to implement, and it requires specialized expertise and infrastructure. Blockchain technology is still not widely adopted in the healthcare industry, and it may be difficult to find providers that are able to use it (Agbo et al. 2019). Blockchain technology raises legal and regulatory issues, as different countries have different laws and regulations regarding data privacy and security (Agbo et al. 2019).

Blockchain technology has the potential to revolutionize the medical tourism industry by making it easier for patients to receive care from providers in other countries, but more research and development are needed to fully realize its potential (Haleem et al. 2021b).

12.6.3 *Artificial Intelligence*

Artificial intelligence (AI) is the simulation of human intelligence in machines that are programmed to think and learn like humans. In the context of medical tourism, AI can be used to improve the accuracy of diagnoses and treatment plans, which can help patients receive more effective care (Klumpp et al. 2021).

AI can be used in medical tourism to make the entire process simpler and easier for patients to navigate. AI can be used to personalize treatments and optimize services to match the needs of each individual patient. For example, AI can be used to find the most reputable medical providers to meet a patient's needs, as well as help to identify the best options for treatment and cost (Khan and Alotaibi 2020).

AI can also be utilized to provide more accurate diagnoses. By using data from medical records and other sources, AI can help identify illnesses and medical conditions and suggest potential treatments based on the patient's individual characteristics (Klumpp et al. 2021). This can help to reduce the risk of misdiagnosis, as physicians can be alerted to potential issues that may have otherwise gone unnoticed.

AI can also be used to provide personalized follow-up care. By monitoring a patient's progress, AI can help identify the best treatments and suggest the best courses of action for each individual (Klumpp et al. 2021). This can help to ensure that each patient receives the best possible care, while also reducing the time and cost of treatment.

There are several advantages of using AI in medical tourism. AI can be used to analyse large amounts of medical data, such as imaging and lab results, which can help improve the accuracy of diagnoses (Lee and Yoon 2021). AI can be used to analyse patient data and create personalized treatment plans, which can be more effective than generic treatment plans (Lee and Yoon 2021). AI can be used to monitor patients' conditions and alert healthcare providers to potential issues, which can help improve patient outcomes. AI can be used to automate certain processes, such as scheduling appointments and ordering lab tests, which can reduce the costs associated with medical tourism (Basu et al. 2020).

However, AI also has some challenges and limitations such as AI can be complex and difficult to implement, and it requires specialized expertise and infrastructure. AI algorithms may perpetuate biased data, leading to inaccurate predictions and recommendations (Kelly et al. 2019). AI is not yet widely adopted in the healthcare industry, and it may be difficult to find providers that are able to use it (Kelly et al. 2019). AI also raises privacy and security concerns, as it involves the processing and storage of sensitive patient information (Kelly et al. 2019).

Thus, AI has the potential to revolutionize the medical tourism industry by making it easier for patients to receive more effective care, but more research and development are needed to fully realize its potential.

12.6.4 Robotic Surgery

Robotic surgery is becoming increasingly popular in the medical field. It is a form of minimally invasive surgery, meaning that it is less invasive than traditional open surgery and offers many advantages (Lanfranco et al. 2004). Robotic surgery can provide a shorter hospital stay, less pain, less blood loss, a lower risk of infection and faster recovery times (Lanfranco et al. 2004). Plus, it enables surgeons to perform more precise and delicate operations.

For example, robotic surgery carried out by 'da Vinci' surgical system (Azizian et al. 2020). This robotic system is controlled by a surgeon who sits at a console and directs the robot's surgical instruments (Azizian et al. 2020). The da Vinci system provides the surgeon with a 3D view of the surgical site, as well as better precision, range of motion and access than traditional instruments (Azizian et al. 2020). The robot also allows the surgeon to control the movements of the surgical instruments with small, delicate motions of the hands (Azizian et al. 2020).

Robotic surgery is already being used to treat many conditions, such as prostate cancer, gallbladder disease and pancreatic cancer, and is becoming increasingly popular for other applications (Lanfranco et al. 2004). Robotic surgery offers the potential to reduce complications, improve outcomes and reduce the costs associated with surgery (Lanfranco et al. 2004).

Improvements of robotic surgery in medical tourism can be in several ways. Robotic surgical systems can be programmed to make very precise movements, which can reduce the risk of complications and improve patient outcomes. Robotic surgery can reduce the recovery time associated with certain procedures, as it can minimize the trauma to the patient's body (Lanfranco et al. 2004). Robotic surgery can make it easier for patients to receive complex procedures that may not be available in their home countries. Robotic surgery can reduce the costs associated with medical tourism, as it can minimize the need for follow-up care and reduce the risk of complications (Zemmar et al. 2020).

However, robotic surgery also has some challenges and limitations. Robotic surgical systems can be complex and difficult to use, and they require specialized expertise and infrastructure (Morris 2005). Robotic surgical systems are not yet widely available, and it may be difficult to find providers that are able to use them (Morris 2005). Robotic surgery relies on remote monitoring and digital images, which may not be enough to make a proper diagnosis, especially in some cases. Robotic surgery raises privacy and security concerns, as it involves the processing and storage of sensitive patient information (Morris 2005).

Collectively, robotic surgery is becoming increasingly popular in the medical tourism industry and is expected to continue to grow as technology improves and more patients and healthcare providers adopt it.

12.6.5 Medical Devices and Wearables

Medical devices and wearables are becoming increasingly important in the field of medical tourism as they provide patients with a convenient and accessible way to monitor their health and communicate with medical providers. Wearable devices such as fitness trackers, smartwatches and health monitoring devices can be used to collect data on a patient's physical activity, sleep patterns and vital signs (Vijayan et al. 2021). These data can then be used to inform treatment decisions and monitor the patient's progress during their recovery (Vijayan et al. 2021).

In addition to their role in monitoring patient health, medical devices and wearables can be used to facilitate communication between patients and medical providers (Dias and Cunha 2018). For example, wearables can be used to remotely monitor patients after they have returned home from a medical tourism trip, allowing medical providers to ensure that patients are recovering as expected and adjust treatment plans as necessary (Dias and Cunha 2018).

Medical devices and wearables can also improve the quality of care provided in medical tourism, as they can aid in the detection of health issues early on, enabling medical professionals to take timely interventions (Dias and Cunha 2018). For example, wearables can be used to detect early signs of chronic diseases such as diabetes or heart disease. These devices can also help medical providers to provide more accurate diagnoses and develop more effective treatment plans (Dias and Cunha 2018). They can also provide patients with more control over their health, which can help to improve patient engagement and increase the chances of a successful outcome.

12.6.6 Internet and Social Media

The rise of the internet and social media has enabled patients to find medical services abroad quickly and easily, without having to worry about language barriers or cultural differences.

Social media is also playing a large role in the promotion of medical tourism as providers and hospitals can efficiently reach out to a large number of potential customers, giving them access to detailed information about the services they offer (Neil Lunt et al. 2011). This has allowed patients to make informed decisions about the quality, safety and cost-effectiveness of the medical services they wish to receive.

The internet has also allowed medical tour operators to gain access to a range of information in a short period of time (National Research Council (US) 2000). This includes reviews, contact details, pricing and other important information which can help patients make informed decisions. Additionally, patients can now easily compare the quality and safety of services provided at different hospitals and locations, which can help them to make the most cost-effective choice (National Research Council (US) 2000).

The Internet and social media also have some challenges and limitations. The Internet and social media can provide limited information about healthcare providers and facilities, and it may be difficult to ensure the accuracy and reliability of the information provided (Tonsaker et al. 2014). They may not be widely accepted in certain countries, and it may be difficult to find providers that are able to use them. Along with that, they raise privacy and security concerns, as they involve the processing and storage of sensitive patient information (Tonsaker et al. 2014). The Internet and social media can be a source of misinformation, which can be dangerous for patients. As there is a chance for unreliable information over the Internet and social media sites, it is always suggested to confirm the authenticity, accuracy and reliability of the information from the official channels (National Research Council (US) 2000).

12.6.7 Cloud Computing

Cloud computing has become an increasingly popular technology in recent years, as it offers businesses and individuals the opportunity to access data and applications remotely. From this perspective, cloud computing is revolutionizing the healthcare industry, as it enables medical service providers to share data and collaborate with each other with ease (Shen et al. 2019).

Medical tourism is a growing phenomenon, as more people are looking for cost-effective and reliable healthcare options in foreign countries. This is where cloud computing comes in, as it enables medical service providers to access patient records, medical history and other important data from a remote location, making it easier for medical tourists to receive quality care. Moreover, cloud computing allows for a much faster and more reliable transfer of data and applications, which allows for more efficient and comprehensive healthcare services (Shen et al. 2019).

Cloud computing also provides a great deal of security for medical data, as it is stored on a secure server that is only accessed by authorized personnel (Kuo 2011). Furthermore, cloud computing can provide medical service providers with the necessary tools to monitor patient conditions and access medical records in real time, thereby allowing for faster diagnosis and treatment and ultimately a better quality of care (Shen et al. 2019; Kuo 2011).

Cloud computing can be used to store and share medical data, such as patient information, imaging and lab results, which can help improve the accuracy of diagnoses and treatment plans (Kuo 2011). It can be used to connect healthcare providers in different locations, which can make it easier for patients to receive care from providers in other countries (Shen et al. 2019; Kuo 2011). It can be cost-effective, as it can reduce the need for expensive infrastructure and IT staff. Cloud computing can be easily scaled up or down to meet changing needs, which can help improve the efficiency of healthcare delivery (Shen et al. 2019; Kuo 2011).

Cloud computing has the potential to revolutionize the medical tourism industry by making it easier for patients to receive more effective care, but more research and development are needed to fully realize its capability.

12.7 Drawbacks of Involving Technologies in Medical Tourism

Though the healthcare technological interventions in medical tourism result in enormous benefits, these applications can often yield to several technical blunders, leading to poor patient outcomes and impacting healthcare business organizations.

12.7.1 Patient Decision-Making

Taking decisions based on information available on the internet can be risky as the information may not be accurate or reliable. The internet can be a source of misinformation, and it can be difficult to verify the credibility of the sources.

When considering medical tourism, patients should be cautious about making decisions based solely on information found on the internet (Tonsaker et al. 2014). They should be aware that the information may not be accurate or reliable, and that it may not take into account all of their individual needs and circumstances. It is important to research and verify information from multiple sources and to consult with a healthcare professional before making any decisions (Tonsaker et al. 2014). Patients should also be aware of the potential risks and benefits of any medical procedure and be sure to ask their healthcare provider any questions they may have.

Additionally, patients should be aware of the potential risks of sharing personal and medical information online. They should ensure that their personal and medical information is protected and only share it with authorized individuals (Ozair et al. 2015).

The internet can be a valuable tool for researching medical tourism options, but it is important to be cautious and to verify information from multiple sources before making any decisions (Shen et al. 2019). It's always recommended to consult with a healthcare professional and consider all the potential risks and benefits of any medical procedure before making a decision.

12.7.2 Collective Decision Is Important When Opting New Technology

Ignoring internal conflicts when requesting new technology can lead to significant challenges and problems in the medical tourism industry. These conflicts can include disagreements among healthcare providers and staff, as well as resistance from patients and families (Ramsay 2001). Collective decision-making is important when opting for new technology because it ensures that all stakeholders have a say in the decision-making process (Ramsay 2001). This includes not only the individuals who will be directly impacted by the technology, such as patients and medical providers, but also those who will be responsible for implementing and maintaining the technology, such as IT staff and administrators (Ramsay 2001). By involving all stakeholders in the decision-making process, it is possible to identify and address any potential issues or concerns that may arise.

Collective decision-making can also help to ensure that new technology is implemented in a way that is consistent with the overall goals and objectives of the organization. For example, when implementing new technology in a medical setting, it is important to consider how the technology supports the delivery of high-quality, patient-centred care (Powell-Cope et al. 2008). By involving all stakeholders in the decision-making process, it is possible to ensure that the technology is aligned with the organization's mission and values, and that it will be used in ways that support the organization's overall goals and objectives.

Moreover, collective decision-making can also be a way to foster innovation and creativity. By involving multiple perspectives and viewpoints, it is possible to identify new and innovative ways to use new technology (Ramsay 2001). The collective decision-making process can also help to ensure that the technology is customized to meet the specific needs of the organization, which can help to increase the chances of success and maximize the benefits of the technology. Overall, involving all stakeholders in the decision-making process can help to ensure that new technology is implemented in a way that is efficient, effective and sustainable (Ramsay 2001).

Ignoring internal conflicts can lead to a lack of buy-in from stakeholders, decreased use of the new technology and ultimately, poor patient outcomes (Hughes 2008). By proactively addressing potential conflicts, healthcare providers can ensure that new technology is adopted and used effectively in the medical tourism industry (Hughes 2008).

12.7.3 Is New Not Always Better?

Believing that newer automatically means better is a common misconception in the medical tourism industry (Neil Lunt et al. 2011). Just because a technology is newer or more advanced, it does not necessarily mean it is better or more effective. Newer technologies may be untested, unproven or have unknown risks and side effects (Thimbleby 2013).

When introducing new technology, it is important to consider several aspects. The clinical evidence supporting its use and its effectiveness compared to existing options. The costs and benefits of the technology, including both the financial and clinical outcomes. The level of expertise and training required to use the technology safely and effectively. The compatibility and integration with existing systems and infrastructure. The potential risks and side effects associated with the technology (Thimbleby 2013).

It is important to critically evaluate new technology and weigh the potential benefits against the potential risks and costs (Neil Lunt et al. 2011). Healthcare providers should also consider the specific needs and preferences of their patients and how the new technology may impact their care.

The Newer does not always mean better in the medical tourism industry (Neil Lunt et al. 2011). It is important to critically evaluate new technology and weigh the potential benefits against the potential risks and costs before making a decision to adopt it. Also, it is important to consider the specific needs of patients and how the new technology may impact their care.

12.8 Summary and Conclusions

Technology has played a significant role in the development and expansion of the medical tourism industry. Advancements in telemedicine, virtual reality, blockchain technology, artificial intelligence, robotic surgery, medical devices and wearables, medical mobile applications, cloud computing and the internet and social media have all enabled patients to access information, schedule appointments and receive care remotely. These technologies have the potential to improve the efficiency and effectiveness of healthcare delivery, increase collaboration among healthcare providers and reduce costs. However, it is important to consider the potential challenges and limitations that these technologies may bring, such as lack of coordination and communication, limited information, quality assurance, legal and regulatory compliance, technical compatibility, limited follow-up care, lack of training, privacy and security concerns. Additionally, it is important to be cautious when taking decisions based on the information available on the internet and not to believe that newer automatically means better. Furthermore, it is crucial to address internal conflicts when requesting new technology, authenticate medical research data and have an effective claims and billing management system in place.

12.9 Future Directions

The future of technology in medical tourism is expected to continue to evolve in ways that improve the quality, accessibility and affordability of healthcare services for patients who travel to other countries for medical treatment. One area of focus is likely to be the use of **virtual and augmented reality** technologies, which can be used to create immersive, interactive experiences for patients and medical professionals. These technologies can be used for a variety of purposes, such as virtual consultations, virtual tours of medical facilities and virtual simulations of medical procedures.

Another important area of focus for the future of medical tourism is the use of **big data and analytics**. With increasing amounts of medical data being collected and stored electronically, it will be possible to use advanced analytics techniques to identify patterns and trends in the data, which can then be used to improve the quality and efficiency of healthcare services. Additionally, the integration of wearable devices and **IoT technology** can enable remote monitoring of patients and enable virtual follow-ups, this will enable medical tourism to be more responsive to the needs of patients, especially those that have chronic conditions.

In terms of security, **cybersecurity** is going to be a key area of focus in the future of medical tourism. As more and more data are shared and stored electronically, it will be important to ensure that these data are protected from unauthorized access and breaches. With sensitive patient data and medical records at risk, it is important that security measures are implemented to ensure that patient data are protected.

Acknowledgements Authors would like to acknowledge JSS Academy of Higher Education & Research and thank them for providing them the opportunity and the resources required for drafting this book chapter. Their acknowledgements are also due to The Special Interest Group in Patient Care Management (SIGPCM).

References

Agbo CC, Mahmoud QH, Eklund JM (2019) Blockchain Technology in Healthcare: a systematic review. Healthcare(Basel) 7(2):56. https://doi.org/10.3390/healthcare7020056

Azizian M, Liu M, Khalaji I et al (2020) 3—The da Vinci surgical system. In: Abedin-Nasab MH (ed) Handbook of robotic and image-guided surgery. Elsevier, pp 39–55., ISBN 9780128142455. https://doi.org/10.1016/B978-0-12-814245-5.00003-7

Basu K, Sinha R, Ong A, Basu T (2020) Artificial intelligence: how is it changing medical sciences and its future? Indian J Dermatol 65(5):365–370. https://doi.org/10.4103/ijd.IJD_421_20

Bouri N, Ravi S (2014) Going mobile: how mobile personal health records can improve health care during emergencies. JMIR Mhealth Uhealth 2(1):e8. https://doi.org/10.2196/mhealth.3017

Bozkurt Y, Karayel E (2021) 3D printing technology; methods, biomedical applications, future opportunities and trends. J Mater Res Technol 14:1430–1450., ISSN 2238-7854,. https://doi.org/10.1016/j.jmrt.2021.07.050

CDC (2022) Medical tourism: travel to another country for medical care. U.S. Department of Health & Human Services. https://wwwnc.cdc.gov/travel/page/medical-tourism

Cesario SK (2018) Implications of medical tourism. Nurs Womens Health 22(3):269–273., ISSN 1751-4851. https://doi.org/10.1016/j.nwh.2018.03.008

Chang C-C (2022) The role of individual factors in users' intentions to use medical tourism mobile apps. Tour Hosp 3:896–907. https://doi.org/10.3390/tourhosp3040057

Dias D, Cunha JPS (2018) Wearable health devices-vital sign monitoring, systems and technologies. Sensors (Basel) 18(8):2414. https://doi.org/10.3390/s18082414

Ehrenstein V, Kharrazi H, Lehmann H et al (2019) Obtaining data from electronic health records. In: Gliklich RE, Leavy MB, Dreyer NA (eds) Tools and technologies for registry interoperability, registries for evaluating patient outcomes: a User's guide, 3rd edition, addendum 2 [internet]. Agency for Healthcare Research and Quality (US), Rockville (MD). Chapter 4. Available from: https://www.ncbi.nlm.nih.gov/books/NBK551878/

European Society of Radiology (ESR), European Federation of Radiographer Societies (EFRS) (2019) Patient safety in medical imaging: a joint paper of the European Society of Radiology (ESR) and the European Federation of Radiographer Societies (EFRS). Insights Imaging 10(1):45. https://doi.org/10.1186/s13244-019-0721-y

Evans RS (2016) Electronic health records: then, now, and in the future. Yearb Med Inform 20(Suppl 1):S48-61. https://doi.org/10.15265/IYS-2016-s006

Gu D, Humbatova G, Xie Y, Yang X, Zolotarev O, Zhang G (2021) Different roles of telehealth and telemedicine on medical tourism: an empirical study from Azerbaijan. Healthcare (Basel) 9(8):1073. https://doi.org/10.3390/healthcare9081073

Haleem A, Javaid M, Singh RP, Suman R (2021a) Telemedicine for healthcare: capabilities, features, barriers, and applications. Sens Int 2:100117. https://doi.org/10.1016/j.sintl.2021.100117

Haleem A, Javaid M et al (2021b) Blockchain technology applications in healthcare: an overview. Int J Intell Netw 2:130–139., ISSN 2666-6030,. https://doi.org/10.1016/j.ijin.2021.09.005

Hong YA (2016) Medical tourism and telemedicine: a new frontier of an old business. J Med Internet Res 18(5):e115. https://doi.org/10.2196/jmir.5432

Hughes RG (2008) Tools and strategies for quality improvement and patient safety. In: Hughes RG (ed) Patient safety and quality: an evidence-based handbook for nurses. Agency for Healthcare Research and Quality (US), Rockville (MD)

Hwang S, Lee D, Kang CY (2018) Medical tourism: focusing on patients' prior, current, and post experience. Int J Qual Innov 4:4. https://doi.org/10.1186/s40887-018-0024-2

Institute of Medicine (US) (1991) Committee on technological innovation in medicine. In: Gelijns AC, Halm EA (eds) The changing economics of medical technology. National Academies Press (US), Washington (DC). (Medical Innovation at the Crossroads, No. 2.) 2, The Diffusion of New Technology: Costs and Benefits to Health Care. Available from: https://www.ncbi.nlm.nih.gov/books/NBK234309/

Javaid M, Haleem A (2020) Virtual reality applications toward medical field. Clin Epidemiol Glob Health 8(2):600–605., ISSN 2213-3984. https://doi.org/10.1016/j.cegh.2019.12.010

Kelly CJ, Karthikesalingam A, Suleyman M et al (2019) Key challenges for delivering clinical impact with artificial intelligence. BMC Med 17:195. https://doi.org/10.1186/s12916-019-1426-2

Kessler AT, Bhatt AA (2018) Brain tumour post-treatment imaging and treatment-related complications. Insights Imaging 9(6):1057–1075. https://doi.org/10.1007/s13244-018-0661-y

Khan ZF, Alotaibi SR (2020) Applications of artificial intelligence and big data analytics in m-health: a healthcare system perspective. J Healthc Eng 2020:8894694. https://doi.org/10.1155/2020/8894694

Klumpp M, Hintze M, Immonen M et al (2021) Artificial intelligence for hospital health care: application cases and answers to challenges in European Hospitals. Healthcare 9:961. https://doi.org/10.3390/healthcare9080961

Kolessar DJ, Hayes DS, Harding JL, Rudraraju RT, Graham JH (2022) Robotic-arm assisted technology's impact on knee arthroplasty and associated healthcare costs. J Health Econ Outcomes Res 9(2):57–66. https://doi.org/10.36469/001c.37024

Kruse CS, Smith B, Vanderlinden H, Nealand A (2017) Security techniques for the electronic health records. J Med Syst 41(8):127. https://doi.org/10.1007/s10916-017-0778-4

Kuo AM (2011) Opportunities and challenges of cloud computing to improve health care services. J Med Internet Res 13(3):e67. https://doi.org/10.2196/jmir.1867

Lanfranco AR, Castellanos AE, Desai JP, Meyers WC (2004) Robotic surgery: a current perspective. Ann Surg 239(1):14–21. https://doi.org/10.1097/01.sla.0000103020.19595.7d

Lee D, Yoon SN (2021) Application of artificial intelligence-based technologies in the healthcare industry: opportunities and challenges. Int J Environ Res Public Health 18:271. https://doi.org/10.3390/ijerph18010271

Lima MR, Wairagkar M, Natarajan N, Vaitheswaran S, Vaidyanathan R (2021) Robotic telemedicine for mental health: a multimodal approach to improve human robot engagement. Front Robot AI 8:618866. https://doi.org/10.3389/frobt.2021.618866

Morris B (2005) Robotic surgery: applications, limitations, and impact on surgical education. MedGenMed 7(3):72

Muschol J, Heinrich M, Heiss C, Knapp G, Repp H, Schneider H, Thormann U, Uhlar J, Unzeitig K, Gissel C (2022) Assessing telemedicine efficiency in follow-up care with video consultations for patients in orthopedic and trauma surgery in Germany: randomized controlled trial. J Med Internet Res 24(7):e36996. https://doi.org/10.2196/36996

National Research Council (US) (1997) Committee on maintaining privacy and security in health care applications of the national information infrastructure. For the record protecting electronic health information. National Academies Press (US), Washington (DC). 4, Technical Approaches to Protecting Electronic Health Information. Available from: https://www.ncbi.nlm.nih.gov/books/NBK233433/

National Research Council (US) (2000) Committee on enhancing the internet for health applications: technical requirements and implementation strategies. Networking health: prescriptions for the internet. National Academies Press (US), Washington (DC). 2, Health Applications of the Internet. Available from: https://www.ncbi.nlm.nih.gov/books/NBK44714/

Neil Lunt RS, Exworthy M, Green ST, Horsfall D, Mannion R (2011) Medical tourism: treatments, markets and health system implications: a scoping review. Directorate for Employment, Labour and Social Affairs, London

Nguyen KH, Wright C, Simpson D, Woods L, Comans T, Sullivan C (2022) Economic evaluation and analyses of hospital-based electronic medical records (EMRs): a scoping review of international literature. NPJ Digit Med 5(1):29. https://doi.org/10.1038/s41746-022-00565-1

Ozair FF, Jamshed N, Sharma A, Aggarwal P (2015) Ethical issues in electronic health records: a general overview. Perspect Clin Res 6(2):73–76. https://doi.org/10.4103/2229-3485.153997

Palanica A, Docktor MJ, Lee A, Fossat Y (2019) Using mobile virtual reality to enhance medical comprehension and satisfaction in patients and their families. Perspect Med Educ 8(2):123–127. https://doi.org/10.1007/s40037-019-0504-7

Powell-Cope G, Nelson AL, Patterson ES (2008) Patient care technology and safety. In: Hughes RG (ed) Patient safety and quality: an evidence-based handbook for nurses. Agency for Healthcare Research and Quality (US), Rockville (MD). Chapter 50. https://www.ncbi.nlm.nih.gov/books/NBK2686/

Ramsay MA (2001) Conflict in the health care workplace. Proc (Bayl Univ Med Cent) 14(2):138–139. https://doi.org/10.1080/08998280.2001.11927749

Reed M, Huang J, Graetz I, Muelly E, Millman A, Lee C (2021) Treatment and follow-up care associated with patient-scheduled primary care telemedicine and in-person visits in a large integrated health system. JAMA Netw Open 4(11):e2132793. https://doi.org/10.1001/jamanetworkopen.2021.32793

Rogers S (2020) How virtual reality could help the travel & tourism industry in the aftermath of the coronavirus outbreak. Forbes. https://www.forbes.com/sites/solrogers/2020/03/18/virtual-reality-and-tourism-whats-already-happening-is-it-the-future/?sh=6c7a1c5928a6

Shen B, Guo J, Yang Y (2019) MedChain: efficient healthcare data sharing via blockchain. Appl Sci 9:1207. https://doi.org/10.3390/app9061207

Snoswell CL, Taylor ML, Comans TA, Smith AC, Gray LC, Caffery LJ (2020) Determining if telehealth can reduce health system costs: scoping review. J Med Internet Res 22(10):e17298. https://doi.org/10.2196/17298

Terashima N (2002) 11—Telesensation, Editor(s): Nobuyoshi Terashima, Intelligent Communication Systems, Academic Press, Pages 127–148, ISBN 9780126853513, https://doi.org/10.1016/B978-012685351-3/50012-3

Thimbleby H (2013) Technology and the future of healthcare. J Public Health Res 2(3):e28. https://doi.org/10.4081/jphr.2013.e28

Tonsaker T, Bartlett G, Trpkov C (2014) Health information on the internet: gold mine or minefield? Can Fam Physician 60(5):407–408

Tyan I, Guevara-Plaza A, Yagüe MI (2021) The benefits of blockchain technology for medical tourism. Sustainability 13:12448. https://doi.org/10.3390/su132212448

Ventola CL (2014a) Socialmedia and health care professionals: benefits, risks, and best practices. P T 39(7):491–520

Ventola CL (2014b) Medical applications for 3D printing: current and projected uses. P T 39(10):704–711

Vijayan V, Connolly JP, Condell J, McKelvey N, Gardiner P (2021) Review of wearable devices and data collection considerations for connected health. Sensors (Basel). 21(16):5589. https://doi.org/10.3390/s21165589

Wong BKM, Hazley SA S'a (2021) The future of health tourism in the industrial revolution 4.0 era. J Tour Futures 7(2):267–272., Emerald Publishing Limited, ISSN 2055-5911. https://doi.org/10.1108/JTF-01-2020-0006

Zemmar A, Lozano AM, Nelson BJ (2020) The rise of robots in surgical environments during COVID-19. Nat Mach Intell 2:566–572. https://doi.org/10.1038/s42256-020-00238-2

Zhang M, Davies TC, Xie S (2013) Effectiveness of robot-assisted therapy on ankle rehabilitation—a systematic review. J Neuroeng Rehabil 10:30. https://doi.org/10.1186/1743-0003-10-30

Chapter 13
Medical Tourism Overview

Medical Tourism: Consequences for Public Health

Kesha Bhadiyadra, Sushman Sharma, Bhupinder Chaudhary, B. S. Dhillon, and Nishi Gandhi

Abstract Medical tourism happens when people travel to a different country to get therapeutic, surgical, or dental services. Medical tourists may visit developing or developed nations for the most prevalent types of medical reasons. Medical tourism, a rapidly growing component of the healthcare industry, has unique issues for both public health and clinical medicine. Patient travels for medical tourism services may have an impact, depending on whether nations such as India, Mexico, Singapore, Malaysia, Thailand, Cuba, or Brazil import medical tourism services. Medical tourists, particularly overseas travelers, have unique health concerns that should be addressed in addition to following standard travel health precautions. People suffering from follow-up care during treatment, language problems, a shortage of staff, hospital accreditation, and poor service quality are some of the consequences that may affect the public during medical care. Some of these requirements, such as follow-up care after treatment and correct paperwork, include the need for appropriate post-procedure care as well as the necessity to ensure that present medical issues have stabilized enough for travel.

Keywords Globalization · Medical Tourism · Consequences · Barriers to growth

---

K. Bhadiyadra (✉) · S. Sharma
Department of Hospital Management, Hemchandracharya North Gujarat University, Patan, Gujarat, India

B. Chaudhary
Department of Hospital Management and Hospice Studies, Jamia Millia Islamia, New Delhi, India

B. S. Dhillon
Hospital Administration, PGIMS Rohtak, Rohtak, Haryana, India

N. Gandhi
Sterling Hospital, Vadodara, India

B. Chaudhary et al. (eds.), *Medical Tourism in Developing Countries*,
https://doi.org/10.1007/978-981-99-8909-6_13

13.1 Introduction

Medical tourism occurs when people travel to a different country to get therapeutic, surgical, or dental services (Singh 2020). Treatment may be considered elective, meaning it depends on individual preferences or wants, or it may be considered obligatory, indicating it is necessary to manage a life-threatening condition. In rare situations, the treatment might not be provided or be prohibited in the patients' native country, or it might be optionally quicker or less expensive overseas (Cosario 2018). It is not uncommon for people to travel abroad in pursuit of improved health and well-being. In the late nineteenth century, patients would travel to other countries like Europe and America for medical procedures and diagnostics because of the lack of facilities available in their own countries (Horowitz et al. 2007). Although traveling for medical care is an old notion, the current concept of health tourism has just emerged in the last 10–15 years. What has changed in the twenty-first century is that individuals are traveling further away, to poorer countries, for invasive and high-tech medical care (Wong and Mun 2014). The following displays depict medical tourism evaluation (Fig. 13.1):

India has long been a popular medical tourism destination. It has developed the most significant international location for medical tourism. It is regarded as a recognized centre for healthcare tourism, particularly for the nearby nations. International patients come from both developed and poor countries. Travel to India for cost-effective access to top-notch healthcare services at the most cutting-edge medical facilities (Lunt et al. 2013; Kelley 2013). In 2012, the worldwide medical tourism industry was valued at USD 10.2 billion, and it is predicted to increase at a 13% CAGR (Compound Annual Growth Rate) between 2022 and 2031, reaching USD 10.4 billion in 2021. According to transparency market research, the medical

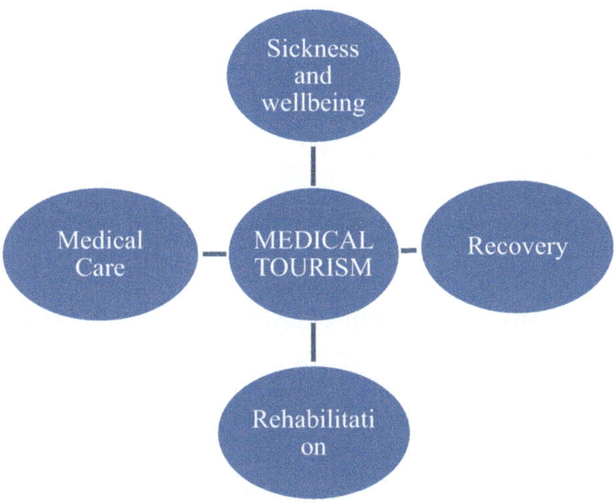

Fig. 13.1 Evaluation of medical tourism services. (Self-made)

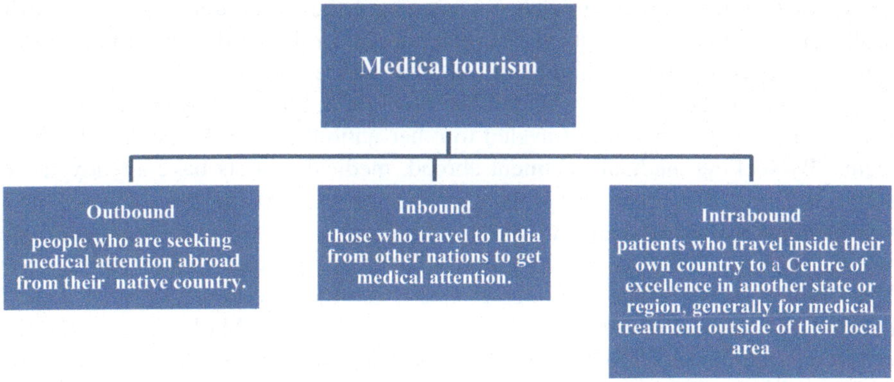

Fig. 13.2 Categories of medical tourism (Asia and Asia 2014; Chen and Wilson 2013)

tourism industry will reach $72.8 billion by 2031, growing at a CAGR of 13.0% between 2021 and 2031 (Transparency Market Research 2022).

13.2 Categories of Medical Tourism Worldwide

The process of traveling to other countries where medical care is available is known as medical tourism. Medical tourism is classified into three types: Outbound, Inbound, and Intrabound (Domestic) (Fig. 13.2).

Medical tourism creates markets both nationally and internationally. Both local and foreign travelers will be medical tourism clients.

13.3 International Medical Tourism Scenario

It is known as "medical tourism" or "health tourism" since it associations travel and healthcare. Traveling abroad to receive medical care is an action that supports the patient's health. Sophisticated remedies for common health conditions are provided in the industry of medical tourism, including check-ups (Malhotra and Dave 2022). The industry of medical tourism globally has experienced rapid expansion and provides a variety of services. Medical tourists seek out treatments that are of the highest caliber and are reasonably priced. The world's export of healthcare services has been able to increase tremendously as the number of individuals using these services is noticeably rising (Kumaran and Reddy 2020). Since more individuals are utilizing healthcare services, the medical industry's ability to export these services globally has been able to expand dramatically. Many people around the world are now able to access healthcare thanks to the trend of choosing healthcare facilities in other affordable locations. The large influx of patients is due to both the rising charge of health treatment in rich countries and the availability of high-quality healthcare at far reduced costs in rising countries. In the predictable future, more patients from across borders are expected (Horowitz et al. 2014).

According to the UNWTO (United Nations World Tourism Organization), more than 14 million persons have traveled to other nations to receive healthcare treatments. By seeking medical treatment abroad, medical tourists have already saved between 30 and 90% of the cost of their procedures. In 2020, the worldwide medical tourism market was esteemed at USD 11.56 billion, and it was expected to increase at a CAGR of 21.1% between 2021 and 2028. It is estimated that it will be USD 53.51 billion in 2028. The total market size is estimated to be between 21 and 53 billion USD, with a 20–25% growth rate (Medical Tourism Market 2022). The list of top international locations for medical tourism now includes Asia as one of the most notable participants. The major healthcare service providers in the Asian region include India, Malaysia, Singapore, and Thailand. Thailand is widely regarded as the most popular Asian destination for cosmetic surgery among Europeans. India and Singapore are known for complicated procedures. India has a cost advantage over Singapore, which has a technological edge (Ile 2017).

Medical tourism has mostly evolved as a result of globalization. The world has no boundaries, there is fierce rivalry, and the environment is changing, making it difficult for both medical tourism suppliers and customers (Helble 2011). The number of people seeking curative care who can afford it has grown tremendously, and the public health care system is unable to accommodate them (Turner 2010a). They are prepared to travel to receive better medical attention and specialized treatment that is not offered in their home nation. Many people might not think it is a smart idea to travel abroad on their own to seek medical treatment. They travel to another nation for medical care for a variety of personal reasons. The number of medical tourism operators or facilitators has increased as a result (Lunt et al. 2013) (Fig. 13.3).

International patients receive 100% of their care through medical tourism, with −25% to −30% declines in emigrants seeking care in their home country. Medical travelers account for −30% to -35% of emergency cases and 35–45% of people are medical travelers.

Through the many types of medical facilitators, there is an overview of the patient's approach to finding, acquiring, and recovering from a medical surgery conducted overseas. The consumer's journey to medical tourism is depicted in the diagram, which shows the process of medical tourism globally (Fig. 13.4).

Operators or facilitators in the medical tourism industry have internal control over the market. These middlemen are the only ones capable of keeping the markets. Both medical travelers and provider groups are significant sources of momentum that have an internal impact on the industry. No less than a complicated network or integrated system is medical tourism. It consists of internal elements as well as outside forces. Medical travelers and provider groups can get in touch with each other directly or through middlemen. The ecology of medical tourism is made up of five key elements (Majeed and Lu 2017; Omisore and Agbabiaka 2016) (Table 13.1). The system of medical tourism is displayed in the following figure (Fig. 13.5):

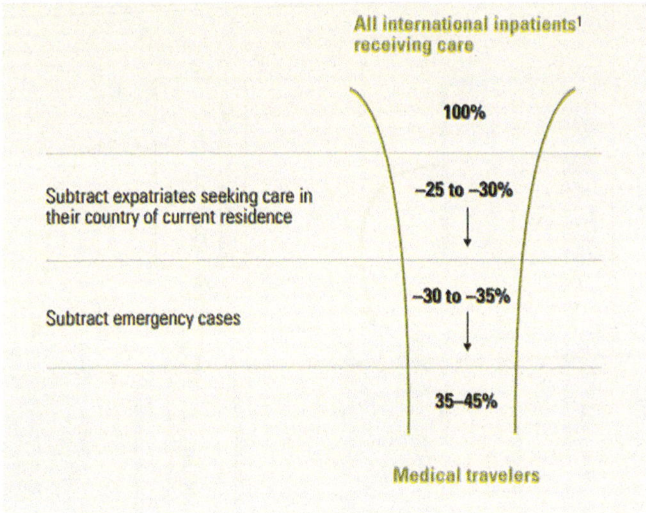

Fig. 13.3 International patients getting care (Ehrbeck et al. 2008)

13.4 National Medical Tourism Scenario

According to the Association of Medical Tourism (MTA), over 50 countries worldwide are encouraging the expansion of health tourism. Various ministries, economic development secretariats, and many more divisions are collaborating on medical tourism. They are going to great lengths to advertise their city, state, or country as a destination for health tourism. The industry of health tourism is influenced to some extent by both the governmental and private sectors (Medical Tourism Association 2022).

The rise of Indian health tourism is primarily the responsibility of the corporate sector. The Ministry of Tourism of the Government of India is largely responsible for supporting marketing and promotions that are essential in the main market. The Indian government has made numerous efforts to market India as a global destination for medical tourism (Jindal 2019). The Indian government's ministry of tourism has launched some excellent initiatives to advance and promote medical travel.

The Indian government's mission statement reads, "To market India as a holistic tourism destination offering a variety of niche tourism products for 365 days a year" (Government of India 2022).

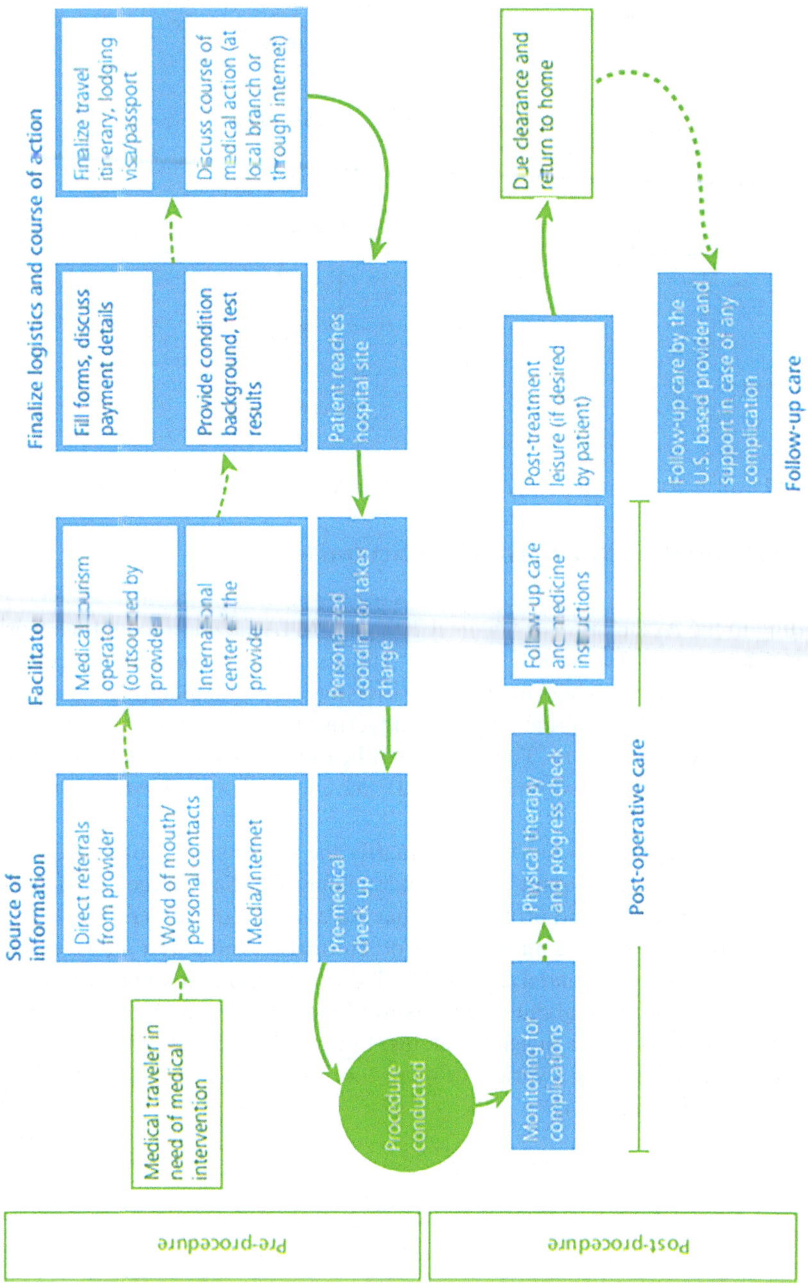

Fig. 13.4 Global medical tourism process (Lisa Purdy 2008)

Table 13.1 Globally market segmentation in medical tourism

Parameters	Section CAGR %	2022 (USD) Billion	2030 (USD) Billion
Global Medical Tourism Market (Medical Tourism Market 2022)	32.5%	10.3	97.9
Top Medical Places World Wide (Shifa International Hospital 2021)	Singapore, Spain, Japan, Dubai, Cost Rica, Abu Dhabi, India, Pakistan, Canada, United Kingdom		
Top Medical Destinations In Asia (Wong and Mun 2014)	India, Thailand, Malaysia, Singapore		
Size of market (Medical Tourism Market 2022)	13.98–53.51 billion approximately		
Number of the cross border (Jadhav et al. 2014)	1.32 million		
Average spending money (health tourism.com 2022)	$ 3000-$ 10,000		
Market growth rate	20%		
Best Hospital For Medical Tourism (2019) (Medical Travel Quality Alliance 2019)	Lebanon, Beirut, Clemenceau Medical Center		
	Turkey, Istanbul, Medical Center of Anadolu		
	Jordan, Amman, The Specialty Hospital		
	Germany, Humberg, Asklepios Klinik Barmbek		
	Thailand, Bangkok, Samitivej Hospital		
	Malaysia, Kuala Lumpur, Medical Center of Prince Court		
	Canada, Toronto, Shouldice Hospital		
	Singapore, Gleneagles Hospital		
	Israel, Loewenstein Rehabilitation Hospital		
	Prague, Proton Therapy Center		

13.5 Medical Visa (MVISA) Concept in Medical Tourism

For those traveling from around the world to India for extended periods to receive specialized medical care, the Indian government has developed the MVISA (Medical Visa). Every medical tourist is given a VISA, which is extendable for an additional year. Anyone receiving this extension may go to India for medical purposes three times per year with a companion, who may be a friend or relative. Only a limited few nations are eligible for visa-on-arrival. Under this arrangement, foreign nationals are permitted a 30-day stay in India for any type of medical operation (Government of India 2022; Amiri 2018).

In 2021, 3,03,526; in 2020, 1,82,945; in 2019, 6, 97,453; and in 2018, 64,0798 foreign tourists visited India on medical visas (Figs. 13.6 and 13.7).

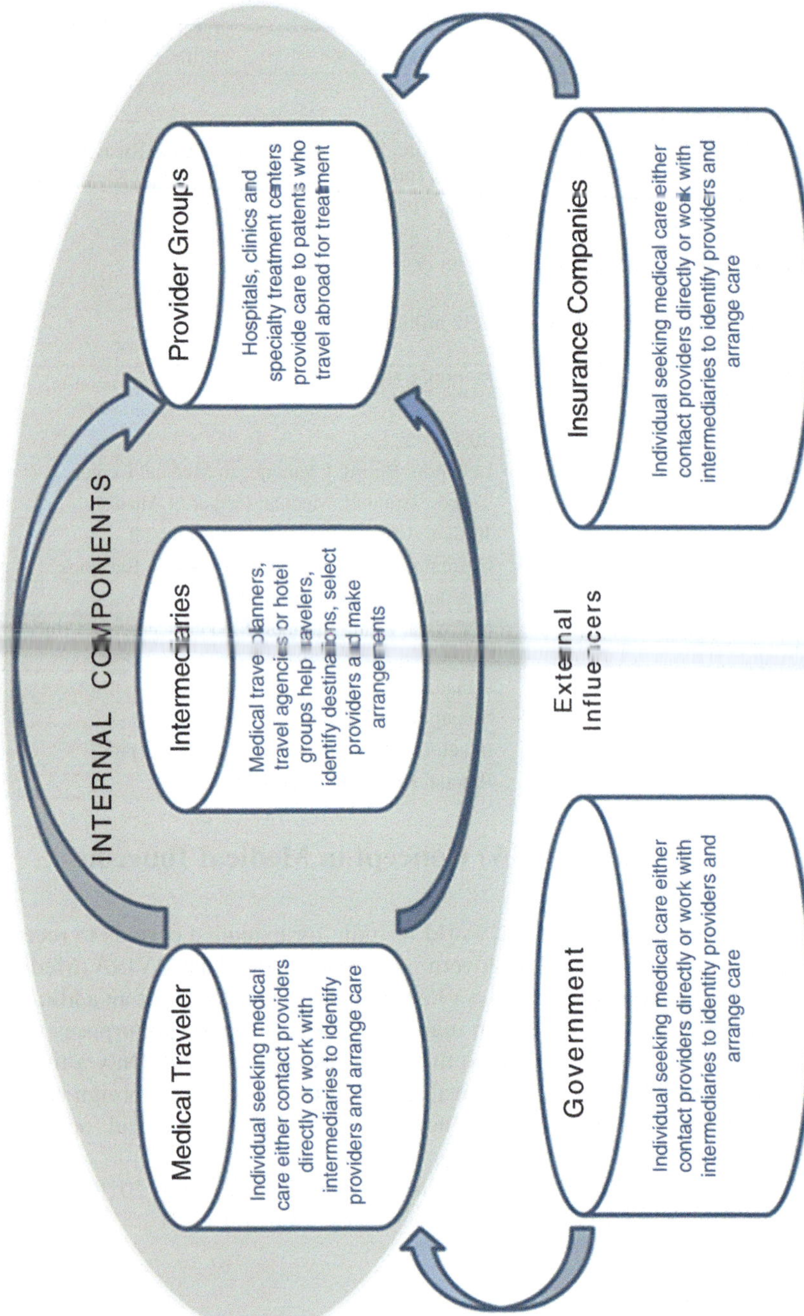

Fig. 13.5 System of medical tourism (Turner 2010b)

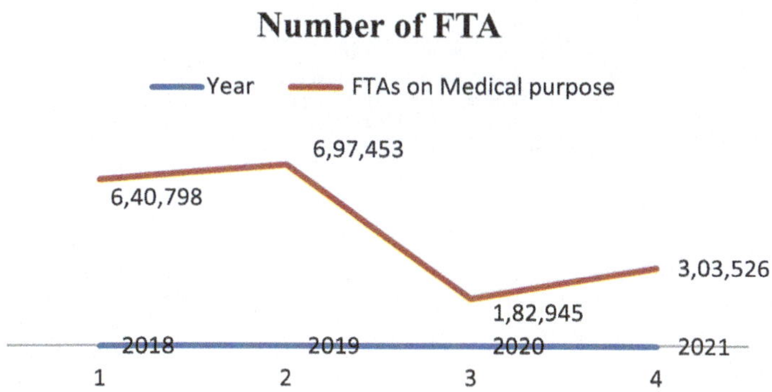

Fig. 13.6 Number of foreign tourists arrival in India on medical visa (Medical Tourism 2022)

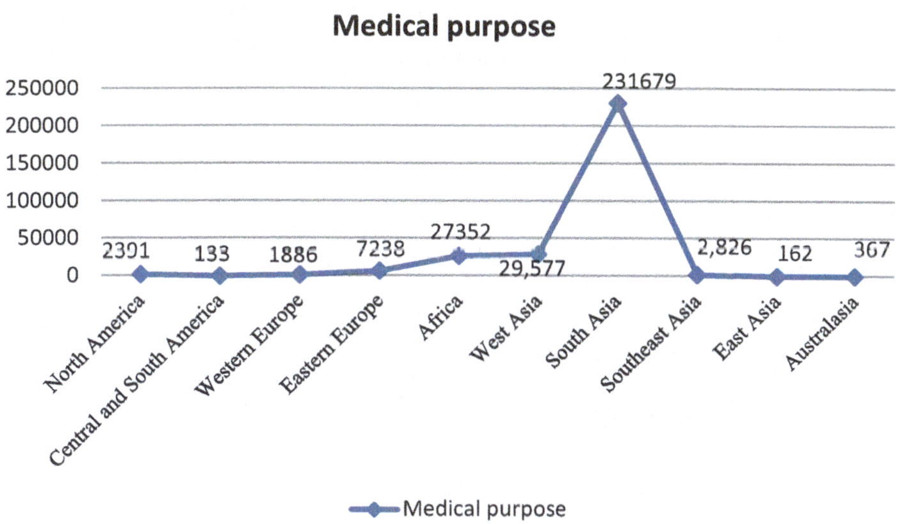

Fig. 13.7 Region-wise foreign tourist arrivals in India on medical purpose (Ministry of Tourism Government of India 2022)

13.6 Medical Tourism: Consequences for Public Health

13.6.1 Hospital Image Issue

Hospital brand image is a very important part of medical tourism because if a hospital holds a market position good, then it has an impact on the patient decision-making process when choosing a hospital (Cham et al. 2016). The patients from other countries had a negative perception of developing nations that predominated in their minds. This makes patients question the sanitation and hygiene of the

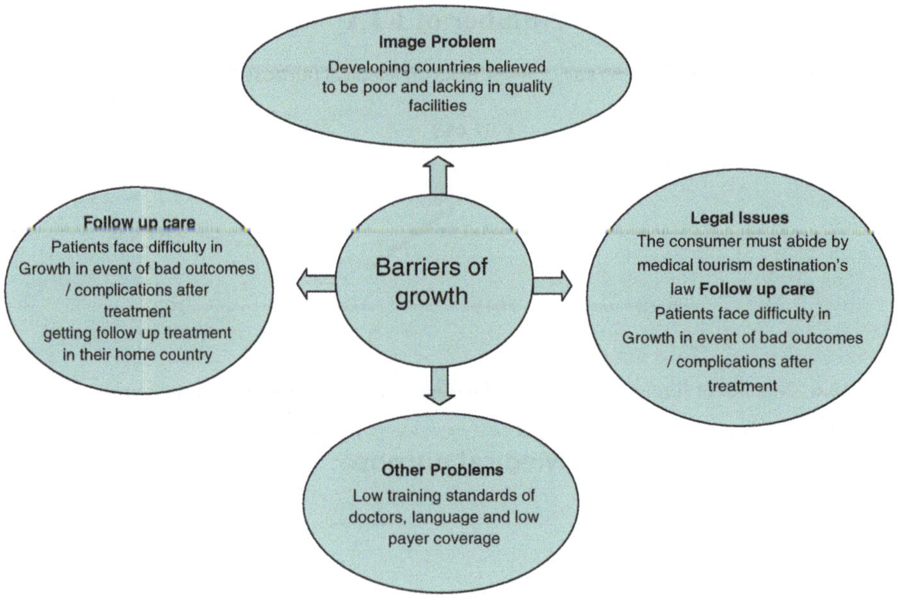

Fig. 13.8 Medical tourism: barriers to growth (Rokni et al. 2017; Shailesh 2016)

facility. Developed nations have health concerns. Many patients stay away from such undeveloped nations because of their negative implications (Burns 2015).

13.6.2 Follow-up Care

After receiving medical treatment in India, patients are discharged, but there is not sufficient follow-up care provided. Even getting in touch with the medical professionals who treated the patients is challenging. Medical tourism companies rarely take the time to get in touch with such patients to get feedback on their posttreatment care. The rise of medical tourism is being hampered by several challenges, which must be resolved. India is currently up against fierce competition from nations like Thailand, Singapore, and Malaysia (Oberoi and Kansra 2019) (Fig. 13.8).

13.6.3 Legal Considerations

Visitors and patients must adhere to the laws of the nation in which the hospital is located. Patients will receive service guarantees as a result (Wahed 2015).

13.6.4 Cultural and Verbal Communication Problems

Patients and visitors may find it easier and more convenient if these cultural and verbal barriers are removed. India has a wide variety of languages as well as beliefs, values, and cultures (Alsarayreh and Matarneh 2013). The experience in the poor world, where the culture shock alone can be distressing, is a long way from the comfort of undergoing a major surgery close to home with family by your side. When traveling so far from home to an unfamiliar location, people often feel apprehensive. One of the biggest challenges is building strong customer relationships and interacting with patients and their families (Almutairi et al. 2020).

13.6.5 Shortage of Staff

The characteristics of each country's national healthcare system will undoubtedly determine the overall medical travel demand. Additionally, those qualities will determine how medical tourism affects the national healthcare system. The policy in this area will eventually be impacted by the dual relationship between medical tourism and the healthcare system. Additionally, identifying labor shortages, particularly in specific medical specialities or geographical locations, is crucial (Whitmore 2015). Over the next decade, one of the most critical challenges confronting the health sector will be the aging population (Age Platform Europe 2018; European Union 2020). In the late 2000s, there were significant worries about anticipated doctor shortages brought on by an aging population and an aging medical profession (European Union 2020).

Many countries are concerned about the general practitioner shortage, especially in rural and remote areas. Many countries still struggle to attract enough medical students to fill unfilled spots for general practitioner training (Radovcic and Nola 2018).

13.6.6 Waiting Time in Medical Tourism

The waiting period is the time that elapses between the time the patient decides to a process and his name is located on a waiting list and when they receive the service for which they are waiting. Long wait times are typically caused by disorganized service, a shortage of healthcare staff, and a lack of physician collaboration. Emergencies, which must be given priority over urgent patients, are mostly to blame for variances in waiting times (Sasirekha and Sankar 2022). During the busiest vacation times, seasonal variation in capacity is one factor. Because of the seasonal reduction in services, waiting times increase. The accessibility of health professionals and resources, including healthcare, is another crucial factor (medhalt 2017).

13.6.7 Issues of Accreditations in Medical Tourism

Accreditation is defined in the perspective of medical tourism as "the action or process of officially recognizing someone as having status or being qualified to do a particular activity." The Joint Commission International (JCI) is regarded as the industry benchmark for healthcare worldwide. JCI's primary duties include measuring, identifying, and disseminating to the globe the best practices in patient safety and quality. It offers direction and aids healthcare organizations with a creative fix. It aids healthcare organizations in various environments in enhancing performance and results. Being JCI accredited and certified nowadays is equivalent to receiving the gold seal of approval. In total, 882 organizations have received JCI accreditation globally (Joint Commission International 2022).

International certification is a crucial step in ensuring that hospitals are accessible worldwide. This would subsequently draw clients from throughout the world. The Joint Commission accreditation for hospital organizations has a global division called Joint Commission worldwide. Similar to this, the United Kingdom has an accreditation program called the Health Quality Service. A National Accreditation Body For Hospitals (NABH) and healthcare has been established in India (Radovcic and Nola 2018).

13.6.8 Concerns Surrounding Service Delivery Competency and Service Quality

Mobile tourists are concerned about the quality of healthcare services as well as medical experts' certification and skills. The extreme lack of skilled professional "caregivers" is even the main issue. The problem is made worse by the fact that the majority of patients and their families lack the expertise necessary to evaluate the level of quality and complexity of the variables at play. The hospital must concentrate on indicators to communicate various aspects of care and therapy. It is critical to address people's negative perceptions of populations, bureaucracy, and sanitation. (The Indian of Tourism and Travel Management Institute 2011).

13.6.9 Importance of Health Insurance in Medical Tourism

People are becoming more globally mobile in a globalized environment. Uninsured individuals may face major penalties if they do not obtain coverage. There could be issues such as receiving less preventive care and delayed care, which could lead to very serious illnesses requiring advanced treatment. These uninsured individuals may also face substantial financial consequences. There may be a variety of reasons for failing to obtain insurance. The main reasons for this can be numerous;

sometimes they are unaware that they would rather pay the fees, and a few of them attempt to obtain coverage but are unable to do so because the coverage is too expensive (Radovcic and Nola 2018; Najar 2022).

These are the obstacles to growth in medical tourism, as well as the consequences for the public.

References

Age Platform Europe (2018) Human rights do not diminish with age' A global awareness-raising campaign against ageism. [Online]. Available: https://www.age-platform.eu/publications/ageing-europe-looking-lives-older-people-eu-eurostat-2019-report

Almutairi AG, Al Mashrafi S, Al Kalbani T (2020) Implications of language barriers for healthcare: a systematic review 1 1. Oman Med J 35:2. https://doi.org/10.5001/omj.2020.40

Alsarayreh MN, Matarneh A (2013) "Communication problems among tourists and community form the tourist perspective "A case study form Karak governorate"," *research gate*, no. January, 2013

Amiri M (2018) Medical tourism in India current scenario. Res Gate. no. March 2017

Asia S, Asia E (2014) "Medical Tourism in India * Manpreet Kaur * Assistant Professor, Guru Gobind Singh College for Women, Sec 26, Chandigarh t Keywords : Health tourism, Medical tourism, Medical care," pp. 64–66

Burns LR (2015) "Medical tourism opportunities and challenges : illustration from US–India trade *," no. April, doi: https://doi.org/10.1179/2047971914Y.0000000091

Cesario SK (2018) Implications of medical tourism. Nurs Womens Health 22(3):269–273. https://doi.org/10.1016/j.nwh.2018.03.008

Cham TH, Lim YM, Aik NC, Guan A, Tay M (2016) Antecedents of hospital brand image and the relationships with medical tourists' behavioural intention. no. November, doi: https://doi.org/10.1108/IJPHM-02-2016-0012

Chen LH, Wilson ME (2013) The globalization of healthcare: implications of medical tourism for the infectious disease clinician. 57:1752–1759. https://doi.org/10.1093/CID/cit540

Ehrbeck T, Guevara C, Mango PD (2008) Mapping the market for medical travel. Health Care (Don Mills). [Online]. Available: https://www.lindsayresnick.com/Resource_Links/MedicalTravel.pdf

European Union (2020) Ageing Europe. [Online]. Available: https://ec.europa.eu/eurostat/documents/3217494/11478057/KS-02-20-655-ENN. pdf/9b09606c-d4e8-4c33-63d2-3b20d5c19c91?t=1604055531000

European Union (2020) Health at a Glance: Europe. [Online]. Available: https://health.ec.europa.eu/system/files/2020-12/2020_healthatglance_rep_en_0.pdf

Government of India (2022) Wellness & Medical Tourism _ Ministry Of Tourism _ Government of India. [Online]. Available: https://tourism.gov.in/wellness-medical-tourism#:~:text=The Ministry of Tourism has also been eligible for the MDA

"Medical tourism statistics and facts _ health-tourism," (2022). https://www.health-tourism.com/medical-tourism/statistics/

Helble M (2011) The movement of patients across borders : challenges and opportunities for public health. *world Heal. Organ.*, no. July 2010, pp. 68–72, , doi: https://doi.org/10.2471/BLT.10.076612

Horowitz MD, Rosensweig JA, Jones CA (2007) Medical tourism_ globalization of the healthcare marketplace—PMC. [Online]. Available: https://www.ncbi.nlm.nih.gov/pmc/articles/PMC2234298/?report=printable

Horowitz MD, Rosensweig JA, Jones CA. "Medical tourism: globalization of the healthcare marketplace," no. May 2014, 2007, [Online]. Available: https://www.ncbi.nlm.nih.gov/pmc/articles/PMC2234298/

Ile FL (2017) Medical tourism market trends—an exploratory research. *Proc. 11th Int. Conf. Bus. Excell.*, no. August, doi: https://doi.org/10.1515/picbe-2017-0114

Jadhav S, Yeravdekar R, Kulkarni M (2014) Cross-border healthcare access in South Asian Countries : learnings for sustainable healthcare tourism in India. Procedia - Soc Behav Sci 157:109–117. https://doi.org/10.1016/j.sbspro.2014.11.014

Jindal P (2019) Medical tourism in India : an analysis. Int J Innov Technol Explor Eng 7:465–471

Joint Commission International (2022) JCI-Accredited Organizations _ Joint Commission International. [Online]. Available: file:///C:/Users/king/Desktop/New folder (2)/JCI-Accredited Organizations _ Joint Commission International.html

Kelley E (2013) Medical tourism. *World Heal Organ*, no. October, [Online]. Available: https://www.researchgate.net/publication/259486257_Medical_Tourism_in_Asia_Thailand_Singapore_Malaysia_and_India/link/5487aac80cf2ef34478ecceb/download

Kumaran MMSS, Reddy C (2020) Medical tourism: history, global scenario and Indian perspectives. Med Tour

Lisa Purdy MF (2008) Evolving medical tourism in Canada exploring a new frontier. Deloitte. https://www2.deloitte.com/content/dam/Deloitte/ca/Documents/life-sciences-health-care/ca-en-health-care-life-sciences-evolving-medical-tourism-exploring-a-new-frontier.pdf

Lunt N, Smith R, Exworthy M, Stephen T, Horsfall D, Mannion R (2013) Medical tourism: treatments, markets and health system implications: scoping review. pp. 1–55, [Online]. Available: https://www.oecd.org/els/health-systems/48723982.pdf

Majeed S, Lu C (2017) Changing preferences, moving places and third party administrators: a scoping review of medical tourism trends (1990-2016). J Tour Cult Territ Dev:56–83

Malhotra N, Dave K (2022) An assessment of competitiveness of medical tourism industry in India : a case of Delhi NCR. Int J Glob Bus Compet 17(2):215–228. https://doi.org/10.1007/s42943-022-00060-0

medhalt (2017) Long waiting times_ medical tourism can save you _ MedHalt Blog. https://www.medhalt.com/blog/long-waiting-time-medical-tourism

Medical Tourism (2022) Government of India Ministry of Tourism

Medical Tourism Association (2022) "Medical Tourism Association _ a global platform for the healthcare ecosystem,". [Online]. Available: https://www.medicaltourismassociation.com/

Medical Tourism Market (2022) Medical tourism market size, growth _ research report [2028]. [Online]. Available: https://www.fortunebusinessinsights.com/industry-reports/medical-tourism-market-100681

Medical Travel Quality Alliance (2019) "MTQUA Top 10 world's best hospitals for medical TouristsTM for 2019 – World's Best Hospitals,". https://worldsbesthospitals.net/worlds-best/

Ministry of Tourism Government of India (2022) "India tourism statistics 2022," [Online]. Available: https://tourism.gov.in/sites/default/files/2022-09/India Tourism Statistics 2022%28English%29.pdf

Najar PA (2022) Medical tourism and health insurance are image constructs of destination: a study of India," no. September

Oberoi S, Kansra P (2019) Factors influencing medical tourism in India: a critical review. Res Gate., no. July

Omisore HI, Agbabiaka EO (2016) Factors influencing patronage of medical tourism in metropolitan Lagos, Nigeria. Int J Sci Technol Res 5:04

Radovcic Z, Nola IA (2018) Medical tourism globe-trotting : Features, impacts, and risks. Int J Healthc Manag:1–7. https://doi.org/10.1080/20479700.2018.1428388

Rokni L, Avci T, Park SH (2017) Barriers of developing medical tourism in a destination: a case of South Korea. 46(7):930–937, [Online]. Available: https://www.ncbi.nlm.nih.gov/pmc/articles/PMC5563875/pdf/IJPH-46-930.pdf

Sasirekha K, Sankar P (2022) A study on the challenges and outlooks of medical tourism in india with reference to chennai region. 6(5). [Online]. Available: https://journalppw.com/index.php/jpsp/article/view/8438/5507

Shailesh K (2016) Prospects of medical tourism in India. [Online]. Available: https://shodhganga.inflibnet.ac.in/handle/10603/78276

Shifa International Hospital (2021) Top 10 countries for medical tourism in 2021. https://shifainternationalpatients.com/blog/medical-tourism-in-2021/

Singh S (2020) Medical tourism in India. no. May , doi: https://doi.org/10.2139/ssrn.3405227

The Indian of Tourism and Travel Management Institute (2011) A study of problems and challenges faced by medical tourists visiting India. [Online]. Available: https://tourism.gov.in/sites/default/files/2020-04/Med.pdf

Transparency Market Research (2022) "Medical Tourism Market _ Global Analysis Report 2031," [Online]. Available: https://www.transparencymarketresearch.com/medical-tourism.html

Turner L (2010a) medical tourism' and the global marketplace in health services : u. s. patients, international hospitals, and the search for affordable health care. Int J Health Serv 40(3):443–467. https://doi.org/10.2190/HS.40.3.d

Turner L (2010b) 'medical Tourism' and the global marketplace in health services: U.S. Patients, International Hospitals, and the search for affordable health care. Natl Libr Med 40(3):443–467. https://doi.org/10.2190/HS.40.3.d

Wahed H (2015) Ethical and legal issues in medical tourism. Res Gate., no. August. https://doi.org/10.31436/iiumlj.v23i2.130

Whitmore R (2015) Medical tourism's impacts on health worker migration in the Caribbean: Five examples and their implications for global justice. researchgate., no. May. https://doi.org/10.3402/gha.v8.27348

Wong B, Mun K (2014) Medical tourism in Asia : Thailand, Singapore, Malaysia, and India. no. July 2012, , [Online]. Available: https://www.researchgate.net/publication/259186257_Medical_Tourism_in_Asia_Thailand_Singapore_Malaysia_and_India/link/5487aac80cf2ef34478ecceb/download

Chapter 14
Regulatory Policies and Medical Ethics of Medical Tourism in Developing Countries

Sursinh Barad, Kesha Bhadiyadra, Sushman Sharma, and Bhupinder Chaudhary

Abstract Medical tourism (also called medical travel or health tourism) refers to the practice of traveling across international borders to obtain healthcare. The main motivation that attracts foreign patients is the low cost of medical treatment. Other factors included excellent medical facilities and cultural and religious similarities. Medical tourism also helpful for developing country and help to strengthening of health services to developing countries. Therefore, The Ministry of India, Tourism and Government has taken several steps to promote as a Medical and Health Tourism like New category of "Medical Visa" has been introduced, Guidelines for accreditation, FRRO Registration of Medical Patients, The dead body transfer or funeral process for Foreigner. Also developing countries have built regulatory policies, medical ethics, and many acts to help in medical tourism like Transplantation of Human Organ Act, Consumer Protection Act for strengthening of healthcare sector. Accreditation in different segments of the healthcare sector, such as hospitals and laboratories, is also helpful in building trust among patients, improving the quality of care and streamlining processes in the healthcare sector. It also aids in enhancing medical tourism and maintaining medical ethics. This chapter is going to be helpful and provide guidance to Hospital who are going to develop Medical Tourism as well as patients who are going to plan to take medical treatment in developing countries.

Keywords Medical tourism · Transplantation · Accreditation · Regulatory process

S. Barad (✉)
Synergy Superspeciality Hospitals, Rajkot, Gujarat, India

K. Bhadiyadra
HNG University, Patan, Gujarat, India

S. Sharma ·
Department of Hospital Management, Hemchandracharya North Gujarat University, Patan, Gujarat, India

B. Chaudhary
Department of Hospital Management and Hospice Studies, Jamia Millia Islamia, New Delhi, India

B. Chaudhary et al. (eds.), *Medical Tourism in Developing Countries*,
https://doi.org/10.1007/978-981-99-8909-6_14

14.1 Introduction

The last few years witnessed dramatic development in medical tourism, particularly in developing countries. This wave of transformation can be seen from the fact that millions of patients, especially from developed countries travel to places like Malaysia, Thailand, and India for medical procedures and medical treatments (Lunt et al. 2011). Medical tourism has developed due to lower costs in treatment for greater access to quality and recognized medical treatment (Horowitz et al. 2007; Gray and Poland 2008; Ormond 2011). There was a study on the factors that promote medical tourism in Malaysia (Musa et al. 2012). The main motivation that attracts foreign patients was the low cost of medical treatment. Other factors included excellent medical facilities and cultural and religious similarities.

14.1.1 The Meaning of Medical Tourism

Medical tourism (also called medical travel or health tourism) refers to the practice of traveling across international borders to obtain healthcare.[1] Medical tourism has been portrayed as a popular mass culture, which involves patients' international travel to a private hospital to obtain medical care and at the same time enjoy a holiday in the destination country (Crooks et al. 2013; Cohen 2012; Lunt et al. 2011).

14.2 Regulatory Policies by Govt. of India

The Ministry of Tourism has taken several steps to promote India as a Medical and Health Tourism Destination, which are as follows:

(a) The Confederation of Indian Industry, on advice from government, has prepared a guide on select Indian hospitals of the country for health tourism purposes. It has been placed on the website of the Ministry of Tourism, i.e., www.incredibleindia.org for wider publicity.
(b) Indian Healthcare Federation, a non-governmental organization affiliated with medical and health tourism has been specifically promoted at various international platforms such as World Travel Mart, London, and ITP Berlin. Similarly, website on tourism has been produced by the Ministry of Tourism and has been widely circulated for publicity in target markets.
(c) New category of "Medical Visa" has been introduced, which can be given for specific purpose to foreign tourists coming to India for medical treatment. The

[1] "Medical Tourism-What is Medical Tourism", accessed March 3, 2013, www.news-medical.net/health/Medical-Tourism-What-is-Medical-ourism.aspx.

Government of India issues medical visa to every medical tourist and this visa can also be extended for over a year. This extended time of visa enables the patients to visit three times a year and these patients can also be accompanied by a relative or friend at the time of medical tour to India.

(d) Guidelines for accreditation of allopathic, Ayurvedic, and Panchakarma centers have been circulated to all state governments for implementation. These have been placed on the website of Ministry of Tourism, i.e., www.incredibleindia.org for wider publicity.

(e) Yoga/Ayurveda/wellness has been promoted over the last 2 years in the print, electronic, internet, and outdoor medium under the Ministry of Tourism's "Incredible India Campaign."

(f) Market Development Assistance (MDA) Scheme in the Sector: The Ministry of Tourism has included the promotion of Medical Tourism as a new initiative. The Marketing Development Assistance Scheme (MDA), administered by the Ministry of Tourism, Government of India, provides financial support to approved tourism service providers.

14.2.1 Guidelines for Medical Tourism by the Government

1. To ensure that the hospital in India to be visited is licensed or not. The hospital must be recognized by a commission, any national or international healthcare auditing agency like National Accreditation Board for Hospitals and Healthcare Providers (NABH) by QCI or by a Joint Commission International (JCI).
2. To check the cost and quality of patient care.
3. To get all possible details about the doctors before selecting them that includes their credentials, achievements, and qualifications. It is advisable to search for hospital credentials on the internet.
4. It is crucial to know about treatment procedure well in order to have realistic expectations from the surgery. Patients should also be clear about post-operative care, recovery period, and physical therapy.
5. Make sure to meet the treating doctor in person before undergoing any procedure. Personal examination such as diagnostic tests of a patient is first performed by the majority of hospitals to assess the possibility of conducting procedure.
6. Make sure to carry all the essential documents along with their copies by the patient and store the originals in a safe place.
7. To carry all the health records and medical reports that are relevant to the medical procedure or surgery such as prescriptions, X-rays, health histories, immunization records, MRIs, and photographs.
8. Passport and visa required along with debit cards, credit cards, and travelers check. Also bring one or two major debit and credit cards, and some local currency.

Make sure to carry your driver's license that remains valid till the time you are traveling.[2]

14.2.2 *Procedure for Visa*

14.2.2.1 Medical Visa

The Government of India recognizes and categorizes medical tourism as niche tourism. The government support toward medical tourism is evident by the introduction of a special category of visa catering to such a segment in the form of medical visa. A new category of "medical visa" has been introduced, which can be given for specific purpose to foreign tourist to India for medical treatment. The Government of India issues a medical visa to every medical tourist; this visa can also be extended for over a year. This extended time of visa enables the patients to visit three times a year and these patients can also be accompanied by a relative or friend at the time of a medical tour to developing countries.

The hospital has to send an invitation letter or request letter to Indian Embassy of the related country for permission of medical visa with mention of proper patient details, attendant (caretaker) details with passport number, disease name or provisional diagnosis, treatment plan of care, and approximate duration of stay for treatment or surgery in country on the bases of this types of request embassy has granted the medical visa. If a foreigner visits on a tourist visa or any normal visa and suddenly requires emergency hospitalization, they must transfer their visa to a medical visa.

Medical Visa is valid up to a period of 1 year or the period of treatment whichever is lesser. However, the prescribed period can be extended where required for another year by the Ministry of Health Affairs on the recommendation of Foreign Regional Registration Offices and State Governments. In ordinary circumstances, only a maximum of three entries are permissible, the only exception to this being emergency cases where special permission is to be sought by Foreign Regional Registration Offices or State Governments. A maximum of two attendants/family members including the spouse can also apply for an MX visa. Further impetus was the launch of an e-visa facility for 43 countries in relation to medical tourism.

The conditions for grant of this kind of visa has been specifically laid down to ensure people who are immigrating to India are doing so in pursuance of receiving treatment. The person is to possess a requisite medical record stating recommendation or reference of specialized treatment that is sought based on preliminary medical treatment in the home country; second, the treatment should be significant in character, for example, neurosurgery, heart surgery, joint replacement, or plastic surgery.

---

[2] https://www.ima-india.org/ima/left-side-bar.php?pid=503#:~:text=The%20government%20of%20India%20issues,of%20medical%20tour%20to%20India

The development of medical visa casts a duty upon hospitals and healthcare centers to not entertain tourists who seek medical treatment but have not applied for the medical visa and are visiting under the general tourist visa.

14.2.2.2 Conversion of Visas

Foreign nationals on a business visa or an employment visa in India can apply to convert their visas to a medical visa if they fall ill, are unable to travel, and require specialized medical treatment in India. A change of visa may be required if the individual falls out of status, for example, if he is on an employment visa and the visa expires. Such individuals will be granted medical visa provided they fulfill all the criteria to be eligible for a medical visa and can provide a medical certificate from a government or government-recognized hospital. In such cases, qualifying members of the principal applicant could apply for a medical attendant visa (MX), which is usually granted to co-terminate with the principle applicant's medical visa. The medical visa and MXV will bear an endorsement stating that employment or business is not permitted.

Medical visa is a result of the government's recognition of the importance of medical tourism in India. It enables individuals to enter the country to procure medical treatment on valid visas.[3]

14.2.3 FRRO Registration of Medical Patient by Hospital

Hospital has to inform District Collector Office and reregister under FRRO (Foreign Reginal Registration Officers FFRO) and fill the Form "C."

[3] https://legalformatsindia.com/the-legal-regime-of-medical-tourism-in-india/

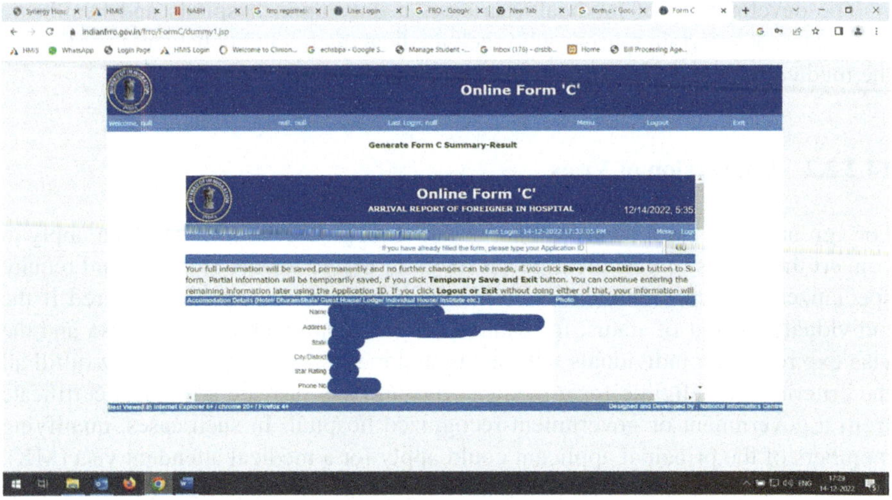

The application is aim to build centralized online registration for foreigners who come for medical treatment www.indiaFRRO/Form"C."[4]

For NRIs (non-residents of India) or OCI (overseas citizens of India) holders, there is no need for a medical visa; they can directly come for treatment on a routine visa.

14.2.4 The Dead Body Transfer or Funeral Process for Foreigner

If a foreigner dies during treatment, legal procedures and decision-related rights are transferred to the next of kin, relative(s), or family member(s) of the deceased, who may wish to transport the body to their country for funeral purposes or have the funeral near the current country.

In both cases, "NOC" is required from local police station.

If the next of kin, relative(s), or family member(s) of the deceased wish have the funeral near the hospital, the hospital must provide a Death Certificate with a no objection certificate (NOC) from the Local Police Station. They also need to inform the Embassy, and, in accordance with religious needs, the kin, relative(s), or family member(s) can proceed with the funeral process.

Transportation of dead bodies from patient country:

If the next of kin relative(s)/family member of the deceased wish to transport the dead body to patient's own country for funeral purposes, the consulate issues a **"No Objection Certificate"** in this regard.

---

[4] https://indianfrro.gov.in/frro/FormC

14.2.4.1 Requirements

Death certificate from hospital with cause of death.

Burial/cremation permit.

- Letter from local police department—NOC (no objection certificate).
- Letter from public health office indicating "no communicable disease."
- Embalming certificate, coroners out of province certificate, name, address, telephone number, etc. of the consignee.
- NOC from embassy.
- Flight details.[5]

14.2.5 *Organ Transplant of Foreign Patients*

Transplantation of Human Organ Act (THOA) 1994 was enacted to provide a system of removal, storage, and transplantation of human organs for therapeutic purposes and for the prevention of commercial dealing in human organs. Since organ and tissue transplants are so difficult to obtain owing to long waiting lists, many patients tend to seek foreign options and engage in medical tourism for organ transplants.

ACT and RULES under THOA:

- Transplantation of Human Organs and Tissues Rules in India, 2014
- THOA amendment in India 2011
- Transplantation of Human Organs (amendment) Rules in India, 2008
- THO Rules, 1995 in India (original rules)
- THOA 1994
- THOTA 1994 with 2011 amendment and 2014 rules[6]

The national network division of National Organ and Tissue Transplant Organization (NOTTO) would function as the apex center for all India activities of coordination and networking for procurement and distribution of organs and tissues and transplantation in the country.

Also, State Organ and Tissue Transplant Organization (SOTTO) is also involved in state-level regulations.[7]

---

[5] https://www.cgitoronto.gov.in/page/transport-dead-body/

[6] https://notto.gov.in/act-end-rules-of-thoa.htm

[7] https://sotto.nic.in/

14.2.6 Medical Malpractice Laws in India

Medical malpractice laws, such as the Clinical Establishment Act in India, focus on the Consumer Protection Act, 1986 (the "CPA"). There are various laws which are set up under the CPA and are applied by Indian courts when dealing with medical malpractice cases, and the relevant factors are taken into consideration while awarding compensation, among other issues.

14.2.7 Consumer Protection Act

Briefly stated, a "consumer" who hires or avails of any "services" for consideration is entitled under the CPA to sue for any "deficiency in service" (not being services rendered free of cost or of a personal nature) and claim compensation. "Deficiency" is usually construed to mean any fault, imperfection, shortcoming or inadequacy in the quality, nature and manner of performance of any service.

14.2.8 Filing Actions that Can Be Taken under CPA

In case of any malpractice by a doctor or hospital, the aggrieved person can seek recourse through the consumer disputes redressal established under the CPA to establish malpractice and claim compensation.

Depending on the value of the services and/or the compensation claimed, the aggrieved person would have to approach (a) the District Consumer Dispute Redressal Forum (pecuniary limit of up to INR 2,000,000 or approx. USD 40,000); (b) the Consumer Disputes Redressal Commission of each Indian State or province (the "State Commission") (which enjoys pecuniary limit above INR 2,000,000 but up to INR 10,000,000, i.e., between approx. USD 40,000 to 200,000); (c) or the National Consumer Disputes Redressal Commission, New Delhi (the "National Commission") (pecuniary limit of any amount above INR 10,000,000 or approx. USD 200,000).

14.2.9 When there Is a Violation of Duty and Action

Having established the duty and standard of care, the aggrieved patient has to prove that there was a breach of the applicable duty and that the doctor had fallen below the accepted standard of care. The violation of the duty should then be linked to "action," i.e., a link should be established between the act of negligence and the injury suffered by the patient.

Indian courts have applied the "but for" test in order to establish causation. In Geetu Sapra v. B. L. Kapoor Memorial Hospital [(2006) 3 CPJ 1], the "but-for" test was applied to establish that if not for the defective equipment in the hospital, the patient would have not suffered the injury. In Samira Kohli v. Prabha Manchanda [(2008) 2 SCC 1] which deals with "informed consent," the Supreme Court held that a doctor can be held negligent if proper consent is not taken and the failure to take consent is sufficient to determine causation.

14.2.10 Hospitals Could Be Held Liable

In India, corporate hospitals (as opposed to government or village hospitals, which are unlikely to attract medical tourism) have been held liable by applying the tort law principle of" vicarious liability" for any malpractice or "deficiency in service" on the part of the doctors or nurses employed in such hospitals. Indian courts have ruled that a hospital cannot escape liability merely by arguing that it only provides infrastructural facilities and services of nursing and support staff to the consultant doctor and that the hospital cannot perform or recommend an operation on its own [Rekha Gupta v. Bombay Hospital Trust and Another (2003) 2 CPJ 160].

14.2.11 Compensation under the CPA

If it is determined that a doctor or hospital had been negligent, the aggrieved person is entitled to claim damages or compensation under the CPA. While determining the amount of compensation to be awarded under the CPA, Indian courts normally take into consideration the following key factors:

- Pain and suffering endured by the patient (including the duration and intensity) as a result of the negligence of the doctor;
- Loss of earnings or future earnings; and
- Expenses incurred for the medical treatment.

Recently, the National Commission in Kunal Saha v. Sukumar Mukherjee and Others [Original Petition No. 240 of 1999] awarded compensation of INR 13,465,750 (approx. USD 270,000) to the plaintiff, out of which the hospital was directed to pay a sum of INR 4,040,000 (approx. USD 80,800) and the remaining amount by the defendant doctors. The National Commission apportioned liability based on the degree of negligence of each doctor and the hospital. In this case, the hospital was found to be one of the main negligent parties.

14.2.12 Execution Proceedings and Remitting Compensation Abroad

Under Indian law, upon award of final compensation (i.e., all appeal remedies have been exhausted), if the defendant has not voluntarily rendered compensation, the aggrieved party is entitled to commence proceedings to execute the award. In such proceedings, the court is empowered to seize and sell (by public auction) any property belonging to the defendant to ensure that the aggrieved person is paid due compensation. Courts are also empowered to imprison the defendant for any non-payment of the award.

In cases involving foreigners, since the proceedings are in India, a concern relates to actual remittance and receipt of the awarded compensation amount by foreigners abroad. In this regard, it is pertinent to note that India's foreign exchange laws have been substantially liberalized over the years. It is now possible for bankers to rely on court orders to allow the defendants to remit the compensation amount to the aggrieved person abroad.

14.2.13 Criminal Negligence of Doctors

In India, in addition to an action under the CPA, a doctor can also be liable under penal laws for criminal negligence. This happens if such a doctor is shown to have been rash and negligent, resulting in the death of the patient [Section 304A of the Indian Penal Code]. A person convicted under Section 304A may be subject either too simple or rigorous imprisonment for a term of up to 2 years, or with fine, or with both.

India is equipped with skilled professionals, comparatively lower cost of medical treatment, and supported by various government initiatives. These factors are conducive to the development of medical tourism in India. The entire rationale behind medical tourism is driven by cost considerations, safety aspects, ethical practices, credibility, and legal issues arising from medical negligence and malpractice, which are often sidelined. The growth of medical tourism in India, therefore, will be incumbent on the effectiveness of the regulatory framework. This protects the interests and rights of patients and monitors hospitals and healthcare institutions.[8]

[8] https://legalformatsindia.com/the-legal-regime-of-medical-tourism-in-india/

14.2.14 National and International Health Accreditation

National and international healthcare accreditation is the process of certifying a level of quality for healthcare providers and programs across multiple countries. These organizations such as the National Accreditation Board for Hospitals and Healthcare Organizations (NABH), Canadian Council on Health Services Accreditation, Joint Commission International, United Kingdom Accreditation Forum, etc., certify a wide range of healthcare programs such as hospitals, primary care centers, medical transport, and ambulatory care services.[9,10]

Joint Commission International is similar to the Joint Commission in the United States. Both are US-style independent private sector not-for-profit organizations that develop nationally and internationally recognized procedures and standards to help improve patient care and safety. They work with hospitals to help them meet Joint Commission standards for patient care. The different international healthcare accreditation schemes vary in quality, size, cost, intent, and the skill and intensity of their marketing. They also vary in terms of cost to hospitals and healthcare institutions making use of them.[11]

14.3 Ethical Aspect of Medical Tourism

Traveling outside their home country for medical care, medical tourists may encounter unfamiliar ethical and legal issues. While some countries currently presenting themselves as attractive medical tourism destinations provide some form of legal remedies for medical malpractice, these legal avenues may be unappealing to the medical tourist.

If problems arise, patients might not be covered by adequate personal insurance or might be unable to seek compensation via malpractice lawsuits. Hospitals and/or doctors in some countries may be unable to pay the financial damages awarded by a court to a patient who has sued them, owing to the hospital and/or the doctor not possessing appropriate insurance cover and/or medical indemnity.

Since medical tourism is aimed at attracting foreigners, local masses in developing economies do not get equal access to healthcare facilities. The cost of medical services in these countries is sometimes beyond the reach of the local population, resulting in a lack of ethical fairness toward the locals. Also, technologies like stem cell treatment are banned in the USA owing to the unethical perspective from which it is viewed. Hence, the credibility of such a practice is again questionable to a

---

[9] Joint Commission International Accreditation and Certification Web, Joint Commission International, retrieved 19 July 2011

[10] Medical Tourism Magazine, Medical Tourism Association, February 2008

[11] Facts about Joint Commission International. Joint Commission. 2008-12-11. Retrieved 2010-09-15

certain extent. Legal and ethical issues have marred the popularity of medical tourism to a large extent.[12]

However, to its credit, the sector has continued to grow at a steady rate. A prospective medical tourist should also be aware of possible legal issues. There is presently no international legal regulation of medical tourism. All medical procedures have an element of risk. The issue of legal recourse for unsatisfactory treatment across international boundaries is a legally undefined issue at present. Medical tourism has received an increasing amount of attention from the media, there has been remarkably little commentary about medical tourists who have fallen victim to medical malpractices abroad (CII-McKinsey 2002).

14.4 Ethical Issues in Medical Tourism

14.4.1 Lack of Attention to Local Patients

In the bid to luring the international patients, the local patients are feeling the dearth of good quality medical equipment and resources that are directed to the former. It has been found that the funds invested by the medical industry are directed toward the health care of the international patients.

Moreover, the quality of the treatment and surgical procedures that are sometimes termed as illegal in a country are still conducted keeping in mind the money involved. These question the ethical policies of the medical tourism industry.

14.4.2 Providing Hospital Documents in the Local Language

Also, certain medical tourism facilities only provide documents in their own regional language, leaving the foreign patient confused. These facilities are likely to lack translation services and have no concept of cultural competency. You should certainly avoid hospitals or clinics such as these as it is necessary to ensure the presence of an interpreter to ensure that you can understand all the legal formalities properly. Violations of ethics also entail providing insufficient legal documents to the patient (such as malpractice laws and consent forms), which leads to a lack of information for the medical tourist.

[12] India: Accreditation a must, International Medical Travel Journal 2015

14.4.3 Overcharging a Medical Tourist

Since catering to the foreign patient, who can usually afford to pay more for a treatment than a local citizen, has become common practice for certain unethical doctors, they tend to do whatever they can to overcharge the medical tourist. This could be in the form of overprescribing hospital tests, charging more than the market price for treatment, and refusing to take care of post-operative complications.

14.4.4 Quality Concerns

Medical tourism industry is concerned with the treatment quality it provides. They lure the customers to invest in the policies. Moreover, spas and health care facilities in different countries do provide the best solutions.

However, serious health care conditions need to be investigated, if the practitioners or healthcare facilities are certified or not. Many such serious operations have been recorded to cause side effects such as infection or incomplete process. Hence, a single wrong decision made during such health tourism can cause you a bomb, affecting your health as well.[13]

14.4.5 Organ Transplant Surgeries

Organs and tissues transplant are surrounded by many controversies. Developing countries like India, Singapore and Thailand, doctors give more importance to medical tourists, obviously for personal financial gain and ignore the condition of the serious patients in their own country. This has created a double level of healthcare, where medical tourists receive high-quality treatment, while local people have a hard time finding specialist care.

Since organ and tissue transplants are so difficult to obtain owing to long waiting lists, many patients tend to seek foreign options and engage in medical tourism for organ transplants. However, the source of these organs is usually a mystery to most patients. There have been several issues regarding the legality of organ and tissue transplants in many countries. There were many reports of organs being obtained from prisoners without their consent or acquired by illegal means. As a patient, you should check with your treating facility to authenticate where the organs are coming from to ensure they are not engaged in any unethical practices.

It is essential for you to make sure that your selected healthcare facility does not have a dual-quality healthcare system, where foreigners are treated in a better way only to get financial gain. In some countries, healthcare facilities also follow a

---

[13] Guide to understanding ethical issues in medical tourism (drprem.com)

dual-pricing system, where treatment to local residents is offered at extreme fewer prices than what foreign patients are charged. This is an unethical practice, as medical tourists have to pay more than the market rate.

In some countries, regulatory bodies established by the government or health association implement standard guidelines and price bands for treatment, in some countries there are no such checks and facilities charge medical tourists at their own will.

You should inquire about the price differences between local and foreign patients and this would be beneficial to protect yourself from such an incident. Certain unethical doctors try to provide more facilities to foreign patients because they generally can afford to pay more than the local patients do. Foreign patients are usually had to pay more for services, and you might have to pay for unwanted services or tests. In addition to this, some medical tourism facilities provide documents in their local language, so that a medical tourist could not understand those guidelines.

Many facilities lack translation services or have no concept of cultural aptitude and you should try to avoid such healthcare facilities. It is important for you to determine that the healthcare facility you have chosen will provide all documents at least in English or provide the services of an interpreter to ensure that you can understand all legal formalities.

It is important for you to discuss all these concern before setting out your journey and make sure that the government departments or healthcare associations control the prices to demonstrate equality for all patients.

References

CII-McKinsey (2002) Health Care in India: the road ahead. CII, McKinsey and Company and Indian Healthcare Federation, New Delhi

Cohen IG (2012) How to regulate medical tourism (and why it matters for bioethics). Dev World Bioeth 12(1):9–20

Crooks VA, Turner L, Cohen IG et al (2013) Ethical and legal implications of the risks of medical tourism for patients: a qualitative study of Canadian health and safety representatives' perspectives. BMJ Open. accessed February 27, 2013, http://bmjopen-2012-002302

Gray HH, Poland SC (2008) Medical tourism: crossing borders to access health care. Kennedy Inst Ethics J 18(2):193–201

Horowitz MD, Rosensweig JA, Jones CA (2007) Medical tourism: globalization of the healthcare marketplace. Medscape Gen Med 9(4):33

Lunt N, Smith R, et al (2011) Medical tourism: treatments, markets and health system implications: a scoping review (OECD: Directorate for Employment, Labour and Social Affairs), 7

Musa G, Thirumoorthi T, Doshi D (2012) Travel behaviour among inbound medical tourists in Kuala Lumpur. Curr Issue Tour 15(6):525–543

Ormond M (2011) Medical tourism, medical exile: responding to the cross-border pursuit of healthcare in Malaysia. In: Minca C, Oakes T (eds) Real tourism: representation, practice, care and politics in contemporary travel. Routledge, London, pp 143–161

Chapter 15
Accreditation of Healthcare Institutions: Assuring Quality services for Medical Tourism in India

Anil Kumar Chillimuntha, Eliah Srikakolli, and Sushman Sharma

Abstract Quality of patient care is how a hospital delivers care for the patients and they ensure safe, effective, efficient, and equitable medical services, which conform to accreditation standards. Accreditation is a formal process to ensure delivery of safe, high-quality healthcare based on standards and processes devised and developed by healthcare professionals for healthcare services. The concept of Accreditation dates back to the 1860s when Florence Nightingale collated hospital statistics and analyzed them. In India, healthcare accreditation dates back to 2005 when they launched an independent accrediting agency called NABH. In the healthcare arena, there are two umbrella accreditation organizations, which are called "the accredited of the accreditors." These two are "The International Society for Quality in Health Care" (ISQua) and "United Kingdom Akkreditering Form" (UKF). These umbrella organizations endorse many of the global accreditation organizations.

For medical tourism patients, accreditation is an assurance of providing high standards of safety and quality medical care. The quality of medical services cannot be experienced prior to availing the treatment modalities; usually, international patients select hospitals based on their quality accreditation. Maximization of patient care quality and minimization of risks associated with medical care are the two important constituents to build safer hospitals. These twin key concepts can be accomplished through the accreditation of healthcare institutions. Medical tourism patients are ensured to get standardized healthcare services regardless of whether the patient is in the USA, Canada, United Kingom, Singapore, or in India. Evidently, standardization through accreditation is a great risk reduction methodology and strategy proven effectively across different nations globally.

A. K. Chillimuntha
Department of Management, Metas Adventist College, Surat, Gujarat, India

E. Srikakolli
North East Adventist University (NEAU), Khliehtyrshi, Shillong, Meghalaya, India

S. Sharma (✉)
Department of Hospital Management, Hemchadracharya North Gujarat University, Patan, Gujarat, India

B. Chaudhary et al. (eds.), *Medical Tourism in Developing Countries*,
https://doi.org/10.1007/978-981-99-8909-6_15

Keywords Accreditation · Medical Tourism · Quality · Standardization

"Quality of Patient Care" is one of the main axioms for patients and a prerequisite for availing services in the emerging quality accreditation realm of the Indian healthcare system, which is challenging and highly competitive. Quality of patient care is how a hospital delivers care for the patients and they ensure safe, effective, efficient, and equitable medical services, which conform to accreditation standards. Quality accreditation has become an important buzzword among healthcare providers today.

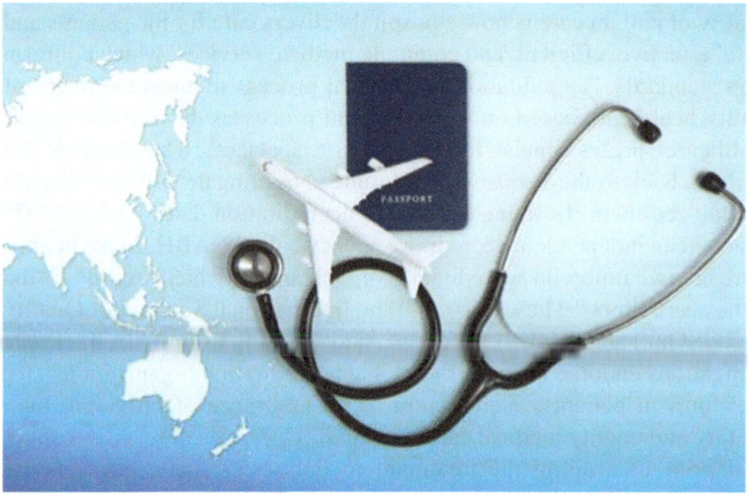

15.1 What is Accreditation?

Every healthcare organization keeps a set of internal standards, rules, and regulations to run the unit operations smoothly. But accreditation ensures that the organization follows a set of standards prescribed by a recognized external agency. It's like an external stamp of approval that the organization is practicing the best industry standards. According to ISQua, "accreditation is a formal process to ensure delivery of safe, high-quality health care based on standards and processes devised and developed by health care professionals for health care services. It is also a public recognition of achievement by a healthcare organization, of requirements of national healthcare standards."

It actually strengthens the organization and proves that it delivers a high quality of healthcare to patients. Accreditation is therefore an external review that portrays the adherence to levels of standards set by an externally well-recognized quality accreditation organization. The organization must prove its compliance to a battery of industry experts who will do an on-site rigorous review of all the implemented structures, processes, policies, and procedures and ensures strict adherence to national and international legal compliances.

The quality mark ensures that the member healthcare organization adheres to and follows laid-out norms and standards and renders quality services. Quality accreditation encompasses everything from patient care to how the healthcare institution ensures effective, efficient, and equitable service delivery to patients by conforming to the prescribed standards and objective elements.

15.1.1 History of Accreditation

The concept of Accreditation dates back to the 1860s when Florence Nightingale collated hospital statistics and analyzed them, which has laid thrust on quality assurance of yesteryears. Her study of these statistics indicated that each hospital has different mortality rates, and they differ from each other based on their patient care and medical practices. In the year 1914, Dr. Earnest Coleman started the "end result system." He promoted hospitals to track the patients who were given medical treatment and to get feedback about the effectiveness of the treatment given. Later in 1919, the hospital standardization program was proposed by the American College of Surgeons (ACS) and found an excellent response from the medical community. They published an article titled "Standard of Efficiency," which is the earliest prototype of quality standards for hospital accreditation. In 1924, ACS published the hospital standardization program, which has become the precursor for healthcare safety and patient care standards. Therefore, we can say that the hospital accreditation system was first developed and established in the USA nearly 100 years ago by the American College of Surgeons. There was an initial thaw in the spreading of this concept but took pace in the 1980s and 1990s, especially in the Western world.

In the year 1951, the Joint Commission on Accreditation of Hospitals (JCAH) came into existence, and they returned the standard of efficiency as a "Hospital Accreditation Program." JCAH was later rechristened in 1987 as the Joint Commission on Accreditation of Healthcare Organizations (JCAHO). In the year 2008, a novel Accreditation program "Qmentum" was launched by Accreditation Canada, who's another healthcare quality accreditor. Qmentum harnessed and used the clinical appraisal tool through an organized assessment system of evaluation.

In recent years, in order to improve the basic health service quality, accreditation has been adopted by many low- and middle-income countries too. The concept of universal health coverage (UHC) driven by the World Health Organization and with a push from different national insurance companies has accelerated the use of healthcare quality accreditation. Accreditation also appeals to various governments since they give a way to fund healthcare services to the ones who provide a high standard of quality healthcare services. This concept of government funding to hospitals that have accreditation helped in the spread of accreditation across the world.

In India, healthcare accreditation dates back to 2005 when they launched an independent accrediting agency called National Accreditation Board for Hospitals and Healthcare Providers (NABH). It's responsible to make healthcare standards for the safety and quality of patient care by adhering to evidence-based treatment.

15.1.2 International Accrediting Agencies

In the healthcare arena, there are two umbrella accreditation organizations, which are called "the accredited of the accreditors." These two are "The International Society for Quality in Health Care" (ISQua) and "United Kingdom Akkreditering Form" (UKF). These umbrella organizations endorse many of the global accreditation organizations such as Joint Commission International (JCI), Australia Council on Healthcare Standards (ACHS), Accreditation Canada, National Accreditation Board for Hospitals & Healthcare Providers (NABH), Trent Accreditation Scheme, Malaysian Society of Quality in Health (MSQH), Central Board for Accreditation of Healthcare Institutions (CBAHI), and many more like this in various countries. Both ISQua and UKF are international organizations that develop benchmark standards for patient safety and also for providing quality patient care in hospitals. These umbrella organizations ensure that accreditation is a continuous quality improvement process and not a one-time certification process.

15.1.2.1 The International Society for Quality in Healthcare (ISQua)

ISQua is an independent not-for-profit organization. It's an international acorn that was established in the year 1985 with the purpose of promoting quality and safety in healthcare institutions through international collaboration. It's a global independent umbrella organization that is called the accreditor of the accreditors and is responsible to do the accreditation of various national and international healthcare organizations that in turn accredit various hospitals in different countries. They strive to constantly enhance healthcare quality and safe patient care. ISQua doesn't survey or accredit any individual institutions. It has a wing that does external evaluation, namely "International society for quality in healthcare external Evaluation Association (IEEA)" for international accrediting bodies.

15.1.2.2 The United Kingdom Akkreditering Forum (UKAF)

The UKAF is also an independent umbrella organization that is London-based and was founded in the year 1998. It is also called an accreditor of accreditors. It's an autonomous body and a pioneer organization in accreditation. It accredits certification bodies and training organizations and is operating in over 25 countries and is a major independent accreditation organization in the world. It's similar to ISQua in developing standards for safe practice and quality patient care. This organization also doesn't survey or accredit individual hospitals. It has pioneered novel approaches to healthcare accreditation by providing benchmarking through measurable evaluation of Confirmity Asessment Body (CAB) performance which are measured year on year to ensure achievement of levels of excellence. It accredits certification bodies and training agencies and provides auditor registration schemes too.

15.1.3 National and International Accrediting Agencies

There are many certification agencies that get healthcare institutions accredited after a rigorous survey of standards and their practices. The noncompliances are identified and intimated to them. The healthcare unit does the closure of their noncompliances and is evaluated for certification. There are many certification agencies in each country that are accredited by the "accreditor of accreditors."

15.1.3.1 Joint Commission International (JCI)

The joint commission is a US-based accreditation system founded in the year 1951. It accredits more than 22,000 healthcare institutions and programs. The Joint Commission International is an independent not-for-profit organization that accredits and certifies healthcare organizations. The certification is recognized globally for quality healthcare and patient safety. JCI identifies, measures, and shares best practices globally. It helps in improving the performance and outcomes of healthcare organizations. It continuously contributes to increased safety and quality through education, publication, and advisory services. It provides accreditation and certification to healthcare units globally in more than 100 countries. As patients move across the care continuum, JCI strives to develop and maintain international standards.

15.1.3.2 National Accreditation Board for Hospitals & Healthcare Providers (NABH)

NABH is an independent body established in the year 2005 and headquartered in New Delhi, India. It's a constituent board of the Quality Council of India. It's the principal accreditation program for healthcare organizations in India. The sole purpose is to design, develop, and monitor the standards for healthcare units in accordance with international standards. NABH is an institutional member of ISQua and a member of the accreditation council of ISQua. NABH is also on the board of the Asian Society for Quality (ASQua) in healthcare.

The first edition of standards was released in 2006. Currently, the fifth edition of standards is in use. NABH now has 10 chapters with 105 standards and 683 objective elements. The healthcare organizations are assessed for these standards and objective elements, which are patient-centered and organization-centered and are revised every 3 years. More than 838 hospitals are accredited by NABH. To accomplish these standards, healthcare institutions need to have a process-driven approach (David & Valas, 2017). There is a continuous accreditation availed from ISQua to ensure international standards are adhered to by NABH. This shows that the hospitals accredited by NABH have international recognition.

15.1.3.3 Trent Accreditation Scheme (TAS)

The Trent Accreditation Scheme is a British accreditation scheme to maintain and continually monitor medical services. The scheme was ended in 2010. It's replaced by many subsidiary independent schemes such as QHA Trent Organization. As of today, in January 2023, the QHA Trent has ceased its operations too.

15.1.3.4 Australia Council on Healthcare Standards (ACHS)

ACHS was established in 1974 and is an independent not-for-profit organization based in Sydney, Australia. It has been a member of ISQua since 1999 and was continually accredited since 2001. It is Australia's largest and leading accreditation provider, which has carved an admirable niche. They have developed an enviable reputation for developing healthcare standards and represent the government, consumers, healthcare professionals, health bodies, and stakeholders of the industry. After receiving international recognition, ACHS started in 2005 an international accreditation system called as ACHS International (ACHSI). It is now providing its services in 18 countries. In 2013, the Australian federal government came up with National Safety and Quality Health Services (NSQHS) standards. ACHS became an accrediting organization for these 10 mandated standards of the nation. EQuIPNational includes not only NSQHS standards but has additional complimentary five standards added. It monitors clinical and non-clinical processes. EQuIP6 will be the premier accreditation standard for international audiences. ACHS is the only accreditation program that has a depository of 805 participating organizations covering 22 specialties for which clinical indicators are tracked through its national clinical indicator program (CIP).

15.1.3.5 Accreditation Canada

Accreditation Canada is an independent, not-for-profit nongovernmental organization established 60 years ago and is headquartered in Ottawa, Canada. It operates globally as an affiliate of the Health Standards Organization (HSO). Accreditation Canada delivers a high-impact assessment program for healthcare, community services, and social services, which are empowered by HSO for public and private healthcare. They are present in more than 15,000 locations in over 38 countries including all provinces of Canada. It has more than 900 expert peer surveyors who are experienced and trained.

HSO develops world-class standards, which are evidence-based and accepted in the medical fraternity. HSO is recognized as a standards development organization

(SDO) by the standards council of Canada. HSO is the only standards development organization that solely focuses and specializes globally on evidence-based and social service standards. It has around 120 standards and evidence-based assessment methodologies. Accreditation Canada fulfills all third-party standards of ISQua, the standards council of Canada, and the Asia Pacific Accreditation Cooperation (APAC).

15.1.3.6 Malaysian Society of Quality in Health (MSQH)

The MSQH was established in the year 1997 for advocating, promoting, and supporting healthcare quality improvement. It has been tremendously performing the task of improving safety and establishing internal standards. It's internationally recognized by ISQua. Since 2014, it has initiated patient-for-patients safety movement. This is to strengthen and improve patient and family engagement in the delivery of medical services.

15.1.3.7 Temos International Healthcare Accreditation (TIHA)

TIHA was founded in 2010. It helps clinics, hospitals, and medical travel coordinators achieve their best performance. TIHA-accredited clients deliver the highest quality patient care to national and international patients. It has innovatively raised the bar of quality and avoids the "one size fits all" approach. It has introduced a tailor-made standard. TIHA is the only accreditation body that incorporated a chapter on "Sustainability in healthcare settings" based on United Nations 2030 Sustainable Developmental Goals.

15.1.4 Impact of Accreditation on the Quality of Healthcare

Accreditation appeals to hospitals and healthcare facilities since it provides external validation of quality medical services. Such proof can have an impact on consumer behaviour, thereby generating increased revenue for accredited hospitals. Patient experience and satisfaction improve significantly.

While going through the accreditation process, there's a significant improvement in the systems and processes of an organization, thereby streamlining the operations. Healthcare organizations also obtain a fair review of their practices through a transparent review by assessors and accordingly provide a document to move forward to upgrading their existing quality. It provides better operational efficiency and creates the best process flows. To achieve accreditation, the staff are trained to deliver high standards of patient care. Therefore, it significantly improves the overall quality of care in a healthcare setup and even improves patient outcomes.

It improves the quality of care and creates trust in patients and all stakeholders in the community at large. It creates increased community confidence in the healthcare organization. Quality accreditation of a hospital elevates confidence and trust in the services rendered. The patient can choose and select a hospital based on the accreditation status.

Accreditation provides a proactive approach to risk mitigation and risk management, which result in safer practices and lesser mistakes, which helps in reducing the liability insurance of a healthcare organization. An accredited healthcare institution gains a competitive advantage by having a leg up by increasing patient satisfaction, thereby increasing footfall due to word-of-mouth marketing by satisfied customers (Debata et al. 2015). Accreditation also helps an organization to receive shared and updated policies and procedures with best practices. In short, we can say healthcare accreditation is a method of risk reduction and quality optimization.

15.2 Medical Tourism

Medical tourism is defined as a process of traveling out of the country of residence for the purpose of receiving quality medical care. In the past, people from less developed countries traveled to developed countries in pursuit of treatment that was not available in their own home country. Today, there's an opposite shift happening where patients are traveling from developed nations to less developed countries to receive medical services. These qualitative and quantitative shifts in patient mobility are due to the delivery of quality care at a very low cost. The prime objective of medical tourists is to avail quality medical care at a very reasonable cost (Wang, 2012).

Medical tourism is truly a direct by-product of globalization and its practices. Due to the fast integration of cultures, economic globalization, increase in cooperation between countries and due to easy cross-border travel, there's an extensive distribution and circulation of services and products across the globe. To benefit from the global market, many industries including the healthcare industry have expanded their horizons and blossomed globally. This resulted in a niche segment where the patients travel across borders to avail quality healthcare services (Mishra & Sharma, 2021). There are excellent healthcare facilities provided across different continents of the world. Today, medical tourism is a multibillion-dollar industry.

Medical tourism is rapidly developing and making a huge impact. Healthcare is also transforming the way it is delivered in different countries. It's based on the healthcare budget, which is allotted by different national governments. The growth of this industry will be impacted as individuals, insurance companies, and governments explore ways to provide high-quality and low-cost medical care.

India is emerging as one of the most favored nations for medical travel destinations. There's a humongous potential of generating huge foreign exchange, employment, and valuable soft power for the country. This positions India as a healing center of the world. The popular medical treatments availed through medical tourism are services such as Hip and Knee Replacements, Kidney Transplants, Cardiac

Surgery, Laparoscopic Surgery, Oncosurgery, Cosmetic Surgery, and Dental Surgery. In Table 15.1, we can see the various classifications of systems of medicine and different medical specialties offered for medical travel patients and which country is strong and weak in those areas.

Many patients in need of acute emergency services are also opting for medical tourism due to long waiting times in their home country while medical tourism destinations eliminate these waiting times and provide quality healthcare services.

India is at a significant advantage due to the availability of world-class doctors trained or worked abroad and is now available at affordable prices when compared to other countries of the world as shown in Table 15.2. We can see the low cost in India when the cost is compared between prices of medical procedures across major destination countries. Secondly, the doctors, nurses, and hospital staff can speak fluent English. Thirdly, there's good availability of top-of-the-line medical and diagnostic equipment. Fourthly, in India, there are nearly 1000 nursing institutes mostly attached to teaching hospitals and produce nearly 10,000 nurses annually, which contributes hugely toward manpower availability for hospitals. Lastly, due to the cost-effective tourism rates and good exchange rates, the budget-conscious traveler can avail first-class service and opt for luxury amenities without any financial constraints (Financial Express, 2022).

The scope of medical tourism has widened, and newer modalities and hospitals catering to these needs have emerged. The medical tourism industry is dynamic and volatile. Many factors such as economic climate, national policies, political instability, travel embargoes, advertising practices, geopolitical shifts, and new innovative pioneering treatment modalities are contributing to the consumption and production of healthcare services in different countries. Medical tourism, therefore, fills a valuable niche created by many countries due to their inefficient bureaucracy and unaffordable healthcare.

Table 15.1 Classification of services offered by medical tourism industry

	Wellness tourism	Alternative systems of medicine	Cosmetic surgery	Advanced and life savings healthcare
Services offered	SPAS, Stress Relief, Rejuvenation Centres	Ayurvedic Siddha treatment for diseases e.g.: Arthritis, Rheumatism	Dental Care, Plastic Surgery, Breast Enhancement, Tummy reduction, Skin Treatment	Open Transplants, Cardio Vascular Surgery, Eye treatment, Hip Replacement, Invitro Fertilization
Profit margin	Low	Low	Medium	High
Key competitors	Thailand, South Africa	–	South Africa, Cuba, Thailand	Singapore, Taiwan, Jordan, Thailand
India's strength	Low - Thailand has captured a significant share of the market	High: - Kerala is popular for this services	Low- South Africa and Thailand lead in plastic Surgery	High - India has strong image on medical tourism

Source: https://www.researchgate.net/publication/334209046

Table 15.2 Cost comparison between prices of medical procedures across major destination countries in USD

Medical procedure	India	Thailand	Malaysia	Singapore	Turkey	South Korea
Heart Bypass	7900	15,000	12,100	17,200	13,900	26,000
Angioplasty	5700	4200	8000	13,400	4800	17,700
Heart Valve Replacement	9500	17,200	13,500	16,900	17,200	39,900
Hip Replacement	7200	17,000	8000	13,900	13,900	21,000
Hip Resurfacing	9700	13,500	12,500	16,350	10,100	19,500
Knee Replacement	6600	14,000	7700	16,000	10,400	17,500
Spinal Fusion	10,300	9500	6000	12,800	16,800	16,900
Dental Implant	900	1720	1500	2700	1100	1350
Lap Band	7300	11,500	8150	9200	8600	10,200
Gastric Sleeve	6000	9900	8400	11,500	12,900	9950
Gastric Bypass	7000	16,800	9900	13,700	13,800	10,900
Hysterectomy	3200	3650	4200	10,400	7000	10,400
Breast Implants	3000	3500	3800	8400	4500	3800
Rhinoplasty	2400	3300	2200	2200	3100	3980
Rhytidectomy	3500	3950	3550	440	6700	6000
Liposuction	2800	2500	2500	2900	3000	2900
Abdominoplasty	3500	5300	3900	4650	4000	5000
Lasik (both eyes)	1000	2310	3450	3800	1700	1700
IVF Treatment	2500	4100	6900	14,900	5200	7900
		Low Price		Moderate Price		High Price

Source: Report of Medical Tourism Association (2019)

15.2.1 *Medical Tourism Scenario in India*

The world over the market share of medical tourism is 439 billion dollars with 11 million medical travelers each year and is growing at the rate of 25% each year. The number of international travelers to India has increased from 4.3 lacs in 2016 to 7 lacs in 2019 with a market share of approximately 5–6 billion dollars. As per the Ministry of Tourism in India, the market share of medical tourism is 9 billion dollars in 2020 with an estimated two million travelers from 78 countries. It's estimated that by 2026, the market share will increase to 13 billion dollars. India is adopting to digital transformation which will be the bridge towards healthcare delivery of tomorrow (Deloitte Global, 2021).

The medical tourism index (Anon 2016, 2020) ranks the perceptions of Americans on 46 international destinations. It provides an insight into how healthcare consumers view 41 criteria having three dimensions such as destination attractiveness, Safety, and Quality of Care. India stands at number 10 in this ranking. India was ranked 5 in the year 2016 but has unfortunately dropped to rank 10 by 2021 (Anon 2021).

NABH has positioned India in the global arena as a provider of safe and high-end quality patient care with world-class medical services and has augmented the confidence levels of international medical travellers.

15.3 Relationship Between Accreditation and Medical Tourism

For medical tourism patients, accreditation is an assurance of providing high standards of safety and quality medical care. The quality of medical services cannot be experienced prior to availing the treatment modalities; usually, international patients select hospitals based on their quality accreditation. The key motivators in medical tourism are premium standards of patient care and cost-effectiveness. Among these two, accreditation of the chosen hospital is a prime important factor in choosing and selecting treatment destinations (Bagga et al, 2020). Quality of care is the key differentiator. The higher the number of quality accreditations the destinations have, the better will be the nation's standing on the international tourism map. Accreditation ensures that a healthcare cost-effective regimen doesn't mean the inferior quality of care, thereby providing patients with informed patient choice and informed decision-making in preference of overseas treatment (Medhekar et al. 2019). Empirical analysis by research also confirms that medical tourism has a positive and fruitful effect on the host nations (Beladi et al. 2019).

Accreditation elevates the patient's confidence levels and trust in the hospital. It ensures that the hospital renders quality patient care services and assures the best standards of care with benefits. It's also a quality index guaranteeing evidence-based practices. It also bridges the huge gulf and mismatch between patient expectations and service delivery. It tries to eliminate the gray areas of inadequacy and institutes world-class standards with impeccable service delivery, staff professional accountability, and clinical excellence (Wang 2012).

We find there's a greater concentration of medical tourism in southern and western parts of India due to the healthcare accreditation of hospitals with JCI. We find Indian cities like Delhi, Chennai, Mumbai, Bangalore, Ahmedabad, and Kochi cater to most of the populations from Asia and Africa. Table 15.3 shows the major players in the Indian Medical Tourism Industry, who cater patients from different countries.

As per Table 15.4, there are 37 Joint Commission International (JCI)-accredited hospitals in India and 716 National Accreditation Board for Hospitals & Healthcare Providers (NABH)-accredited hospitals in India as of 2020.

Table 15.3 Major players in Indian medical tourism industry

Sl. no.	Name of hospital	Number of beds	Turnover	Percentage revenue from international patients	Major international markets
1	Escorts Hospital	326	2180	11.9	SAARC, East African Countries, Afghanistan
2	Apollo Hospitals	1500	2010	15	Middle East
3	Indraprastha Apollo Hospital	650	1650	7.3	Nepal, Bangladesh, Sri Lanka, Gulf and Africa
4	Hinduja Hospital	351	1350	3	African and SAARC Countries
5	Jaslok Hospital	376	1080	10	Japan, Middle East and African Countries

Source: https://www.researchgate.net/publication/334209046

Table 15.4 Hospitals with JCI accreditation in major Asian medical tourism destinations

Sl. no.	Medical tourism destination	No. of JCI accredited hospitals
1	Thailand	60
2	India	37
3	Indonesia	30
4	Malaysia	16
5	South Korea	11
6	Singapore	4
7	Total JCI Accredited Hospitals World-wide	960

Source: Compiled from Joint Commission International (JCI) Website

The patient clinical outcomes in these hospitals are at par with internationally recognized facilities. These outcomes lead to patient satisfaction and further growth of medical tourism. India not only has these quality accredited hospitals but also robust allied sectors such as strong diagnostic, rehabilitative services, pharmaceutical, and medical device industries along with a greater focus on medical research and development.

15.3.1 Key Dimensions of the Medical Tourism Industry

There are many factors that influence the development and growth of medical tourism in a particular region. As per Fig. 15.1 we can see the factors influencing growth of medical tourism. The infrastructure available for accommodation, transportation, accessibility, culture and exoticness, sociocultural and political environment, the safety of tourists, weather, language, and communication are vital factors contributing to the growth of medical tourism destinations. Government support with tourism-friendly policy intervention and modeling 14 regulatory framework promotes the medical tourism industry. The marketing, branding, and image of medical tourism destinations also contribute greatly to the growth of this sector.

The study done by Malhotra and Dave (2022a, b) shows that the competitiveness of a nation as a medical tourism hub is influenced majorly by cost and quality accreditation. Affordability of medical care and service quality are important attributes that contribute to the growth and development of medical tourism destinations. Many other factors contribute such as the specialties and modalities of treatment, available medical infrastructure, technological upgradation, medical innovation, doctor's skill, and competence, administrative efficiency, standards of care, and service quality influence the growth of medical tourism destinations. There's huge importance laid on the credibility and trust of the hospital, which is brought about by certification through accreditation.

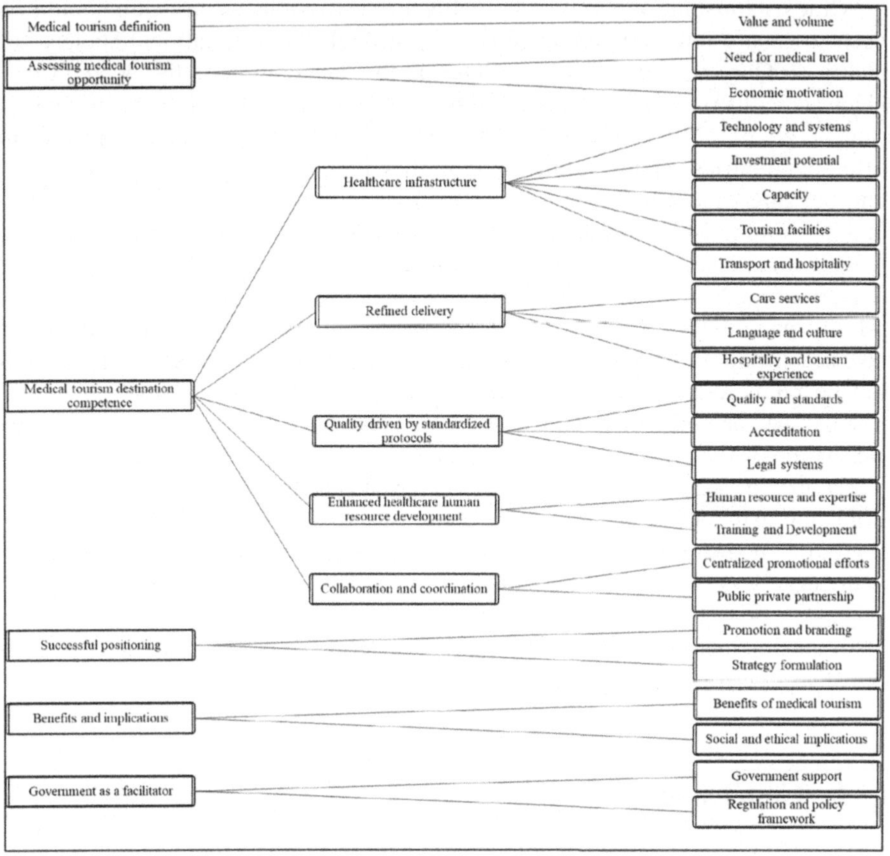

Source: Malhotra & Dave (2022)

Fig. 15.1 Factors influencing the growth and development of medical tourism destination

15.3.2 Need for Accreditation for Medical Tourism

With growth seen globally across borders for quality healthcare destinations, showcasing an alternative for a Western country citizen, the inevitable question arises "how safe are these healthcare destination hospitals?" and "will I receive the same quality standard care as I would receive in an American hospital?" So, therefore, the practical solution for this is to obtain an internationally recognized accreditation. This will assure the clients of medical tourism confidence and trust in quality care delivery for them.

While establishing international healthcare institutions tie-up, care should be taken to ensure international accreditation through the international society for quality (ISQua) for all hospitals. ISQua is the "accreditor of the accreditors," which accredits international accrediting Organizations such as JCI, Accreditation Canada, NABH, Malaysian Society for quality in health, and many more from different countries. Many countries claim they have a national accreditation system, but care should be taken to see if that accreditor is accredited with ISQua. Patients coming across borders would like to avail healthcare services from hospitals that have accreditation to ensure quality standards are followed during the delivery of medical services. The different agencies who solicit patients and provide for patients to take informed decisions also market only the hospitals that have accreditation. This is what is evidenced today, where patients flock to accredited hospitals and tend to skip unaccredited hospitals. As healthcare becomes global, the accreditation and regulatory standards also need to become transnational.

The idea of accreditation is to offer interested stakeholders a process of quality evaluation externally against a set of consensus standards of healthcare delivery. Therefore, medical tourism patients are ensured to get standardized healthcare services regardless of whether the patient is in the USA, Canada, United Kingdom, Singapore, or in India. Evidently, standardization through accreditation is a great risk reduction methodology and strategy proven effectively across different nations globally.

15.4 Conclusion

Maximization of patient care quality and minimization of risks associated with medical care are the two important constituents to build safer hospitals. These twin key concepts can be accomplished through the accreditation of healthcare institutions. This organizational framework is designed to quantify the quality of patient care and analyze and isolate and mitigate the risks. Global medical tourism beneficiaries perceive hospital accreditation as an attestation of quality. The patients feel accreditation is an endorsement of medical excellence delivery and safeguards from the dearth of oversight.

Accreditation minimizes the surge of risks associated with medical tourism. Therefore, it is considered globally a risk-alleviating and risk-mitigating tool. It provides performance judgment and gives an organization an instrument to model strengths and weaknesses and domains for improvement. The increasing aging population, rising cost of medical care, sensitivity to quality assurance, and long waiting periods for availing treatment in the international landscape will make medical tourism a sought-after service provided international healthcare accreditation ensures a safer and quality patient care environment at lower costs.

References

Anon (2016) International healthcare research center report on Medical Tourism Index 2016–17. https://www.healthcareresearchcenter.org

Anon (2020) International healthcare research center report on Medical Tourism Index 2020–2021

Anon (2021). https://www.financialexpress.com/lifestyle/travel-tourism/medical-value-tourism-in-india-what-makes-the-country-a-leading-medical-tourism-destination/2338644/lite/

Aziz A, Yusof RM, Ayob M, Bakar NTA (2015) Measuring tourist modelling intention through quality in Malaysian medical tourism industry. Procedia Econ Financ 31:280–285. https://doi.org/10.1016/S2212-5671(15)01179-X

Bagga T, Vishnoi SK, Jain S, Sharma R (2020) Medical tourism: treatment, therapy, and tourism. Int J Sci Technol Res 9(3):4447–4453

Beladi H, Chao CC, Ee MS, Hollas D (2019) Does medical tourism promote economic growth? A cross-country analysis. J Travel Res 58(1):121–135. https://doi.org/10.1177/0047287517735909

David SN, Valas S (2017) National Accreditation Board for Hospitals and Healthcare Providers (NABH) Standards: a review. Curr Med Issues 15:231–236

Debata BR, Patnaik B, Mahapatra SS, Sree K (2015) Interrelations of service quality and service loyalty dimensions in medical tourism: a structural equation modelling approach. BIJ 22(1):18–55. https://doi.org/10.1108/BIJ-04-2013-0036

Deloitte Global (2021) Digital transformation and health care delivery model convergence. Retrieved from https://www2.deloitte.com/content/dam/Deloitte/global/Documents/Life-Sciences-Health-Care/gx-digital-transformation.pdf

Financial Express (2022) Medical value tourism in India: what makes the country a leading Medical Tourism Destination. Financial Express

Malhotra N, Dave K (2022a) Dimensions and drivers of medical tourism industry: a systematic review of qualitative evidence. Int J Bus Glob. https://doi.org/10.1504/IJBG.2022.10042738. (in press)

Malhotra N, Dave K (2022b) An assessment of competitiveness of medical tourism industry in India: a case of Delhi NCR. JGBC 17:215–228. https://doi.org/10.1007/s42943-022-00060-0

Medhekar A, Wong HY, Hall JE (2019) Factors influencing inbound medical travel to India. J Health Organ Manag. https://doi.org/10.1108/JHOM-08-2018-0234

Mishra V, Sharma MG (2021) Framework for promotion of medical tourism: a case of India. Int J Glob Bus Compet 16(1):103–111. https://doi.org/10.1007/s42943-021-00027-7

Report of Medical Tourism Association (2019) Accessed on June 12, 2023 and Accessed at https://www.medicalindiatourism.com/treatment-cost.html

Wang HY (2012) Value as a medical tourism driver. Manag Serv Qual: An International Journal 22(5):465–491. https://doi.org/10.1108/09604521211281387

Chapter 16
Communication: An Inevitable Aspect of Medical Tourism in India

Hetal S. Patel, Dilip C. Patel, Sushman Sharma, and Ritesh S. Patel

Abstract Communication is an essential part of human life, which makes human beings different from other creatures on this universe. It is through communication that the whole world is connected, and thus, it has become a global village in this twenty-first century. In the field of medical tourism, one cannot ignore the role of communication. In fact, communication is the heart of medical tourism that makes it possible. Medical tourism in India is an emerging concept nowadays, and it will not be possible without proper communication. The process of communication begins at the initial stage of medical tourism when the patient and his/her relatives start thinking of opting for that. From that point onward, in all the stages of medical tourism, proper communication needs to take place. Taking from the application to travel to another country for medical treatment to the return from the host country, communication is an important factor. It is only through proper and effective communication that the patient and his/her relatives are convinced to travel to another place for medical treatment. The medical tourists are apathetic towards medical tourism in India because of the problems they would have to face due to lack of translators at the hospitals. Good interpreters fluent in using various languages are rarely available at good and reputed hospitals, which impacts negatively on the enhancement of medical tourism in India. Therefore, it is the need of the time now to find a way out to cope with this lacuna to enhance the scope of medical tourism in India.

H. S. Patel
Department of English, Hemachandracharya North Gujarat University, Patan, Gujarat, India

D. C. Patel
Department of Sanskrit and Bharatiya Vidya, Hemchandracharya North Gujarat University, Patan, Gujarat, India

S. Sharma (✉)
Department of Hospital Management, Hemchandracharya North Gujarat University, Patan, Gujarat, India

R. S. Patel
Health1 Hospital, Shilaj, Ahmedabad, India

B. Chaudhary et al. (eds.), *Medical Tourism in Developing Countries*,
https://doi.org/10.1007/978-981-99-8909-6_16

Keywords Communication · Language · Wellness centres · Tourism · Barriers and remedies · Ayurveda · Nature cure

16.1 The Process of Communication

Human beings are social animals, and communication is the key to human survival. It is due to communication only that the whole world has become a global village. In simple terms, communication can be defined as a process of exchange of ideas, thoughts, emotions, information, or requirements to the other person/persons so that they are reciprocated. Without reciprocation, the process of communication remains incomplete and one-sided. The process can be explained well through the diagram shown below:

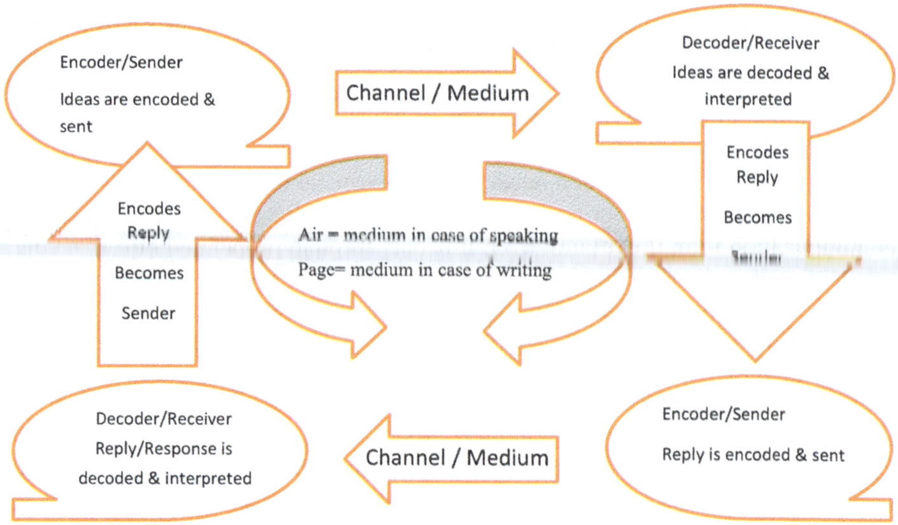

Thus, from the above diagram, it is clear that communication is a two-way process in which it is not possible in the absence of any one of the sender or receiver of the message. It is also necessary that both the sender of a message and receiver of the message need to be familiar with the medium, that must be common for both. Language is one such medium used for communication. Thousands of languages are used in different countries. It is mandatory for proper communication that people need to have a common medium of language. By the word "common," it is meant that the encoding and decoding of the information should be in the same language. If the information/message is produced in a language with which the decoder is unfamiliar, the process of communication remains incomplete because it is not reciprocated/ replied. Therefore, it is required that both the speaker/producer and listener/receiver of message need to know the common medium of the exchange of ideas for proper communication. In addition, both the encoder and decoder need to be present, no communication is possible in the absence of any one of the two. It is rightly said in Sanskrit:

कमि् करषि्यतविक्तार: श्रोता यत्र न वदि्यते।.

नग्नक्षपणके देशे रजक: कर्किरषि्यतिा। (Chowkhamb Krishnadas Academy n.d.)

(If the listeners do not know, what can a speaker do?
In a land where mendicants are naked, what can a washer man do?)

Thus, from ancient times, it has been noticed that the speaker can communicate only when the listeners know the language of the speaker. There are various types of communication among which verbal communication is the most common and effective type. Language is one such mode of verbal communication.

16.2 Scope of Medical Tourism in India

Ancient Indian system of Ayurveda can be the source of attraction for medical tourism in India. Ayurveda believes in the wellness of body and in preventing diseases rather than curing them. Kalidasa has said in Kumarasambhava that:

शरीरमाध्यम खलु धर्म साधनम् । (Patel 2012)

(i.e., A healthy body is the true medium to attain one's true Dharma, i.e., duty.)

Healthy body, free of diseases, is always preferred in Ayurveda. It is also emphasized in Indian system of Auyrveda that a healthy body is the only source of a healthy mind. It is mentioned in Kautilya's *Chanakya Niti* that:

पुनर्वतिं पुनर्मत्रिं पूनर्भार्या पुनर्मही।

एतत्सर्वं पुनर्लभ्यं न शरीरं पुन: पुन:॥ (Anon n.d.-a, p. 75)

(Wealth, a friend, and a kingdom may be regained; but this body when lost may never be acquired again.)

Thus, Indian Ayurveda emphasizes more on prevention of diseases by introducing healthy lifestyle. Keeping this at the center, wellness centers and natural healthcare institutes are established in many states in India, which may attract foreign patients. The world has been developed a lot in the field of technology, but this development has affected badly the average health of people. Many diseases like diabetes, blood pressure, heart diseases are caused due to hectic lifestyle, that can be controlled easily with the help of changing lifestyle mentioned in Ayurveda. Besides this, the wellness centers train people about healthy and nutritious food habits that are helpful in preventing the lifestyle diseases. These healthcare centers, Indian Yoga, and Natural Cure Centers can attract foreign patients who can also visit tourist places of India, which are rich in natural beauty. It is the result of this awareness and attraction for Indian Yoga that the World Yoga Day is celebrated. Thus, India is a country that has its natural tourist places and a rich ancient system of medication that can attract a huge number of people from developed nations.

16.3 Communication and Medical Tourism

Just as language and communication are essential for survival of human beings, traveling and tourism are also equally important in the twenty-first century when the whole world has become a global village. Medical tourism is an emerging factor in India nowadays. India has been a well-known nation in the world for the ancient Ayurveda treatment and natural cure therapy since ages. Some references of this can be found in the inscriptions of King Ashoka that some people ho were experts in Ayurveda migrated to Egyptian Civilization between 273 to 233 B.C. (Shukla and Tripathi 1996, p. 106) There is also a mention that King Alexander took along with him some expert Vaidyas and Ayurveda Acharyas from India. Apart from this, it becomes clear from the study of history of Ayurveda that numerous countries like Mesopotamia, Samaria, Babylonia, Assyria, China, Iran, Thailand, Indonesia, Sri Lanka, and Mauritius were highly influenced by this ancient treatment of Ayurveda. After that, the scope and popularity of Allopathic treatment increased after the industrial revolution in the eighteenth century in Europe. India was a part of British Colony during those days, and therefore, the Allopathic treatment became famous in India also due to its immediate effect. It is a positive impact of this modern method of medical treatment that the average age of human beings is increased notably. Combination of various methods of treatments is also innovatively used to cure some chronic diseases. And therefore traveling from one country to another for medical treatment has also increased in this age of globalization. Traveling has also become easier these days, and thus, the scope of medical tourism is increased.

India is a country of unity in diversity, which attracts foreign tourists, and it has also become a center of attraction for patients from abroad. Multiple languages are spoken in India due to which the number of people knowing multiple languages is high. This benefits in providing the facility of translators to foreign patients who don't have any knowledge/exposure to Indian languages. Thus, knowledge of medical treatments both traditional and modern and people knowing multiple languages can provide a golden opportunity for medical tourism in India. Communication becomes a vital question when people, i.e., patient and relatives of the patient think of coming to India for medical treatment from foreign countries. It has been found out from the authors' visits to various hospitals in Ahmedabad and Nadiyad that generally patients from poor countries come to India for medical treatment. Since most of these countries are not English-speaking countries, people knowing English can rarely be mediators/ translators to these non English foreign patients.

Generally, two kinds of problems of communication are faced during medical tourism in India: (1) foreign patients who do not know any Indian languages and (2) patients who do not know English as well as any Indian languages. It is seen that patients from neighboring countries like Pakistan, Bangladesh, Afghanistan, Sri Lanka, and Indonesia are familiar with Hindi or some of the Indian languages because of popularity of Indian Bollywood movies in these countries, and also at some point of time in history, these nations were a part of India. However, patients from these countries also face communication problems during the legal process of getting visa. In fact, the process of communication in medical tourism begins the moment the patient decides to go abroad for medical treatment. Once the decision is taken, the patient and relatives have to pass through a legal procedure for getting entry in India, which seems to be troublesome for those who do not have any knowledge of English or any Indian languages. Patients also come to India for medical treatment who have no exposure to either any of the Indian languages or English. Such people face communication problems in India that need to be solved for increasing opportunities of medical tourism in India. It is because of these communicational problems that the concept of medial tourism is not so popular as it should be in India.

16.4 Case Study of a Few Reputed Hospitals in Ahmedabad and Nadiad[1]

For studying the scope of medical tourism in India, the authors visited some corporate holistic hospitals in Ahmedabad as well as Civil Hospital at Asarava area of Ahmedabad that is the biggest hospital in Asia where we met the concerned doctors/officers and enquired about the present issues related to medical tourism. Mr. Nilesh Soni in Health1 Hospital, Shilaj, Ahmedabad, informed that he is appointed to take care of the foreign patients who visit the hospital for medical treatment. There is a separate department for foreign patients in this hospital. According to him, foreign patients of Indian origin especially visit the hospital more. Since they are migrants from India, they are usually familiar with the treatment as well as the language used by doctors and the supporting staff. However, language becomes a barrier to those foreign patients who are not familiar with the local Indian languages. Communication becomes quite difficult in such cases where the patient is not familiar either with the local languages or even with English language.

One of the authors of this chapter, Dr. Ritesh Patel himself is a medical practitioner who recently faced communication problem during surgery of a teenage patient from Mozambique who could only communicate in Portuguese. She came along with her mother, and both could neither speak English nor were they familiar with any of the Indian languages. A 16-year-female was admitted for scoliosis correction (spine surgery), was operated on January 16th, 2023 who was postoperatively shifted to ICU for respiratory and metabolic acidosis due to prolonged anaesthesia and blood loss was treated with blood products and ventilation. Recovery was good and she was shifted to room next day. In this case, it was one of the risky surgeries, and the doctors wanted to make both the mother and the patient aware of the medical situation and the seriousness of the surgery. Without the mother's consent, the hospital could not act further. Then, the technical support staff of the hospital had to search for an interpreter who could communicate in Portuguese to both the mother

[1]Visited Health1 Hospital, Shilaj; SGVP Hospital, SG Highway, Ahmedabad and J.S.Ayurved Mahavidyalay, Nadiad on 16th January, 2023.

and the daughter, they found a person who helped them convey the message to the them, and then the doctors moved the patient to operation theater.

Mr. Nilesh Soni informed that on average 2–5% of the total patients are international patients, and the highest number of patients come from Bangladesh, South East Asia, Africa, and Middle East countries. Mostly they come for treatment of cardiac, orthopaedic, oncology, infertility, weight loss and metabolic surgeries, and QI surgeries. According to him, unlike native patients, international patients always expect detailed explanation of their treatment from doctors, paramedical staff, and admin staff, which is not routine in India. This creates problem in proper communication. Even though the hospital provides best facilities with expert doctors and caring supportive staff, cultural and linguistic difference brings difficulty in medical tourism. Many of the international patients come from small villages, and when they visit the hospital, they cannot communicate properly. It is the experience of Mr. Soni that apart from the difficulty in communication, such patients also find it difficult to adjust with the taste of food provided in hospital during and after treatment. He gave an example of a Kenyan patient who eats "Ugali," a local Kenyan food, daily. They could not communicate its recipe to the cook of the hospital. The cook tried to prepare it as much as he could understand, but the patients were not satisfied due to its different taste. Later on, the cook came to know that they don't use spices. This is just one example of the communication gap that takes place with the foreign patients every day, and we have hired separate supporting staff for such patients.

Communication with the junior staff of the hospital becomes a major problem especially with patients from Middle East who do not know English and speak Arabic language only. Same is the case with patients coming from Mozambique who speak Portuguese language only. Therefore, the hospital has to provide the facility of an interpreter/translator in such cases that would help them in communicating the problems faced by the patient that can be addressed by the doctors. The hospital has to take care while appointing the translator that s/he is not only an expert in various foreign languages but is also familiar with the nearby tourist places. Not only that, the interpreter is also expected to have good resources who may help in providing the visitor patients facilities at tourist places. It was stated by Mr. Nilesh that it is very difficult to find qualified well-resourced translators/interpreters in Gujarat as this field is new, and young students are not familiar about that. Apart from this, the universities in Gujarat lack in introducing foreign language departments, only a few State Universities at present have language departments that teach languages other than English like French, German, Urdu, Spanish, Portuguese, Arabic, and many more such languages. He suggested that the universities in Gujarat should think of introducing short-term foreign language teaching courses, which may help in addressing the barriers created due to lack of communication in medical tourism.

On visiting the SGVP holistic hospital, it was found that the foreign patients are attracted more to the Ayurvedic treatment for lifestyle diseases. There was no separate facility for international patients in this hospital. J.S. Ayurveda Mahavidyalaya in Nadiad is one of the oldest Ayurveda colleges in Gujarat that was established in 1938 (Anon n.d.-b). After visiting this college, the authors came to know that international patients frequently visit this Ayurveda hospital, and most of them are either of Indian origin or from Germany. It was also found out that German patients visit this hospital mostly for skin treatment and lifestyle diseases. NRI patients come to address health problems like constipation, lifestyle diseases like weight loss, obesity, and many such diseases. Problems of communication are faced less because both the patients and medical staff know English language. We came to know that Germans have special liking for the Indian Ayurveda system of treatment as there is awareness about Ayurveda treatment in Germany because the famous German scholar Max Muller promoted it among the Germans. Due to the special attempts of Max Muller, Germans accepted it wholeheartedly, which is visible in their attempt to cure diseases with the help of Ayurveda. It is a matter of pride for us and at the same time a matter to ponder over that this Indian system of Ayurveda is promoted in other European nations, which would increase the scope of medical tourism in India. Special facilities are provided to international patients in this hospital of Nadiad. The number of Nonresidential Indians around Nadiad and its surrounding villages is high and these NRIs can be of a great help in promoting the Indian Ayurveda in their residing countries. If the NRI patients bring with them the foreign patients, problems of communication can be reduced.

16.5 Problems Due to Lack of Communication Skills in Medical Tourism

Communication is highly important in medical treatment. There must be a proper rapport between a patient and a doctor for a successful treatment. This rapport can be created only when the patient is able to communicate his/her health problem properly. If the patient is not comfortable with the doctor in communicating to the doctor, even an expert doctor cannot help cure the disease. Such problem of communication between a patient and a doctor becomes vital when either of the two is not familiar with the language of communication. It is because of lack of communication skills only that many foreign patients drop the idea of traveling to India for medical treatment. Sometimes the patients desire to come to India for medical treatment, but the legal formalities that they have to finish while entering into the country compel them to drop the idea due to lack of knowledge of English. It happens many times that patients do come for medical treatment in India, but due to lack of communication and lack of knowledge of the surrounding tourist places, they get their treatment done and go back to their native countries.

16.6 Remedies to the Problems in Communication

Thus, it is a matter of concern for a developing country like India that medical tourism is slow only because of poor communicational facilities even though there is richness of geographical and technical facilities, natural beauty, and variety of medical treatments in India. It is an attempt here to discuss the problems of communication and their remedies to it so that the scope for medical tourism in India increases. The problems that are faced due to communication may be addressed successfully in the manners mentioned below:

- The Government of India should promote universities to increase the rate of Memorandum of Understanding (MoU) with various foreign countries that can help in producing interpreters/translators knowing Indian languages and the languages of the relevant countries who may play the role of mediators and facilitators.
- The campaign for Indian method of medical treatment should be increased in such foreign countries from which patients for medical tourism can be attracted/increased. The Government/hospitals should ensure that language or medium of communication does not hinder the process of medical tourism.
- The corporate hospitals should be encouraged by the Government of India to attract foreign patients by developing a separate section for them in the hospitals so that foreign currency is brought to India.
- Such separate active and effective sections for foreign patients should also be established and promoted in Government Civil Hospitals so that the attempts of humility by Indian Government are noticed globally.
- The number of foreign language departments in universities should be promoted effectively so that young students can learn foreign languages. This will also increase job opportunities for young students fluent in usage of foreign languages.
- Apart from teaching the major foreign languages, the Universities should introduce language teaching courses of those minor foreign languages.
- The language departments in Universities should focus more on the practical aspect of languages, i.e., speaking and listening should be emphasized more.
- The Indian books on Ayurveda should be translated into most of the languages of the world and should be promoted in most of the countries so that more people become aware of this Ayurvedic treatment.
- NRIs residing in various countries should be encouraged to promote the Indian Medical System of Ayurveda so that the local people of the respective countries become aware of it and may be attracted to visit India for medical treatment as well as tourism.

References

Anon (n.d.-a). https://ia601704.us.archive.org/27/items/chanakya-neeti-darpan/chanakya-neeti-darpan.pdf

Anon (n.d.-b). https://nadiadayurveda.org/

Chowkhamb Krishnadas Academy (n.d.) Sanskrit Subhāshita Ratnākara. Chowkhamb Krishnadas Academy, Varanasi

Patel G (2012) Kumarsambhavam-5:13. New Bharatiya Book Corporation, New Delhi, p 142

Shukla V, Tripathi R (1996) Ayurved ka Itihas Evam Parichay. New Delhi, Chokhamba Sanskrit Pratishthan

Chapter 17
Future Prospects for Growth of the Medical Tourism Industry

N. Shalini, R. Sathish, B. J. Divya Rao, and H. K. Mamatha

Abstract Medical tourism, the practice of seeking healthcare services overseas, has emerged as a thriving global industry over the past decade. This chapter explores the key prospects for the continued growth of the medical tourism industry.

The primary driving factor behind the industry's growth is the significant cost savings it offers to patients seeking treatment abroad. Many countries have invested in state-of-the-art medical facilities staffed by skilled healthcare professionals, ensuring high-quality care at lower costs compared to their home countries. Additionally, reduced wait times for medical procedures and growing demand for cosmetic and dental treatments contribute to the appeal of medical tourism.

Supportive government policies, including streamlined visa processes and special healthcare packages, have facilitated the growth of medical tourism. Furthermore, advancements in travel and communication have made it easier for patients to research, book, and communicate with healthcare providers and facilitators efficiently.

Despite promising excellent prospects for expansion, the medical tourism sector still has to deal with issues including inconsistent quality standards among destinations and significant language challenges. Yet, these challenges can be successfully overcome by putting in place appropriate regulatory and accrediting mechanisms.

In conclusion, the medical tourism industry has the potential for future growth. Stakeholders must work together to promote sustainable development and maximize the industry's beneficial effect on global healthcare to take benefit of the potential for economic growth and increased accessibility to healthcare.

N. Shalini (✉) · B. J. Divya Rao · H. K. Mamatha
Department of Health System Management Studies, JSS Academy of Higher Education and Research, Mysore, Karnataka, India
e-mail: shalini.dhsms@jssuni.edu.in

R. Sathish
Department of Oral and Maxillofacial Surgery, JSS Dental College, JSS Academy of Higher Education and Research, Mysore, Karnataka, India

B. Chaudhary et al. (eds.), *Medical Tourism in Developing Countries*,
https://doi.org/10.1007/978-981-99-8909-6_17

Keywords Medical Tourism · Stakes holders · Service Quality · Destination Competitiveness · Future

17.1 Introduction

Health is wealth is a well-known adage, and healthy individuals make healthy nations. The gross disparity in terms of medical facilities, access, and affordability to medical care has formed the basis for people looking at countries that are better placed to provide affordable healthcare. One such concept is medical tourism wherein patients travel beyond geopolitical boundaries to access healthcare.

17.2 History of Medical Tourism

A person traveling from the country of their residence to another temporarily is called a tourist. If they travel to another country with the intent of seeking medical treatment, they can be called a medical tourist, and the process is medical tourism. This is not a new phenomenon, it has been happening in the past, some of the significant examples of medical tourism in the past are:

- People traveled from Greece to the sanctuary of Asclepios, the god of healing (Subbaraman and Reddy 2020).
- Spas built by Romans, which facilitated numerous health-related activities (Unit 9 Health Tourism 2017).
- The city of Bath in England, based on a line of the Roman bath, was a famous destination for health tourists (Unit 9 Health Tourism 2017).
- People traveling to Japan to gain the health benefits of water enriched with volcanic soil (Subbaraman and Reddy 2020).
- India has been a popular destination due to 5000-year-old yoga retreats, centers for meditation, etc. (Subbaraman and Reddy 2020).

17.3 Trends in Medical Tourism

In the present busy world, many people always want to feel healthy and look good, for which they are always engaged in some form of health-beneficial activities, like yoga, meditation, gym, and spas. The health-related activities are provided attractively by combining them with tourism in the form of a package. Package medical tourism is most sought after by the people whose working lifestyle involves too much traveling (Unit 9 Health Tourism 2017) (Fig. 17.1).

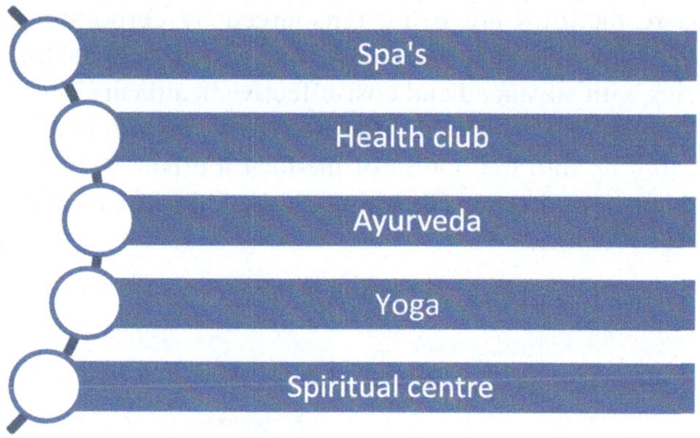

Fig. 17.1 Different types of medical tourism packages

Asian countries like India, Thailand, and Malaysia have formulated various programs and implemented policies that facilitate the establishment of medical hubs of world standard, thus not only building the medical tourism industry but also trying to improve foreign trade (Beladi et al. 2019). Medical tourism has been given importance by many countries after the 2008 financial crisis, to bring an economic boost. Some of examples of positive indications toward medical tourism is (Beladi et al. 2019) are:

- Improvement in the revenue of Thailand from US$340 million to US$622 million from 2010 to 2013 (Beladi et al. 2019).
- Investments toward medical tourism from Latin American countries to get patients from North America (Beladi et al. 2019).
- Eastern European countries have established themselves as popular medical destinations, keeping western European patients a target (Beladi et al. 2019).
- Middle East, Turkey, UAE, and Israel are also emerging as a healthcare-providing hub to get patients from across the globe (Beladi et al. 2019).
- Dubai planned to build world-class hospital facilities to attract people across the globe, thus improving its economy (Beladi et al. 2019).

Developing countries are promoting medical tourism to improve their economy, as MT is becoming a multibillion-dollar industry (Beladi et al. 2019). The Global demand for MT and the cost of health care service are determined by the following factors (Malhotra and Dave 2022).

- Increase in aging population and also growing popuslation (Malhotra and Dave 2022).
- Transformation in digital technology, which is expensive (Malhotra and Dave 2022).
- Varied patterns of diseases (Malhotra and Dave 2022).

The healthcare facilities are being outsourced by corporations and governments to emerging markets due to the increasing disparity in healthcare cost, seen more in countries with advanced and cost-effective healthcare facilities. People in countries with limited healthcare facilities both in the government and private sector and forced to look into the option of medical tourism. Some of the countries that have established and are establishing in medial tourism are (Malhotra and Dave 2022) (Fig. 17.2) ….

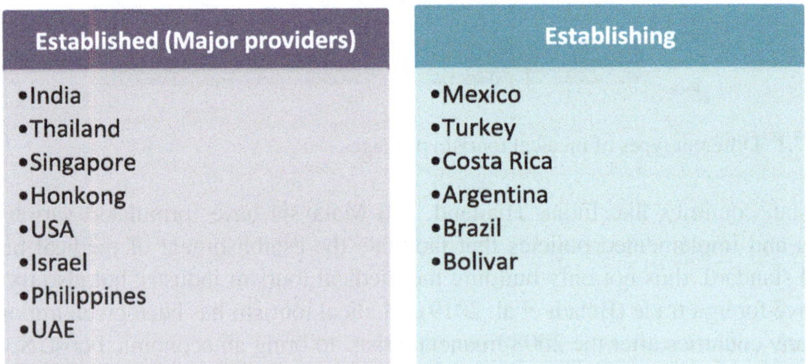

Fig. 17.2 Established and establishing medical tourism countries

17.4 Key Stakeholders of Medical Tourism

The key stakeholders of medical tourism are (Fig. 17.3):

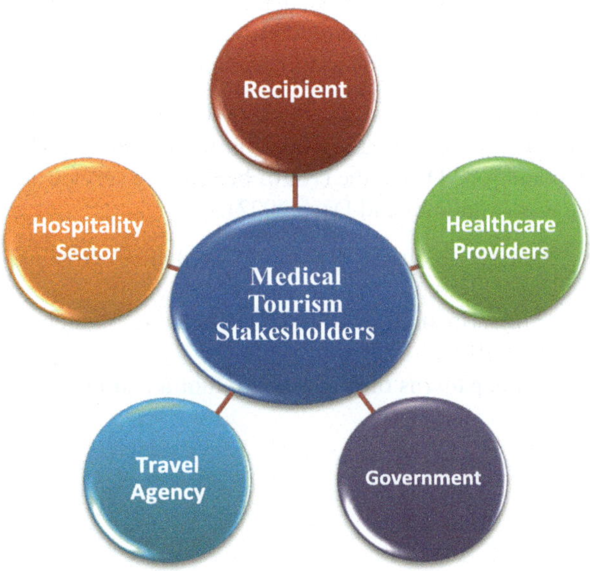

Fig. 17.3 Key stakeholders of medical tourism

17.5 Key Dimensions of the Medical Tourism Industry

The key dimensions of medical tourism are:

- Prime factor.
- Service quality.
- Macroenvironment factors.
- Destination competitiveness (Fig. 17.4).

17.5.1 Prime Factors

Cost in medical tourism can be considered as a hedging factor that ensures that medical services are available, the hospitals can operate at a reasonable cost, visitors can spend more money at shopping malls and on transportation, they can visit nearby famous cities, and stay in the safe and secure location (Sasirekha and Sankar 2022). Most patients travel abroad for treatment that was not offered and affordable in the place of their residence (Cortez 2008). International demand for medical interventions from advanced nations has risen substantially because of the lower healthcare services offered in developing nations (Aziz et al. 2015).

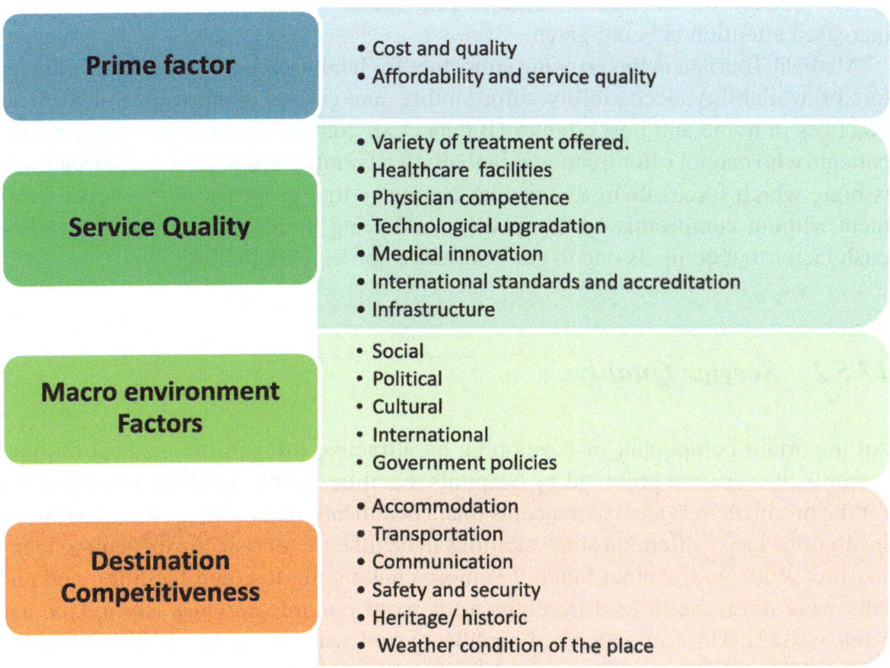

Fig. 17.4 Key dimensions of the medical tourism industry

According to World Bank research, the US's healthcare and insurance prices are much costlier compared to several other countries These differences are pushed in considerable amount by the price of specific medical procedures (Cortez 2008).

For example, according to the World Bank, the cost of knee surgery is around $1500 in leading countries like India and Hungary, but the same costs $10,000 in the United State. The best medical care in India and Thailand offers coronary artery bypass grafts for less than $9000, which includes the travel charges when compared to the United States, which charges approximately $35,000. According to WHO, the price of health treatment in emerging nations is 3–10% of the price in the United States (Cortez 2008).

The lower treatment costs in destinations are the driving factor of medical tourism, 83% of the literature review on medical tourism reports that reduced treatment costs attract medical tourists to several destinations (John and Larke 2016) and are also attractive to travelers from Western countries, specifically who do not have adequate insurance coverage costs at home.

Recent advancements that felicitate medical tourism in developing countries have seen the following dramatic changes (Cortez 2008).

- Quality of medical professionals.
- Improved infrastructure facility.
- Effective utilization of technologies.
- Increased proficiency at marketing their services.

The quality of services is a major pull factor in medical tourism, to which increased attention is being given.

Medical Tourism is the growing substitute for health seekers assessed by the factors of availability, accessibility, affordability, and ethical comparisons of medical practices in home and host country (Bagga et al. 2020). Affordability is crucial for patients who cannot offer treatment in their own country where the cost of treatment is high, which forces them to consider a country that proposes a lower-cost treatment without compromising the quality and saving money. Affordability is a key push factor that compels one to get healthcare abroad (Singh 2019).

17.5.2 Service Quality

An important component of developing an attractive offer in the medical tourism sector is the services provided by hospitals. Facilities in the medical industry stand for the products, services, or concepts that a healthcare institution offers. Healthcare institutions face a dilemma since facilities in healthcare tourism are difficult to identify precisely. On the other hand, it is more challenging to count facilities, and clients view these facilities differently from more tangible services (Sasirekha and Sankar 2022). The competence of healthcare professionals in developing nations is rising to Western levels. Numerous nations are modifying their medical curricula to meet the standards of North America and Western Europe and are increasingly providing instruction in English. By obtaining certification from reputable organizations like the Joint Commission for the Accreditation of Health Care Organizations (JCAHO), hospitals using top-notch implants and consumables have acquired respect for their cutting-edge facilities and diagnostic centers on a global scale. As certification typically means that a service satisfies minimum requirements of proficiency and quality, many hospitals in developing nations fulfill Western standards. Many believe that medical tourism will significantly increase as global norms for healthcare quality, accreditation, and education become more established. Even a program for evaluating the accrediting bodies themselves was developed by a group of nations (Cortez 2008).

The medical technology available in many developing nations has improved, including treatments and innovations that the FDA has yet to have approved. Even some hospitals in undeveloped countries are enhancing biotechnology goods produced by American and European firms. These innovations are openly promoted by foreign hospitals (Cortez 2008).

The Wockhardt Hospitals Group in India, for instance, advertised that it utilized the same medical technology as "hospitals in New York, London, or Sydney (Cortez 2008)."

As nations have privatized and liberalized trade in national healthcare sectors and as bodies like the Joint Commission offer global accreditation, healthcare facilities have become more international. By establishing multinational hospital chains, the global hospital sector promotes medical tourism (Cortez 2008).

The Parkway Group and the Raffles Medical Group, two Singapore-based organizations, have purchased hospitals and formed partnerships with regional healthcare organizations in Malaysia, India, Sri Lanka, and the United Kingdom. Plans for hospitals in Sri Lanka, Nepal, and Malaysia have been announced by the Indian Apollo Hospitals Group (Cortez 2008).

17.5.3 Macroenvironment Factors

Medical tourism benefits society by offering millions of people access to better healthcare at reasonable costs, enhancing their quality of life, and fostering scientific and cultural advancements as well as employment creation. When health tourists choose a destination, the similarity of the cultures is a major factor. In fact, "culture" has long been regarded as an effective determinant in forming the trends of the medical tourism industry. "Culture" has long been regarded as an effective determinant in creating the trends of the medical tourism sector. The "cultural competence" of the healthcare workforce affects how well healthcare providers can provide culturally appropriate services (Rokni et al. 2019).

The lack of competent national public health services, the rising expense of healthcare, and the availability of less expensive alternatives in developing nations have all contributed to the enormous rise of the health services industry globally (Rokni et al. 2019). This has caused the globalization of healthcare, as evidenced by the expansion of cross-border health service delivery, which is thought to be worth more than US$140 billion (World Trade Organization 2001) (Hazarika 2010).

Some nations strive to establish themselves as national medical tourism destinations. Governments actively support the medical tourism sector by engaging national ministries of tourism, health, and state/regional tourism promotion organizations or by launching studies and research. The role of the state in encouraging, developing, structuring, and promoting medical travel differs significantly between countries. Some nations place a strong emphasis on fostering the medical tourism sector by launching efforts aimed at enhancing the nation's comparative advantages, while others either don't care or actively work to prevent it. Examples of such policies to encourage industrial expansion include (Ruka and Garel 2015):

- facilitated visa processes or medical visa categories.
- tax incentives.
- healthcare infrastructure investment,
- special, either state-funded or privately funded organizations that are dedicated to promoting the expansion of the medical tourism sector.
- subsidies.

17.5.4 Destination Competitiveness

A feel-good element, which offers a competitive advantage in destination marketing for drawing in medical tourists, is another aspect that influences the growth of medical tourism. The feel-good factor refers to supplementary services like airport assistance, visa extensions, discounted hotel rates, insurance plan coverage, discounted medical treatment packages, and discounted trip excursions following medical treatment (Sasirekha and Sankar 2022).

Patients' perceptions are impacted by the destination's reputation, image, climate, tourist attractions, infrastructure, and historical context. These elements are crucial in helping patients choose hospitals and nations. Websites are important sources of this information (Tontus and Nebioglu 2018).

17.6 Benefits to the Stakeholders (Fig. 17.5)

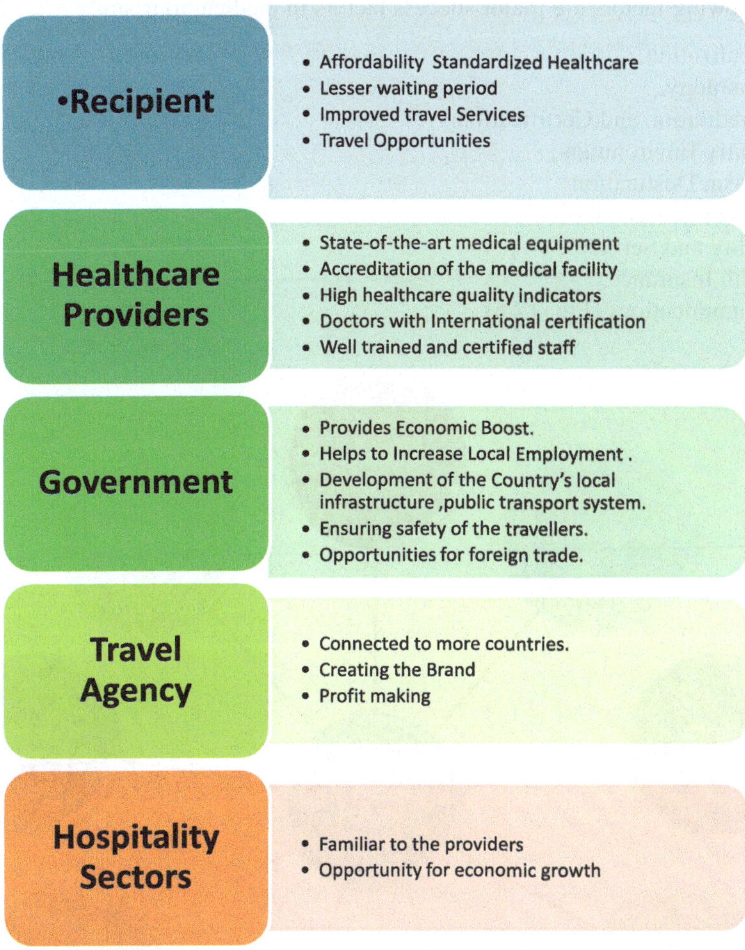

Fig. 17.5 Stakeholders' benefits

17.7 The Future of Medical Tourism Success

The following factors are major success factors in medical tourism:

- Globalization.
- Technology.
- Accreditation and Certification.
- Country Environment.
- Tourism Destination.
- Medical Tourism Costs.
- Facility and Services.
- Health Insurance.
- Communications (Fig. 17.6).

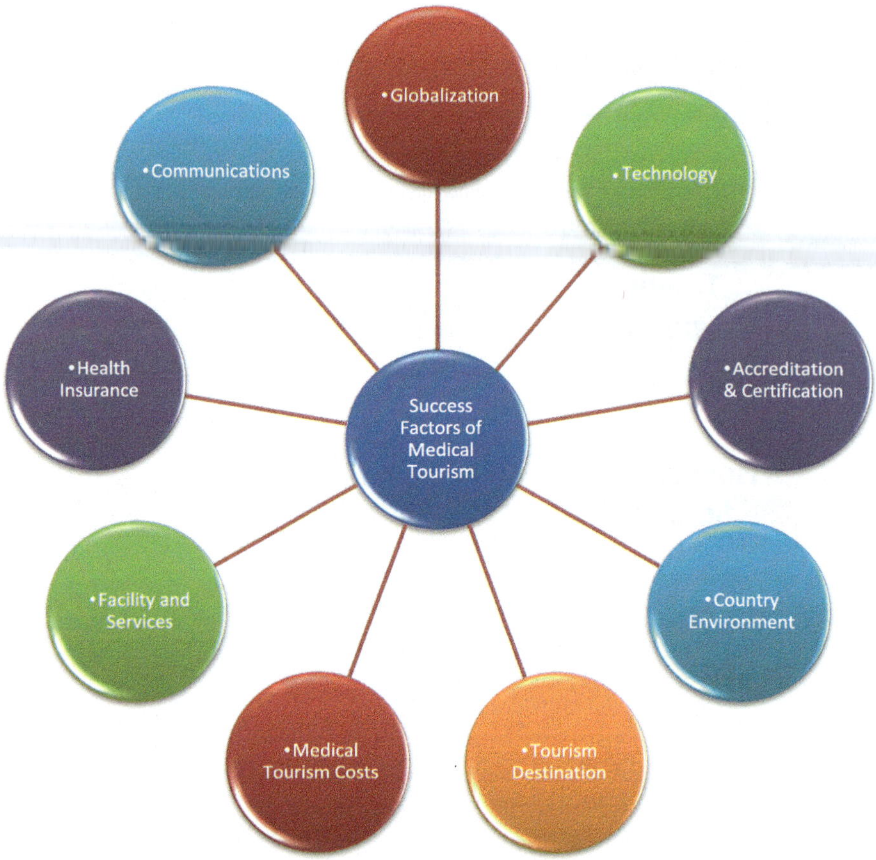

Fig. 17.6 The future success factors of medical tourism growth

The developing countries insist on several suggestions to be successful MT destinations and attract tourists.

- Governments of emerging nations should endorse legislation promoting medical tourism and should mandate licenses for medical tourism service providers (Tontus and Nebioglu 2018).
- To monitor overseas providers through the licensees, related state entities may set record-keeping requirements as part of the licensing system. Through accrediting schemes like JCI, this is possible (Tontus and Nebioglu 2018).
- Even if a patient decides to receive medical care outside of the country, health insurance plans are still required to adhere to HIPAA regulations (Tontus and Nebioglu 2018).
- Patient should decide whether MT is appropriate or not keeping in mind the cost of procedure, cost, and distance of travel staying away from family friends, and other support systems (Tontus and Nebioglu 2018).
- Even if a facilitator is handling the travel arrangements (Tontus and Nebioglu 2018).
- Experts and relevant authorities should certify that the service provider's team is adequately qualified and speaks English with simultaneous translation options. The patient should ensure the quality and accreditation of healthcare providers in foreign places along with the certification of the doctor (Tontus and Nebioglu 2018).
- To provide medical tourists with individualized attention, hospitals should make sure that there are designated information desks for international patients (Tontus and Nebioglu 2018).
- Travel and tourism groups should work with healthcare professionals who are governed by accountable state entities to promote medical tourism (Tontus and Nebioglu 2018).

17.8 Conclusion

Medical tourism is a gain for one and a drain for the other.

Medical tourism is an economic gain for the host nation, which reflects in the rate of foreign trade inflow and output growth, and a drain for the sending countries by undermining fair access to health care also impair the development of health system in these countries.

Health tourism has become and is still thriving because of globalization. This emerging market brings in billions of dollars annually for participating nations and deserves attention and development.

References

Aziz A, Yusof RM, Ayob M, Bakar NT (2015) Measuring tourist behavioural intention through quality in Malaysian medical tourism industry. Procedia Economics and Finance 31:280–285

Bagga T, Vishnoi SK, Jain S, Sharma R (2020) Medical tourism: treatment, therapy & tourism. Int J Sci Technol Res 9:4447–4453

Beladi H, Chao CC, Ee MS, Hollas D (2019) Does medical tourism promote economic growth? A cross-country analysis. J Travel Res 58(1):121–135

Cortez N (2008) Patients without borders: the emerging global market for patients and the evolution of modern health care. Ind LJ 83:71

Hazarika I (2010) Medical tourism: its potential impact on the health workforce and health systems in India. Health Policy Plan 25(3):248–251

John SP, Larke R (2016) An analysis of push and pull motivators investigated in medical tourism research published from 2000 to 2016. Tour Rev Int 20(2–3):73–90

Malhotra N, Dave K (2022) An assessment of competitiveness of medical tourism industry in India: a case of Delhi NCR. Int J Glob Bus Compet 17(2):215–228

Rokni L, Park SH, Avci T (2019) Improving medical tourism services through human behaviour and cultural competence. Iran J Public Health 48(11):1988–1996. PMID: 31970097; PMCID: PMC6961201

Ruka E, Garel P (2015) HOPE: European Hospital and Healthcare Federation report. file:///F:/MT/98_2015_HOPE-PUBLICATION_Medical-Tourism.pdf

Sasirekha K, Sankar P (2022) A study on the challenges and outlooks of medical tourism in India with reference to Chennai region. J Posit School Psychol 6(5):7141–7153

Singh L (2019) Medical tourism motivations: the driving force. J Multidiscip Acad Tour 4(2):77–86

Subbaraman K, Reddy C (2020) Medical tourism: history, global scenario and indian perspectives. Introduction: tourism is the activities of travelers to see the different tourism attractions and (researchgate.net)

Tontus HO, Nebioglu S (2018) Drivers of healthcare globalisation and their effects on medical tourism. e-Review of Tourism Research 15(2/3)

Unit 9 Health Tourism (2017) IGNOU Issue. https://egyankosh.ac.in/handle/123456789/11470

Chapter 18
Current Status of Indian Medical Tourism and Role of Apollo Hospitals Group in Chennai

Barnali Mahanta

Abstract Medical tourism is growing very fast all over the world. In medical tourism, some Asian countries are taking a very forward-looking approach to promoting their healthcare services and facilities as tourist services. Among them, Singapore, Malaysia, Thailand, Turkey, and India are at the forefront. This chapter is specifically about the present status of medical tourism in India and highlights the role of Apollo Hospitals Group in Chennai. In conclusion, Tamil Nadu serves as the center of medical services in the eastern part of the world, and the city Chennai in the particular is called the health capital of India. India attracts a good number of international medical tourists, proving that medical tourism is the first emerging sector in India.

Keywords Medical Tourism · Indian Medical Tourism · Chennai Tourism · Apollo Hospitals

18.1 Medical Tourism

Medical tourism is becoming one of the most lucrative sectors and is growing rapidly in the countries around the world, mainly involving travel and tourism with biomedical procedures. Carrera and Bridges (2006) defined medical tourism as travel that is systematically planned to maintain one's physical and mental health condition. Medical tourism is also known by some other names like Health Tourism, Wellness Tourism, Medical Value Travel (MVT), or Global Healthcare. Furthermore, medical tourism usually refers to the growing practice of travel between countries to obtain medical treatment at low cost, as well as to attract tourists by deliberately promoting its healthcare services and facilities in addition to regular tourist

B. Mahanta (✉)
Department of Tourism Management, Pragjyotish College, Guwahati, Assam, India
e-mail: barnalimahanta@pragjyotishcollege.ac.in

B. Chaudhary et al. (eds.), *Medical Tourism in Developing Countries*,
https://doi.org/10.1007/978-981-99-8909-6_18

services. Currently, dermatology, dentistry, and gynecology medical tourism has seen a high percentage of tourists.

18.2 Current Status of Medical Tourism in India

Since the last decade of the twentieth century, India has become apparent as a major center for medical tourism. As per the Medical Tourism Market Report, India ranks as a top destination because it offers the highest-quality treatment at the lowest cost. According to the Medical Tourism Association, India ranks tenth in the Medical Tourism Index for 2020–2021 out of 46 destinations in the world. In May 30, 2022, India was ranked 54th position at World Travel Tourism index out of 117 countries, but good news is it tops in South Asia. Due to COVID-19 outbreak, it has slipped from 46th position in 2019 to 54th position in 2022 (https://travel.economictimes.indiatimes.com/news/research-andstatistics/figures/india-drops-to-54th-place-on-travel-and-tourism-development-index-top-ranked-in-southasia/91765622). So, in this difficult time, Indian medical tourism extends a helping hand by starting Online Consultation with top Indian doctors. India had gone back a bit due to horrific COVID waves but revived its market due to its credible international recognition, top-class medical technology, comparatively easy M visa procedures, and its multi-faceted medical services with its English-speaking doctors, which attracts an increasing number of medical professionals, medical tourism companies, and medical tourists. According to the Ministry of Tourism in India, 7% of the total foreign tourists are medical tourists. A recent study by the Federation of Indian Chambers of Commerce and Industry (FICCI) has revealed that India is becoming a medical tourism hub and is among the top three medical destinations in Asia. As of now, India has 39 hospitals accredited by the US-based organization Joint Commission International (JCI) and 657 hospitals accredited by National Accreditation Board for Hospitals & Healthcare Providers (NABH). According to recent data, most of the medical tourist arrivals in India come from South East Asia, Middle East, Africa, and SAARC region. Amidst all this, the most medical tourists in India come from Bangladesh and Afghanistan.

Medical tourism is rapidly growing as an industry in India, and India is constantly working on upgradation of medical technology and service facilities to attract patients from all over the world. Data source from American Medical Association (AMA) shows that medical treatment in Europe is still more expensive than in India, while India is also the least expensive compared to other Asian countries. The Indian Medical Tourism business is expected to grow at a Compound Annual Growth Rate (CAGR) of 21.1% from 2020 to 2027 as healthcare is costlier in developed countries.

18.3 India and Medical Tourism

Travel to India is often associated with cultural heritage, alluring beauty, myriad attractions, culinary delights, and delightful diversity, but now a new trend has come and where travelers flock to India for the high-quality healthcare services and low-cost-effectiveness. The medical tourism in India is currently growing as an industry and developing as a leading service provider of various types of medical treatments including cardiology, orthopedics, dental implant, oncology, fertility, hair transplant, cosmetic surgery, organ transplant surgery, and neurosurgery. Currently, India is promoting modern medical science as well as ancient medical system of Ayurveda, Yoga, Unani, Siddha, and Homeopathy, which is also known as AYUSH. Yoga, Ayurveda, Rejuvenation Therapy, and Panchakarma are among the ancient healing therapies in alternative medicine popular today. This makes India the most popular destination for both modern and traditional medicine and therapy. Nowadays, government is promoting India as a medical destination all over the world. In fact, government is keen to promote dental tourism as it accounts for 10% of what medical tourism receives. India's leading public and private healthcare providers are the All India Institute of Medical Sciences (AIIMS), Apollo Hospitals, Fortis Hospitals, National Institute of Mental Health and Neurosciences (NIMHANS), Christian Medical College (CMC), Tata Memorial Hospital, Sankara Nethralaya, Medanta Hospital, Kokilaben Hospital, and Hiranandani Hospital, and and so on. All these hospitals provide various treatments at affordable prices such as heart surgery, cancer surgery, bone-marrow transplant, kidney and heart transplant, cardiac bypass, total hip replacement, and knee replacement along with liver. Andhra Pradesh, Karnataka, New Delhi, Kerala, Tamil Nadu, and Maharashtra lead among Indian states while Chennai, Kolkata, Mumbai, Bangalore, Hyderabad, Goa, Vellore, Alleppey, and Delhi are leading cities.

18.4 Apollo Hospitals Group in Chennai

The Apollo Hospitals Group is India's largest healthcare first corporate chain founded by an Indian entrepreneur and cardiologist Dr. Pratap Chandra Reddy in 1983. It has also franchised in Bangladesh, Kuwait, and Qatar. It is considered one of the best health providers in Asia that manages 70 hospitals, more than 4000 pharmacies, several primary care and diagnostic clinics and telemedicine units in 13 different countries. The Apollo hospital located in Chennai is considered a leading name in the field of medicine and key services provider in various medical procedures including Cardiology, Robotic Surgery, Oncology, Neurology and Neurosurgery, Cosmetic, Dentistry, Orthopedics, Spine Surgery, etc.

The Apollo Hospitals Group has several specialties and super specialties hospitals in Chennai. Below are the glimpses of Apollo Group of hospitals in Chennai:

- The Apollo Hospitals located in Greams Road has been considered the flagship hospital of the Apollo Group and declared as a center for excellence by the Government of India. It provides medical care in over 60 specialties and super specialties. Another hospital located on Greams Road is named Apollo Heart Institute, which specialized in open heart surgery and cardiac catheterization.
- Apollo Children's Hospital was started in 2009 just a mile away from the flagship Apollo Hospital, Greams Road. The 100-bedded offers pediatric care and treatments for newborn babies, children, and adolescents.
- The Apollo Specialty Cancer Hospitals at Teynampet is accredited by NABH and also India's first ISO-certified healthcare provider to provide advanced 360-degree treatment for Oncology, Orthopedics, Neurology and Neurosurgery, Head and Neck surgery, and Reconstructive and Plastic Surgery as well. Apart from treatment, this hospital also offers deluxe, platinum, and super deluxe wards, mainly for its international patients.
- The Apollo First Med Hospital is located at Kilpauk started in 2002, which provides secondary services in various departments and treated more than 1 lakh patients in just 4 years with their great infrastructure and up-to-date technology.
- The Apollo Medical Centre at Karapakkam offers services such as cutting-edge maternity care in Boutique Birthing, Gynecology and Obstetrics, Pediatrics, Neonatology, and Diabetes. The another well-facilitated hospital at Karapakkam is the Apollo Cradle & Children Hospital that exclusively provides services for women and children.

Above these hospitals are easy to reach in terms of proximity and are located close to airport and railway stations for both domestic and international tourist cum patients. International and national tourists visit Apollo Hospitals Group of Chennai every year for full range of medical care, while some pages visit this hospital on the advice of doctors; many others have been selected for quality healthcare. There are some countries where people come for treatment at Apollo Hospitals throughout the year, out of which Kenya, Burundi, Congo, Nigeria, Oman, Iraq, and Bangladesh are at the forefront. The Apollo Hospital Chennai has medical health screening for local people and is also approved by the Department of Immigration and Citizenship of Canada and Australia and Consulate General of United States of America to conduct medical examination of persons who are immigrants or have come for the purpose of holiday. Besides this, Apollo Hospitals have separate wings for its international patients.

Mostly, Apollo Hospitals Group in Chennai has been seen as a major choice for medical tourists from Bangladesh and North Eastern regions in India in terms of private healthcare. Keep in mind the fact the Indian Railway Catering and Tourism Corporation (IRCTC) has collaborated with Apollo Hospitals to facilitate hassle-free travel for patients and their families who travel for medical care. They offer a prepaid preventive health checkup package with charter rail coach service that includes return train ticket, local transportation to hospital, accommodation, and local sightseeing for people from Northeast and Eastern part of the country. IRCTC is also planning to expand these services to neighboring countries like Bangladesh and Sri Lanka by pertaining with airline services and other service providers in these countries. In addition, the Apollo Hospitals Group has an online webpage for its international patients. Additionally, they provide much more than just medical care; they also come bundled with amenities including airport transportation services, semi-private executive rooms in the Apollo suits, tailored cuisine, international language translators, travel-related caretakers to patients on the road to recovery, and sightseeing guides.

Chennai is emerging as a global healing destination in medical tourism. Along with Apollo Hospitals, several hospitals like Madras Medical Mission, Sankara Nethralaya, Sri Ramachandra Hospitals, Lifeline Hospitals, and many others have entered the field and are aggressively promoting medical tourism in India. When one visits the city for medical reasons, one can revitalize the body and soul by doing city sightseeing.

Reference

Carrera PM, Bridges FP (2006) Globalization and healthcare: understanding health care and medical tourism. Expert Review of Pharmacoeconomics and Outcomes Research

Chapter 19
Marketing and Economics of Medical Tourism

Divya Rao, Averil Rebello, N. Shalini, and H. K. Mamatha

Abstract The sector that caters to tourists by offering them information, lodging, transportation, and other services is the tourism industry. Travel for pleasure, leisure, health, or business is also included. Since tourists purchase goods and services they need, tourism is one of the businesses with the quickest growth rates worldwide. Therefore, the tourist sector is crucial to the prosperity of many nations. People who travel across borders to receive treatment for an illness, ailment, or a surgical operation are said to be engaging in medical tourism to find lower-cost, higher-quality healthcare.

The medical tourism industry relies heavily on effectively educating prospective patients about procedures, alternatives, medical facilities, travel arrangements, tourism opportunities, and destination nations. Various promotional materials like flyers, pamphlets, and websites are used to promote medical tourism.

International marketing of its services is important for the medical tourism sector to flourish. The expansion of the medical tourism market in the Southeast Asian countries has resulted as a crucial component for national economic development and the growth of health sector. These nations' national governments actively market their countries as destinations for international patients.

India is well positioned to take advantage of the worldwide potential in the medical and wellness travel industry. The government plays a vital role in the expansion of the emerging medical and wellness tourism sector because it is up against fierce competition on the international market.

Keywords Medical tourism · Health and wellness · Medical value travel

D. Rao (✉) · N. Shalini · H. K. Mamatha
DHSMS, JSSAHER, Mysuru, India
e-mail: divyaraobj.dhsms@jssuni.edu.in

A. Rebello
Yenapoya Medical College, Mangalore, India

B. Chaudhary et al. (eds.), *Medical Tourism in Developing Countries*,
https://doi.org/10.1007/978-981-99-8909-6_19

Objectives
This unit on medical tourism fulfills the following objectives:

1. Need and development of medical tourism.
2. Factors that drive the growth of medical tourism.
3. Marketing of medical tourism.
4. Impact of medical tourism on the economy of the country.

19.1 Introduction

The growth of international trade in medical technology, capital funding, and regulatory frameworks have all contributed to the emergence of new patterns in the supply and consumption of healthcare services over the past few decades. Medical tourism, the practice of moving patients across borders in search of medical care and treatment, has emerged as an important new element of the developing healthcare sector. Medical tourism is defined as the practice of consumers traveling abroad to receive medical treatment. This care may extend to the full range of medical operations; however, the most common ones include dental work, elective surgery, cosmetic surgery, and fertility treatment.

Patients from more affluent, developed nations are traveling to less developed nations more frequently to receive medical treatment, this trend is partially attributed to the accessible, cost-effective therapies in the latter, as well as the accessibility of low-cost flights and online information sources.

Throughout the past few decades, new patterns of healthcare service production and consumption have emerged because of the expansion of international trade in medical technology, capital funding, and regulatory frameworks.

The World Trade Organization's General Agreement on Trade in Services and the free flow of goods and services under its auspices (Smith 2004; Smith et al. 2009) have both accelerated the liberalization of the trade in health services, as have developments in the use of regional and bilateral trade agreements. Health services are now increasingly tradable, global commodities because the healthcare sector is mostly a service industry. The movement of patients across borders in search of medical care and treatment—a practice known as "medical tourism"—has become a substantial new component of this industry.

Access to healthcare overseas is not a recent trend, thus changes must be understood in the context of the past. Since ancient times, people have traveled for health reasons. In the nineteenth century, for instance, there was a trend for the expanding middle classes in Europe to visit spa towns to "take the waters," which were thought to have health-improving properties. Wealthy people from less developed regions of the world traveled to industrialized countries during the twentieth century to access better facilities and highly skilled medical professionals. However, compared to prior types of health-related travel, the changes that are currently occurring in medical tourism are both numerically and qualitatively distinct.

The domestic and international production and consumption patterns of health services may change due to a variety of factors, including the economy, domestic policy changes, political unpredictability, travel restrictions, advertising strategies, geopolitical shifts, and innovative and groundbreaking forms of treatment (Lunt et al. 2011).

19.2 Definitions of Medical Tourism

A wide range of medical services are covered by medical tourism, which has grown to be a popular form of vacationing. It combines relaxation, entertainment, and leisure with health and wellness.

Healthcare tourism as defined by Goodrich & Goodrich in 1987 "the attempt on the part of a tourist facility (for example a hotel) or destination to attract tourists by deliberately promoting its health-care services and facilities, in addition to its regular tourist amenities." (Goodrich and Goodrich 1987).

Medical Tourism Association has defined medical tourism as "Medical Tourism is where people who live in one country travel to another country to receive medical, dental and surgical care while at the same time receiving equal to or greater care than they would have in their own country, and are traveling for medical care because of affordability, better access to care or a higher level of quality of care. 'Domestic Medical Tourism' is where people who live in one country travel to another city, region or state to receive medical, dental and surgical care while at the same time receiving equal to or greater care than they would have in their own home city, and are traveling for medical care because of affordability, better access to care or a higher level of quality of care." (Anon n.d.-a).

19.3 Different Variations of the Term Medical Tourism

World Tourism Organization has defined tourism (1995) as "the activities of persons traveling to and staying in places outside their usual environment for not more than one consecutive year for leisure, business and other purposes." Tourism includes travel for business, medical treatment, and other objectives in addition to leisure travel (World Tourism Organization 1995).

A tourist has been defined as "temporarily leisured person who voluntarily visits a place away from home for the purpose of experiencing a change" (Graburn 1983:21. cf. Graburn 1983).

19.4 Emergence of the Concept of Medical Tourism

People from developing nations traveled to wealthy nations like the USA and Germany to access services not available in their own countries, health tourism began to take off in the beginning of twentieth century. These countries' inadequate technological infrastructure and shortage of qualified personnel were factors contributing to the paucity of local healthcare services. Horowitz and Rosensweig (2008) referred to this movement/tourism as "conventional medical tourism," while Pafford referred to it as the "second wave" of medical tourism (Pafford 2009).

In the 1990s, developing nations began to construct facilities that are comparable to the top medical facilities in industrialized nations. The key forces behind this occurrence were advances in technology that made it possible for new methods and affordable fixes, together with economies of scale in production. People who lack access to affordable local healthcare due to time restrictions or inadequate insurance coverage view foreign health tourism as a feasible alternative (Cohen 2012). The terms "new medical tourism" (Horowitz and Rosensweig 2008), "third wave," (Pafford 2009) and "neo-traditional medical travel," (Cohen 2012) respectively, are used to describe this new trend of migration from rich nations to less developed ones. Recognizing the factors influencing consumer choice is made easier by understanding the main forces influencing this modern kind of healthcare tourism (Aydin and Karamehmet 2017).

19.5 Types of Medical Tourism

A trip that is made for the purpose of receiving medical care, research, or therapy is referred to as medical tourism. During the trip, the traveler makes use of the infrastructure, amenities, and attractions of the destination place. Several ancient records from thousands of years ago provide evidence of the benefits of travel for health.

The term "medical tourism," also known as "health tourism" and "wellness tourism," emerged from the rapidly expanding industry where people from all over the world travel abroad to receive medical, dental, and surgical care while also touring, vacationing, and fully experiencing the attractions of the countries they are visiting. Dental Tourism forms a subset of medical tourism.

Those who travel across borders to acquire medical care for a disease, sickness, or condition are known as medical tourists. These travelers may do so in search of lower costs, better-quality care, greater access to care, or alternative care and hence focus on biomedical procedures mixed with travel and tourism.

Health and wellness tourism refers to travel for receiving rejuvenation and alternative therapies. The complete spectrum of medical procedures may be covered by this care, although the most frequent ones are dental work, elective surgery, aesthetic or cosmetic surgery, and fertility therapy.

19.6 Tourism Types (Pourkhaghan et al. 2013)

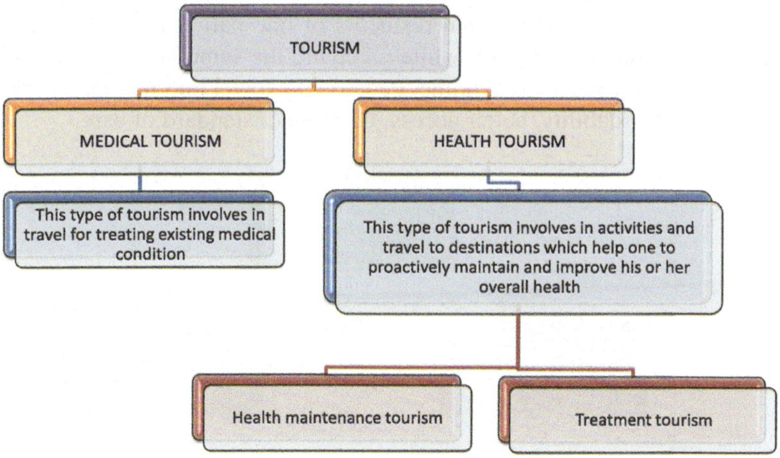

19.6.1 Differences: Medical, Health, and Wellness Tourism (Anon n.d.-b)

Medical tourism	Health and wellness tourism
Reactive form	Proactive practice
The existence of a medical distress	Preventing or maintaining health using alternative procedures
Needs to be investigated, diagnosed, and treated by medical procedures	Without the involvement of specialized clinics, specialized medical personnel, or in-person treatments

19.6.2 Differences between Health and Wellness Tourism (Anon n.d.-b)

Health tourism	Wellness tourism
Traveling by people with an objective of getting health alone	Travel to a different place to productively pursue activities that maintain or enhance their personal health
	Seeking unique, authentic, or location-based experiences may, but typically do not involve specialzsed medical facilities

19.6.3 Inbound v/s Outbound Medical Tourism (Anon n.d.-b)

International medical tourism when residents of one nation travel to another for medical, dental, and surgical care while receiving the same level of care or better than they would have received at home. People may travel internationally for medical care due to affordability, better access, or a higher standard of care.

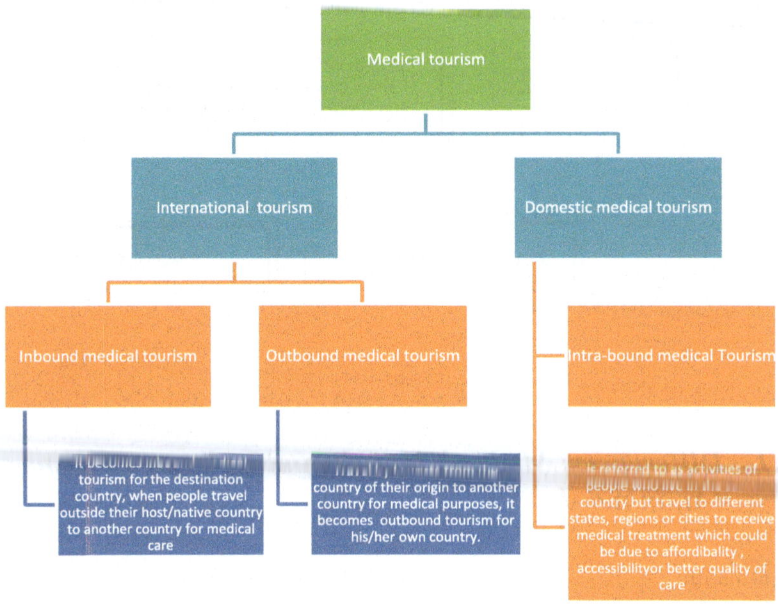

19.7 Current Market Scenario in India (Healthcare 2023a)

India's healthcare industry has grown to be one of the country's largest in terms of both employment and revenue. Hospitals, medical devices, clinical trials, outsourcing, telemedicine, medical tourism, health insurance, and medical equipment are all part of the sector. Due to its expanding offerings, coverage, and rising spending by both public and private entities, the Indian healthcare business is expanding at a rapid rate.

The public and private sectors form the two main components of the Indian healthcare delivery system. The government system concentrates on providing primary healthcare facilities in rural areas while reserving a small number of secondary and tertiary care facilities in major cities. The majority of secondary, tertiary, and quaternary care institutions are run by the private sector, with substantial concentrations in metro areas and larger cities.

India is one of the countries with the fastest expanding medical tourism industries. The medical tourism industry in India is poised to become the next success story after software/IT industry.

Particularly over the past 5 years, the country's healthcare sector has expanded quickly, with a Compound Annual Growth Rate (CAGR) of almost 22% since 2016 (Healthcare 2023a).

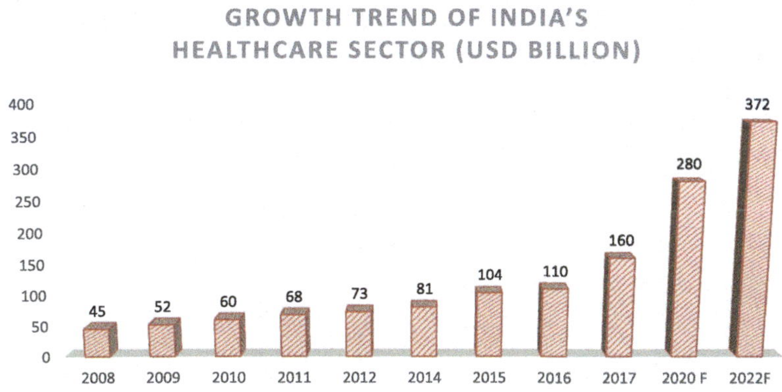

19.7.1 Medical Value Travel

In India, the MVT, or medical tourism, industry is expanding. India's medical tourism industry is expected to be worth USD 5–6 billion by mid-2020 (Healthcare 2023a; Anon n.d.-c). Prior to the COVID-19 outbreak, the valuation was projected to be in the neighborhood of USD 9 billion by 2020 (Healthcare 2023a; Anon n.d.-c). By 2022, it is anticipated that the market would increase to $13 billion (Healthcare 2023b). India was third among the top 10 wellness tourist markets in Asia-Pacific and seventh overall in the top 20 wellness tourism markets in 2017 (Anon n.d.-c; Healthcare 2023b).

Around 37 hospitals in India have received accreditation from the Joint Commission International (JCI), while 513 hospitals have received accreditation from the National Accreditation Board for Hospitals & Healthcare Providers (NABH) (Anon n.d.-c; Healthcare 2023b).

Clinical outcomes at top hospitals in India are on par with those at facilities that are renowned internationally.

India is a popular location for medical tourism for a number of reasons. Patients from all over the world are increasingly traveling to India due to the emphasis on wellness and prevention, strong branding of alternative medicine, and rejuvenation procedures. Ayurveda and yoga-based wellness tourism, in particular, is a quickly developing and expanding sector within India's MVT industry.

19.8 Foreign Tourist Arrival in India According to Purpose

Historically, the majority of medical tourists to India have come from Afghanistan, Pakistan, Oman, Bangladesh, Maldives, Nigeria, Kenya, and Iraq. In the last 4 years from 2018 to 2021, India has received 1,009,583 medical tourists from Bangladesh alone (Sarwal et al. 2021).

In 2021, as per the analysis, 39.4% of foreign tourist arrivals were for the purpose "Indian Diaspora," followed by Medical (21.2%), Business and Professionals (12.1%), and other purpose (9.4%). In 2021, Leisure Holiday and Recreation and Student is lowest, 5.8% and 2%, respectively. 68.4% of arrivals from South Asia were under the category Medical followed by West Asia (61.1%) and Africa (40.0%) (Source: Ministry of Tourism, Market Research Division, Government of India, India Tourism Statistics 2022).

Out of total arrivals from Bangladesh, were for Medical (77.6%), Afghanistan, (53.6%), Maldives (85.8%), and Iraq (94.7%) (Anon n.d.-d).

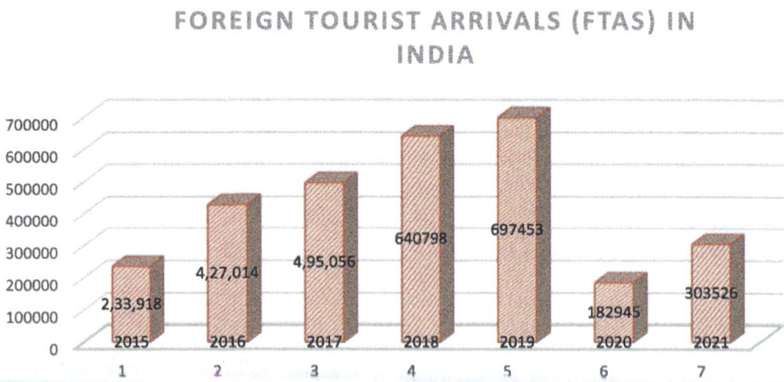

19.9 Market Research and Analysis

Market analysis and research play a very important role in determining what product or service has to be delivered to the specific market segment and also to identify the niche market. Since health tourism is a unique tourism product that combines travel and medical services, market research is extremely important for designing and marketing health tourism goods. It is a highly specialized service that necessitates cooperation between medical professionals and product designers, i.e., developers of tourism products and destination services.

Marketing is the process of persuading customers to select a specific good or service while overlooking alternatives.

An ethical and scientific marketing strategy can increase hospital profits, which indirectly raises the nation's GDP through commercialization of healthcare. Marketing has the power to not only attract patients from other nations but also to increase the revenue from delivery of medical care, boost hospital business, and improve the reputation of the nation rendering the medical services. Medical marketing can be very successful at luring both domestic and international patients and building hospital brands among patients. More importantly, though, it can save lives by raising awareness among patients worldwide about the availability of a particular treatment for life-threatening diseases in a specific hospital of any nation (Das 2017).

The unique characteristics of the services like intangibility, inseparability, heterogenicity, perishability, and ownership make the services completely different from the products. As tourism forms one of the main parts of the service sector, its products have similar qualities. Hence, it is crucial to fully comprehend these qualities and how they are applicable to the tourism industry. A better comprehension of these traits would enable to create, run, and market these services and products successfully (Loveluck 1991).

Another important basis for the customer behavior is based on the extent of contact between the user and the provider indicating the importance of physical presence of the provider for the desired quality especially for the high contact services like tourism, education, and hospitality.

Needs and requirements of the tourist and health tourism industry: in terms of packages and trips, niche market, new concepts, or modification of the existing concept and creating a market for the same (Anon n.d.-e).

Segmentation of the market is usually done on the basis of geographic characteristics, demographic characteristic, psychographic styles, and buying behavior, which makes the market segment very discrete, identifiable, viable, and appropriate (Anon n.d.-e).

19.10 Selection of Destination: Choice Models

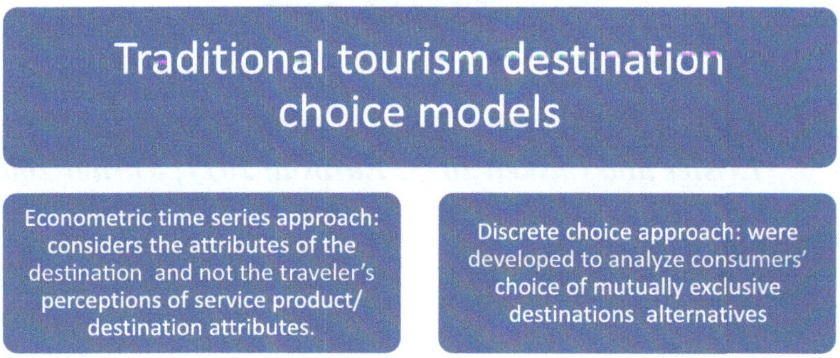
Traditional tourism destination choice models
Econometric time series approach: considers the attributes of the destination and not the traveler's perceptions of service product/ destination attributes.
Discrete choice approach: were developed to analyze consumers' choice of mutually exclusive destinations alternatives

19.11 Factors that Drive the Growth of Medical Tourism

Roger Doswell, a prominent expert on the design of tourist products, stated that the attractions, facilities, and services utilized or visited during a visit are all included in the destination's tourism products. It also consists of everything that occurs to and experienced by the guests (Doswell 1997).

Tourism products are not standardized, as they are primarily a combination of goods and services. Since in tourism, one man serves another, it is exceedingly challenging to consistently deliver the same experience (Anon n.d.-e).

The personal elements and personal experiences of the passengers are discovered to be another factor influencing consumer behavior in destination choosing (Baloglu and McCleary 1999).

19.12 Components of Tourism Markets (Smith 2004; Cook et al. 2002; Connell 2006)

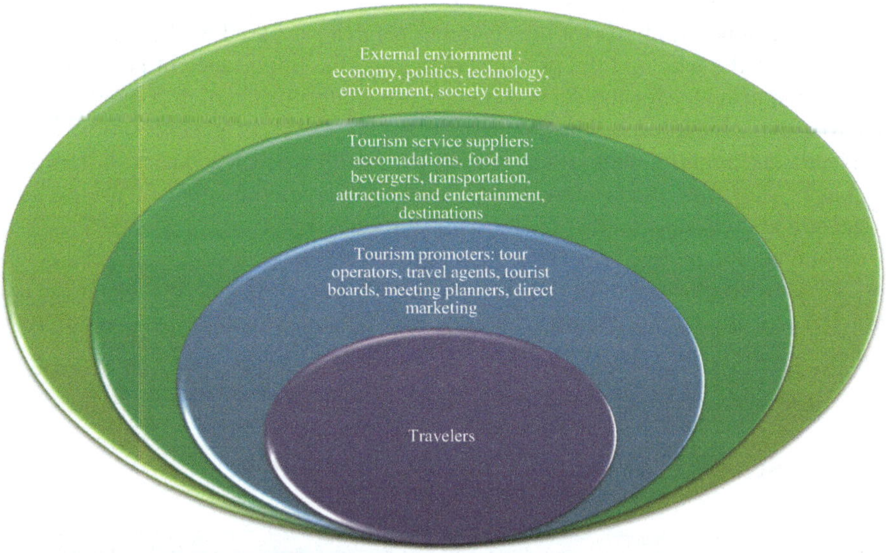

19.12.1 Factors (Smith 2004; Connell 2006; OECD 2012; Eissler and Casken 2013; Eurostat 2011; Turner 2007)

Increased rate of globalisation	•Technological advances •World trade organisation activities-freedom in movement of goods and services •International mobility of medical equipment, health care professionals and patients
Increased health care expenditures	•Expenditures is more in developed countries than in developing countries due to increasing need for medical care of aging population
Increased availibility of global travel	•Increase in airline companies and tecnological advances has decresed the air fare considerably. This is also coupled with the imapct of globalisation .
Increased demand for non essential healthcare services	•Certain health related services like opthalmic, dental etc as well as the wellness related services are considered as non essential services lile cosmetic services are on a rise •Most of theese services are not covered by insurance
Significant differences in health care costs	•Develop countries have higher personnel cost as well as fixed costs when compared to developing countries leading to price diffrence in the cost of care
Increased sophistication of health tourism sector	•Insurance companies as well as the large companies offering health insurance to thier employees consider health care tourism as viable options •Emerging countries are increasing sophistication and professionalism , enforcing regulations and incentive mechanisms leading to increase demand for health tourism
Better information and communication technologies and rise in internet	•One of the main factors facilitating health-care tourism expansion is because of the internet as a massive information source. •The internet provides an opportunity for individuals to identify, analyze, and compare a range of global healthcare service alternatives. The internet is a fantastic resource for communication that enables medical travellers to get in touch with doctors, surgeons, medical facilities, and travel organisations for consultations, appointments, or in-depth information.

19.12.2 Demand-Side Drivers of Mass-Market Medical Tourism

Globalization on all fronts—economic, social, cultural, and technological—is a driving force behind medical tourism.

Tightened eligibility requirements, waiting lists, and altering priorities for health care could all have an impact on consumers' choices in many domestic health systems.

Additionally, consumerism and patient choice are on the rise, even in nations with historically publicly supported healthcare. The availability of information and the growth of several providers who compete on quality and price now meet all needs (Lunt et al. 2011).

Five factors, including familiarity, availability, cost, quality, and bioethical legislation (foreign travel for abortion services, fertility treatments, and euthanasia services), are responsible for the rise in demand for medical services provided abroad, according to Glinos et al. (2006). Expatriates frequently receive medical care when they return to their home country, which is also known as medical tourism.

In the patient's home country, some therapies might not be accessible or might need a wait. The most recent methods and technologies could be included here. It's possible that some therapies are illegal in the nation of origin. The need for privacy and the desire to combine medical operations with typical tourist destinations, hotels, climate, cuisine, and cultural experiences are also considered to be major drivers of market expansion (Lunt et al. 2011; Connell 2006; MacReady 2007; Ramírez de Arellano 2007).

19.13 Supply Side: Models of Service Delivery and Funding (Lunt et al. 2011)

A number of private (and public) providers in developed countries have focused on what they believe to be a lucrative medical tourism industry in terms of delivery and funding.

The approach of emerging medical tourism destinations with an emphasis on quality and customer service has been partially influenced by the experience of numerous private patient hospitals and hospital wings for wealthy patients in the United Kingdom and the United States. To sustain the collapsing private sector in Thailand, where domestic private patients were switching to the publicly supported system, medical tourism services were developed.

The private and corporate insurance systems could be a more attractive source of cash in addition to individual out-of-pocket payments for treatment. Medical tourism service providers have had only a little amount of success thus far in capturing these prospective revenue streams.

It might be argued that the sector is undergoing a legitimization and marketing process with a focus on promoting service quality and competitiveness, and that this process includes focusing on workplace/private/public health insurance systems.

19.14 Need for Medical Tourism: Demand and Supply (Heung et al. 2010)

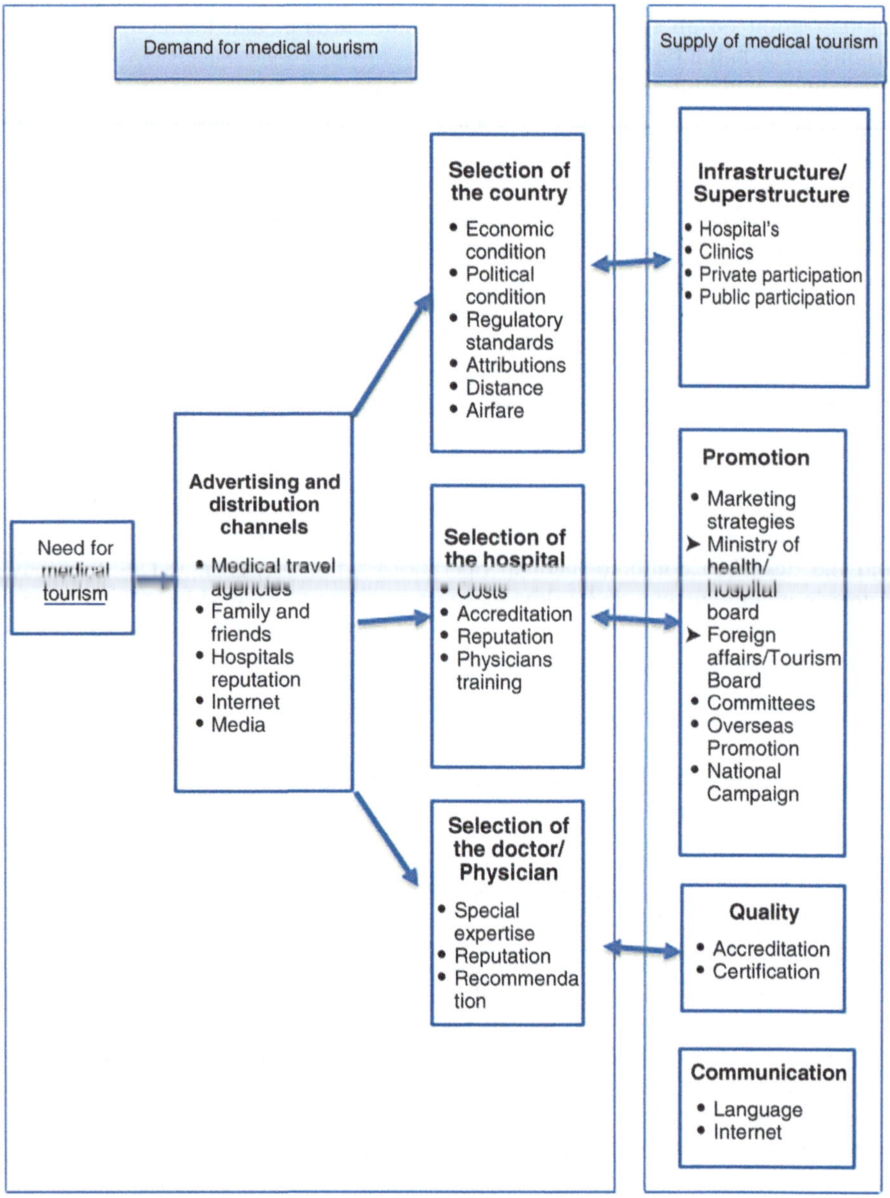

19.15 Push–Pull Model Motivators of Medical Tourism

"Push–Pull model" describes the factors as "people travel because they are pushed into making travel decisions by internal, psychological forces, and pulled by external forces of the destination attributes" (Walker and Walker 2010, p. 43).

Motivation is one of the most practiced notions in medical tourism and is the reason that tourists do what they do. Motivation can be defined as the driving forces within individuals that compel them to act (Jeong 2014). These motivating factors may elicit, guide, and integrate a person's conduct (Yoon and Uysal 2005). Various classifying motivators are available, generally push/pull factors are commonly used (Kanagaraj and Bindu 2013; Kim et al. 2003; Mohammad and Som 2010; Uysal and Jurowski 1994).

Push factors motivates individuals to want to go on a tour, whereas the pull factors aid the person in choosing a suitable location (Goossens 2000).

19.15.1 Factors (John and Larke 2016)

Push factors	Pull factors (Healthcare provider specific)	Pull factors (Destination specific)
Are associated with the attributes of the individual tourists	Are associated with the attributes of the destination country and they can create demand for inbound tourism	Are associated with certain characteristics of a medical tourism destination which influence their choice. They refer to those factors that make a specific medical tourism market attractive to the potential medical tourists.
Recommendation from doctors, family, and friends	Lower medical costs	Infrastructure
Inadequate insurance coverage (Cosmetic, dental, vision, fertility treatments, etc.)	Service quality	Availability of specific treatments (abortion, stem cells therapy)
Desire for privacy and confidentiality of treatments	Language proficiency of the Medical staff	Reputation of the medical professionals in the destination
Prior medical tourism experience	Accreditation of medical facilities	Political and social stability
Proximity of destination	Less waiting time	Favorable exchange rates
Affordability of international travel	Access to treatments/ medications not available in-home country	Food and accommodation facilities
Sociodemographic status (age, gender, income, etc.)	Hospital reputation	Regulatory environment (legal protection)
Cultural similarities	Reputation of the doctors	Social and cultural familiarity
Lack of treatment options in home countries		
Distrust in local healthcare systems		

19.16 Factors Affecting Medical Tourism Destination Attractiveness (Heung et al. 2010; Pocock and Phua 2011; Musa et al. 2012)

The increased competitiveness among the healthcare domain at the national and global levels is one effect of trade liberalization in the healthcare sector. Various nations acknowledge the potential of medical tourism, leading to their governments promoting medical tourism destinations.

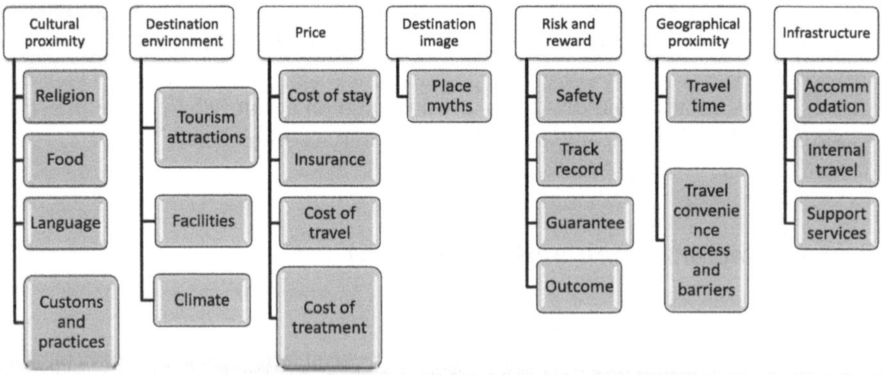
Cultural proximity
Religion
Food
Language
Customs and practices
Destination environment
Tourism attractions
Facilities
Climate
Price
Cost of stay
Insurance
Cost of travel
Cost of treatment
Destination image
Place myths
Risk and reward
Safety
Track record
Guarantee
Outcome
Geographical proximity
Travel time
Travel convenie nce access and barriers
Infrastructure
Accomm odation
Internal travel
Support services

19.17 Marketing of Medical Tourism

Philip Kotler defined marketing as "A human activity directed at satisfying needs and wants through exchange processes." Thus, marketing emphasizes on the concept of consumer orientation and satisfaction leading to the profitability of the organization.

Effectively reaching the target customers is essential for the success of medical tourism. The potential customers must be informed and persuaded that the clinics, physicians, and dentists are not only secure, but also among the most cutting-edge, highly skilled, and modern healthcare providers in the world, all of whom are available for significantly less money than the same services in their home country.

Hence, marketing strategy plays a very important role in the development of the medical tourism market. Marketing strategies are tools that are used to outline the various campaigns and marketing models.

19.18 Types of Marketing Stratergies

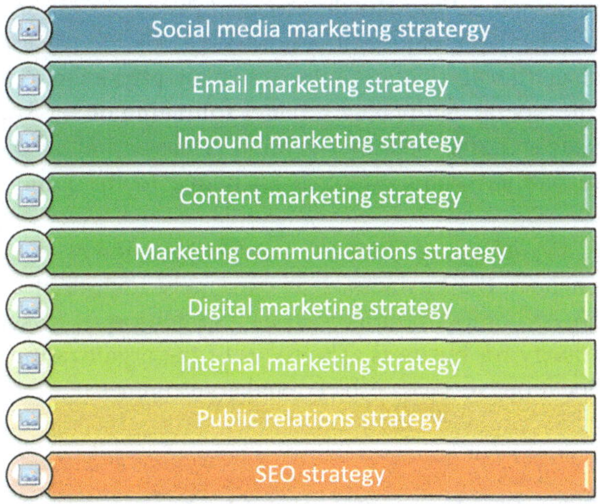
Social media marketing stratergy
Email marketing strategy
Inbound marketing strategy
Content marketing strategy
Marketing communications strategy
Digital marketing strategy
Internal marketing strategy
Public relations strategy
SEO strategy

There isn't once size that fits all marketing strategy. Strategies come in a variety of formats, including word papers, flowcharts, and PowerPoint slides. But, despite their apparent differences, the most successful marketing tactics always share a few characteristics.

19.18.1 Marketing Strategies for Medical Tourism

Education Education is essential for effective marketing. As potential customers won't select anything they don't fully comprehend. To make a choice, a buyer requires options. Hence, the informed potential clients about the independence, accessibility, and caliber of medical services available.

Identifying the ideal customer: the customer can be identified through geography (identified zone or region), demographics (specific therapies for specific age groups, i.e., through demographic profiling), and psychographics (in terms of customer thinking, motivating to action, reactions like happiness or fear, etc., can lead to psychographic profiling of the customer)

19.18.2 Messaging to Educate, Establish Credibility, and Differentiate

Customers are informed about services and the customer experience by successful medical tourism businesses, which aids in decision-making. To create a relationship with potential consumers and encourage them to make a purchase, sales materials should inform them about the services, advantages, personnel, and treatment philosophy.

Most prospective medical tourists do not meet the organization or the physician before they make a decision. Hence, it is necessary to build trust and credibility in the person to select the particular organization or physician. This can be done through the website, social media pages, better following on the social media, written articles for search engine operations, press releases, industry seminars, blogs, etc., can increase publicity and establish an image in the mind of the potential customers.

Differentiating the products from the competitors makes it important for the organization to enhance the business. It is extremely important to understand the competitor, perceived competition as well as recognition of lesser competitors to make the right strategy for business. The focus of the organization has to be on the quality, pricing, location, service delivery, and convenience.

19.18.3 Website Marketing/Digital Marketing

- **No website = you don't exist**
- **Proper english translation is CRITICAL**
- **Well-designed site: strong branding and purpose**
- **Keep it simple/easy to use and understand**
- **Website must include: what you do , differentiation, conact number**
- **Reply quickly**
- **Focus on SEO and key words**
- **Website content marketing: establishing credibility**
- **Keep it fresh**
- **Keep it plain and simple**

The story to tell: public relations marketing:

Referrals continue to be one of the best ways to grow a medical tourism service. Positive public relations have the strongest influence on referrals. The heart-warming anecdote of a patient requiring a unique or specific medical procedure available in the destination that was unavailable in their country in turn leads to creating a brand and better sought after organization.

By providing articles and news items, the organization may establish itself as a trustworthy news source, which generally attracts more attention and greatly raises the perceived credibility of the organization.

19.19 Promotional Strategy for Development of Organization as a Destination (Crooks et al. 2011)

The medical tourism industry relies on effectively educating prospective patients about procedure alternatives, medical facilities, travel arrangements, tourism opportunities, and destination nations. Many marketing tools, including flyers, pamphlets, and websites, are used to promote medical tourism.

Thus, the promotional materials can include (Crooks et al. 2011):

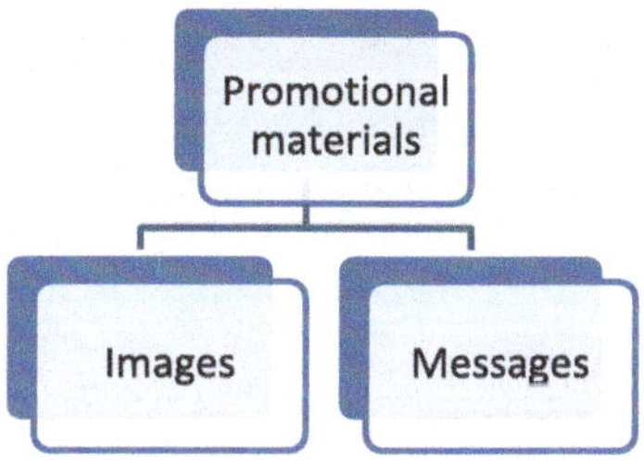

IMAGES (Crooks et al. 2011) may be depicting the organization in lieu of facilities, staff as well as procedures carried out and success stories.

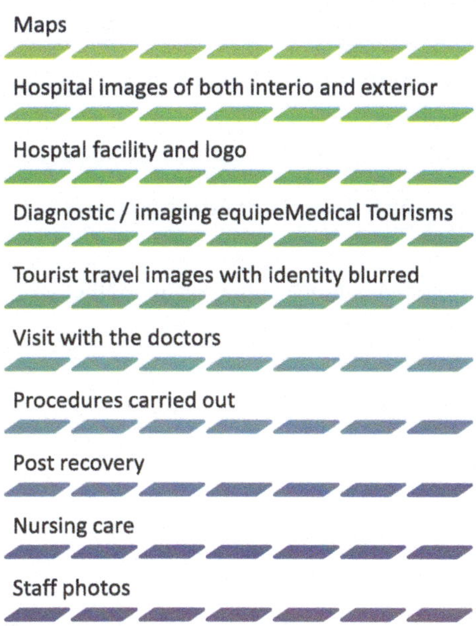

19.19.1 Messages (Crooks et al. 2011)

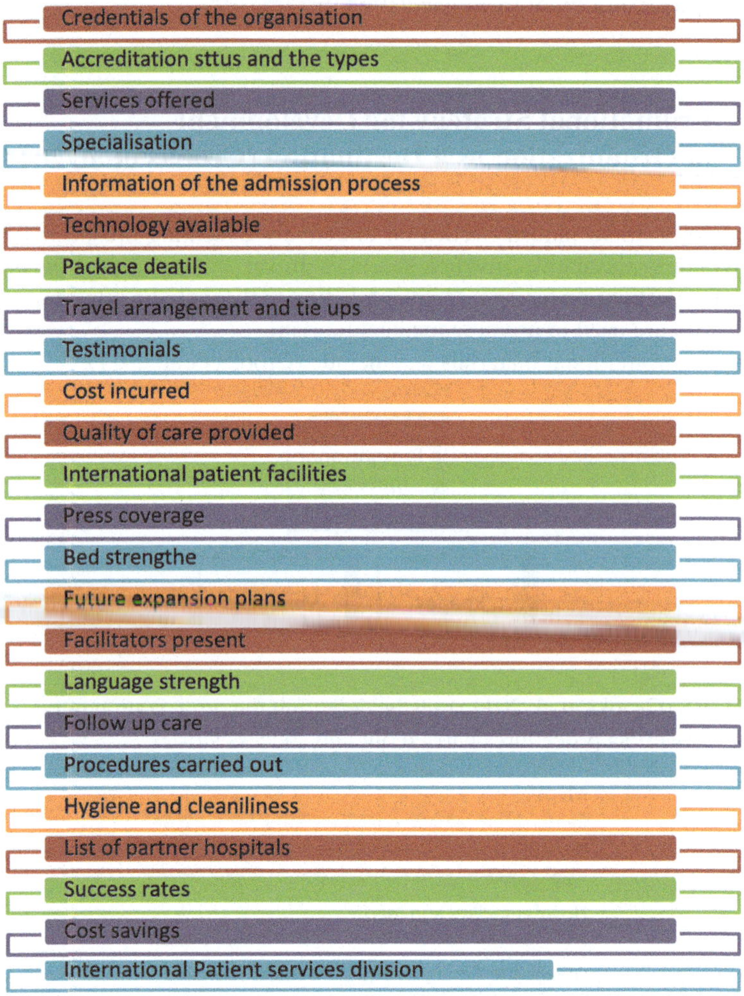

International Patient division can provide assistance like:

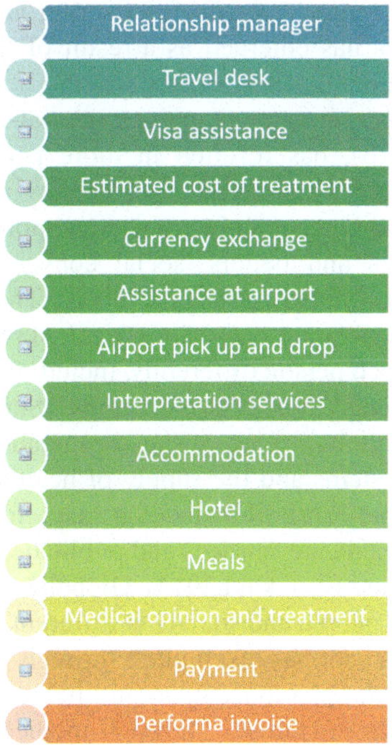
Relationship manager
Travel desk
Visa assistance
Estimated cost of treatment
Currency exchange
Assistance at airport
Airport pick up and drop
Interpretation services
Accommodation
Hotel
Meals
Medical opinion and treatment
Payment
Performa invoice

19.20 Economies of Medical Tourism

Economic impacts of medical tourism:

The Indian patients have not been significantly impacted by the globalization of the healthcare industry, but it has caused the Indian economy to open up, making it easier to obtain the best implants, pharmaceuticals, and equipment. Due to competitive benchmarking system, based on the healthcare systems of industrialized countries, it has led to choice and improved healthcare quality. The foreign exchange collected from the international patients is used to fund medical research and offer financially disadvantaged individuals subsidized care. However, there has been a dramatic change in the economy, causing patients to migrate from an unaffordable to an affordable range. Patients for underdeveloped countries who were unable to afford care can do so now because of health insurance. This change in the dynamics has resulted in patients able to receive more affordable care.

The growth and development of the primary sector, which utilizes natural resources and encompasses agriculture, fishing, forestry etc., secondary sector, which encompasses heavy manufacturing, light manufacturing, energy production, food processing, etc., and tertiary sectors of the economy that encompasses a wide range of activities like health and welfare, tourism, leisure as well as recreation activities, are directly related to the economic development of any given nation. Additionally, this industry has a significant impact on foreign exchange and significantly advances the nation's economy today.

Over the past century, a new pattern of delivering and consuming healthcare-related goods and services has emerged as a result of the internationalization of healthcare services. The liberalization of trade in the healthcare sector has led to increase in the foreign direct investment, entrepreneurial-minded healthcare professionals (Skountridaki 2015), has resulted in more people looking for medical care abroad.

Several elements, including economic growth, technology advancements, political forces, cultural values and beliefs, social conventions, and environmental changes, are responsible for globalization (Lee 2000). These elements of globalization have an impact on healthcare on various levels, both directly and indirectly. Globalization can affect each person differently, including patients who go overseas and healthcare professionals' household earnings (Skountridaki 2015). Patient mobility is one way that globalization at the organizational level can impact the resources of healthcare systems and the supply of healthcare professionals (Saker et al. 2004). At the national level, globalization may change the legal framework governing international healthcare services and public health spending (Mattoo and Rathindran 2006; Vidalis and Kyriakaki 2014). Globalization can consequently lead to a number of changes in people and society at different levels.

Liberalization of health care has taken place through professional mobility, foreign direct investment in the pharmaceutical and healthcare sectors, cross-border healthcare services, and more evidently through medical tourism leading to free travel for health and wellness. Globalization of healthcare services has resulted it in being a business opportunity for some and some others view it as a danger to their professions (Skountridaki 2015). The complete spectrum of medical procedures may be covered by this care, although the most frequent ones are dental work, elective surgery, aesthetic surgery, and fertility therapy.

Medical tourism has the potential to impact a diverse range of people and stakeholders, including the employment prospects for healthcare workers, the prognosis for patients travelling from other countries, national laws governing medical ethics and data protection, and last but not least, the financial prospects for the hospitality industry. Lautier (2014) estimated that in Tunisia, over 19,000 employment opportunities were tied to tourism, whereas medical tourism generated over 37,000 jobs.

According to almost all estimations, medical visitors spend more than other tourists (Connell 2006). A medical tourist in Singapore spends around three times as much as a regular visitor, according to Turner (2007). Researchers looking at the spending habits of medical tourists in Malaysia revealed that their overall spending was 12 times more than that of tourists traveling for leisure (Musa et al. 2012). The cost of the medical care is the primary expenditure of a medical travel trip, followed by international airfares, lodging, scheduled trips, shopping, food, and beverage costs, and domestic transportation (Musa et al. 2012). The list of costs associated with a medical trip reveals that almost half of the costs are related to healthcare services, while the other costs are related to tourism.

In addition, medical tourists frequently travel with at least one accompanying person and remain longer than leisure travellers (Connell 2011, 2006; Lautier 2014; Musa et al. 2012), which considerably increases the overall cost of a medical tourism trip considerably.

Dr. Devi Shetty and Dr. Govindappa Venkataswamy, entrepreneurial doctors, have established healthcare cities and eye hospitals in India (Burns 2015; Rangan and Thulasiraj 2007), are attracting patients from across nations to receive high-quality medical care at reasonable costs (Rangan and Thulasiraj 2007).

The European Commission has established a set of recommendations to promote patient travel with the aim of guaranteeing each European Union citizen the freedom to receive medical care and travel within the European Union for such purposes (Vidalis and Kyriakaki 2014). Significant adjustments were made to public health insurance at the same time to ease patient travel among member states of the European Union (EU). The European Union Directive on international healthcare was adopted in 2011. The European Union Directive gives all European Union residents the right to purchase healthcare services throughout the European Union and to submit a claim for reimbursement to their home country's national health system. However, due to a shortage of financing incentives, fewer patients are claiming their European Union rights (Lunt 2015).

To accommodate the rising number of medical tourists, South East Asian nations including Thailand, Singapore, Malaysia, and India have issued medical tourist visas (Pocock and Phua 2011; Burns 2015).

The following are the financial advantages of medical tourism, which dominates all other tourism-related industries (Anon n.d.-f).

The best travelers from both developed and developing nations come here. Therefore, if medical travel is regarded as a high value-added product, its economic impact on the nation will likewise be substantial.

It boosts revenue from foreign currency exchange.

It boosts employment both directly and indirectly and generates fresh business prospects. Jobs including taxi services, hotels, restaurants, and gift shops include direct work. Contrarily, employment created because of the manufacturing of goods and services required by the health tourism industry is referred to as indirect employment.

It places a strong emphasis on improving infrastructure to draw in medical tourists from abroad and improve the level of living for citizens.

The prestige of the nation in terms of medical tourism will draw in additional visitors, which will subsequently spur economic growth through a multiplier effect.

The expansion of the medical tourism sector will assist a few linked industries, including the hospital, medical equipment, and pharmaceutical sectors. Because of the medical tourism sector, there are more physicians, nurses, and medical technicians. This makes the medical tourism sector one of the most significant for the economy. Medical tourism has many subsectors and has a big impact on the world economy.

19.21 Cost for Patient and One Accompanying Person Travelling (Lunt et al. 2011)

Procedure	Cost UK (£)[a]	Cost procedure India (£)[b]	Cost of flight[c]	Hotel stay[d]	Total cost India	Cost saved per operation (£)	Waiting list[e]	Total saved (£)
CABG	8631	3413	1000	230	4643	3988	97	386,836
Coronary angioplasty	2269	2363	1000	69	3432	−1163	25,241	Not worth it
Total hip replacement	8811	3413	1000	322	4735	4076	28,800	117,388,800
Total knee replacement	6377	5145	1000	161	6306	71	53,911	3,827,681
Femoral hernia repair	1595	819	1000	69	1888	−293	1686	Not worth it
Inguinal hernia repair	1595	717	1000	46	1763	−168	65,064	Not worth it
Total								121,603,317

[a]NHS reference costs 2007-2008
[b]From Fortis Healthcare Mohali (JCI accredited)
[c]From British Airways, two week in advance of flying (i.e. 30th of September)
[d]Used exchange rate £1 = [illegible] Rp [illegible]/night in Mohali (where Fortis is) luxury accommodation (Imperial Hotel Mohali)
[e]Obtained from Hospital Episode Statistics, Main procedures and operations 2007-2008

19.22 Cost for Only Patient Traveling (Lunt et al. 2011)

Procedure	Cost UK (£)[a]	Cost procedure India (£)[b]	Cost of flight[c]	Total cost India	Cost saved per operation (£)	Waiting list[e]	Total saved (£)
CABG	8631	3413	500	3913	4718	97	457,646
Coronary angioplasty	2269	2363	500	2863	−594	25,241	Not worth it
Total hip replacement	8811	3413	500	3913	4898	28,800	141,062,400
Total knee replacement	6377	5145	500	5645	732	53,911	39,462,852
Femoral hernia repair	1595	819	500	1319	276	1686	465,336
Inguinal hernia repair	1595	717	500	1217	378	65,064	24,594,192
Total							206,042,426

[a]NHS reference costs 2007–2008
[b]From Fortis Healthcare Mohali (JCI accredited)

[c]From British Airways, 2 week in advance of flying (i.e. 30th of September)
[d]Used exchange rate £1 = $1.66 rounded to nearest pound
[e]Obtained from Hospital Episode Statistics, Main procedures and operations 2007–2008

19.23 Impacts of Medical Tourism on Host Countries

Positive impacts	Negative impacts
The increase of medical tourism benefits the economies of the host nations. By generating income in the travel and tourist-related industries, and expansion of the local economy.	Medical resources in the host nation's public health care system are depleted as a result of the growth of medical tourism. Because of this crowding-out effect, worker productivity declines, which in turn slows economic growth.
Foreign exchange influx and output growth both indicate the significance of medical tourism to the host economy. The revenue from medical tourism is accepted as an export that can increase a nation's balance of payments by bringing in foreign exchange. The supply of health care services to foreign patients and the related expenditures by patients and their companions on food, lodging, and local tourism activities are examples of potential sources of income for host countries Lautier (2014).	The growth of medical tourism leads to an unfair distribution of public funds in the host nations. Tourists typically seek elective and non-emergency medical procedures, which differ from local health requirements.
Employment prospects in the healthcare industry and allied businesses increase as medical tourism grows. In contrast to public hospitals, private institutions that participate in medical tourism frequently provide health workers with more attractive compensation, better employment conditions, and more promising career possibilities, narrowing the pay gap between domestic and foreign earnings. This makes the working at the home country more attractive resulting in better retention of the skilled workers at home and also bring about those who are overseas to return home	Maintaining a competitive advantage in these medical specialties for which the host country is known for has negative consequences, including excessive investment in high-tech medical equipment and a rise in the number of medical graduates choosing to work in specialties that are in demand from patients abroad while showing less interest in careers in public health.

Positive impacts	Negative impacts
Access to and the standard of domestic medical treatment are improved by medical tourism in underdeveloped nations (Helble 2011). The quality of domestic health systems, particularly in developing nations, is improved by the availability of such cutting-edge facilities and a wide range of medical skills. Also, it encourages local citizens to seek treatment at home rather than overseas, which lessens the outflow of hard currency (Johnston et al. 2010). Promoting medical tourism allows hospitals in nations with tiny populations to achieve economies of scale, fully utilize excess capacity, and justifiably invest in costly modern medical technology because the health business requires a lot of capital.	The cost of local healthcare services may increase due to a thriving medical tourism business, making care for locals less accessible. Private hospitals in the host nation make significant investments in cutting-edge medical technology and luxurious facilities akin to five-star hotels in order to draw in foreign patients. They also provide individualized nursing care, high doctor-to-patient ratios, and quick access to specialists, radiology, and other services.
Foreign direct investment in healthcare institutions in host nations brings in extra funding and may lead to the transfer of technology and knowledge.	Internationally compliant medical equipment that is state-of-the-art adds to foreign debt and companies boosting health care costs to stay profitable. Furthermore, foreign investors who may not be concerned with the Well-being of locals may operate private healthcare institutions in developing nations. As a result, rising health care costs could drive out local residents, particularly those with modest incomes, from the local health system.
	Medical workers—Especially highly qualified and experienced health professionals—In the host country's public health care sector are drawn to the private health care sector because of better pay and career prospects. Although medical tourism can help prevent external brain drain, it can exacerbate internal brain drain.

19.24 Local Benefits of Medical Tourism

The primary motivation for many Emerging Markets to invest in medical tourism is economic growth (Connell 2013; Turner 2007). Medical Tourism offers these nations a great chance to prosper economically by bringing in foreign exchange and the potential for two labor-intensive industries (healthcare and tourism) to provide a steady source of growth (Bookman and Bookman 2007). Additionally, the popularity of Medical Tourism might draw in both domestic and foreign investments to boost economic expansion. Government tax vacations and exemptions from customs taxes on medical equipment permitted hospitals to import expensive equipment that was previously unavailable (Chen and Flood 2013). Thus, the government's initiative to promote Medical Tourism helped the nation's healthcare system progress.

"Brain drain" has also been exacerbated by the growth of Medical Tourism practices in some nations as nurses and doctors opt to seek for employment and better income outside of the country (Bookman and Bookman 2007). There are some evidences of "brain gain" in the nation, though, professionals with advanced degrees who were educated in the West returning to their homeland and beginning to work in their area of specialization. Some of them even become entrepreneurs starting their own companies, creating jobs for people, and training future medical professionals too.

19.25 Local Challenges in the Industry

Medical Tourism can contribute to both the challenges and the solutions in the destination nations. Medical Tourism's trickle-down impact has not yet been proven, despite the fact that some people think it can be a good source of funds for the local healthcare (Connell 2011).

Providers in Emerging Markets nations frequently emphasize their ability to provide timely and affordable modern medical services. However, because they are pricey and more geared toward international healthcare customers, most local patients are unable to utilize these services (Pocock and Phua 2011). For additional information, see the significance of proper physical infrastructure in the development of Medical Tourism.

Providers in Emerging Markets nations frequently emphasize their ability to provide timely and affordable modern medical services with adequate physical infrastructure making it an ideal destination for international healthcare customers leading to deficiency of services to the local population because of the expensive nature of these services (Pocock and Phua 2011).

19.26 Issues that Restricted the Progress

- Expensive air travel.
- Lack of direct flights.
- Transfers at airports could make patients more anxious, especially if they are already susceptible from their disease.
- Insufficient transport infrastructure.
- Lack of adequate Internationally accredited hospitals.
- Security and public safety of the medical tourists.
- Developing the country as a niche market in Medical Tourism.
- Government role in the development of medical tourism sector in the country.

Privately operated hospitals and clinics design their own business models and operating frameworks to suit their institutions. In Medical Tourism, the well-established medical providers (mostly privately held) who can afford to invest in cutting-edge medical technology, hire medical specialists, (re)build new structures, and achieve international accreditation and affiliation thrive while the rest are left behind. These factors lead to unfavorable effects on the healthcare business in the country.

Firstly, it negatively impacts the reputation of the nation as a potential travel destination by widening the quality gap between public and private healthcare.

Secondly, it leads to local brain drain. The expansion of the private healthcare industry attracts more young and seasoned specialists, endangering the public healthcare system.

Finally, focusing on the diaspora can make it more difficult for Medical Tourism stakeholders to recognize the chance to draw in the vast majority of patients from abroad.

Local issues in the Medical Tourism sector must be resolved since they prevent the nation from attaining its full potential (Beladi et al. 2019).

19.27 Barriers for Development

Barrier is defined as "A factor that impacts or hinders smooth implementation thus affecting performance towards desired objectives/goals." There may be many hindrances for the development of medical tourism for various destinations. Some of them may be summarized as follows: (Heung et al. 2010).

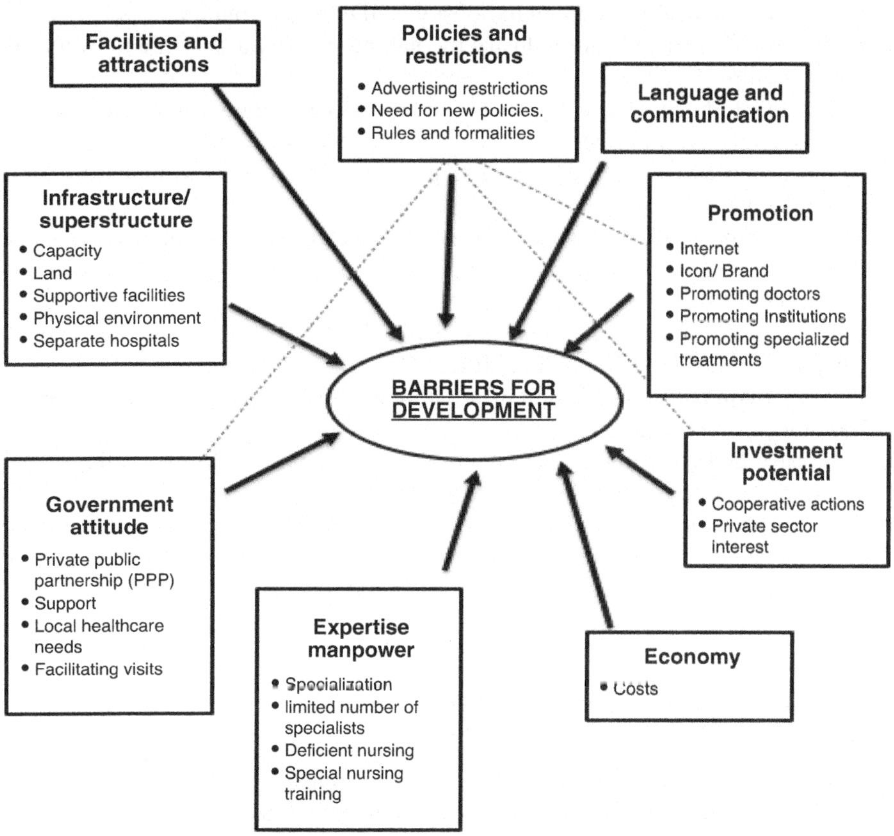

19.28 Role of Government to Promote Medical Tourism (Anon n.d.-g)

With the government acting as a catalyst, medical tourism is the ideal approach to promote the country as "The Global Destination for medical tourism". Traditionally, the medical tourism industry has been mostly supported by the private sector.

Government initiatives can be in terms of:

- Allocation of funds for the development of human resources for health and medical education.
- Extension of the e-medical visa facility to the citizens of different countries.
- Establishment of new medical colleges.
- Establishing a board for medical and wellness tourism to promote the same in the country as well as abroad.

- increase public health spending to boost the GDP of the country,
- revolutionize the healthcare industry by making it easily accessible to everyone in the country,
- Govt looks to boost medical tourism via various campaigns leading to creation of a comprehensive online repository of every type of health-care worker in the nation which assist external parties like patients, employers to matching their requirements.
- The government can strategically invested in the growth of medical tourism by coming up with various alternative therapies and schemes to attract the patients to their country.
- Emphasis on accreditation of hospitals and their listing to ensure that the country can provide world-class health facilities.
- All major companies and hospitals are now focused on building state-of-the-art hospitals.
- They have tied up with reputable doctors locally to prevent further collapse and facilitate the local citizens healthcare needs.
- The Government can announce loans to boost the infrastructure and announce working capital or personal loans to companies operating in the tourism industry to restart after the hit they took in the COVID-19 phase.

19.29 Road Ahead (Anon n.d.-g)

The challenge before the tourism marketer is to transform routine into a unique experience, and this needs creativity as well as imagination.

The healthcare industry, which encompasses providers, payers, and medical technology, is highly diversified and offers opportunities in every area. Businesses are trying to investigate the newest dynamics and trends that will have a beneficial impact on their business because of the increased competition.

Opportunities for those involved in the medical device sector can exist in any nation. With significant capital expenditure for cutting-edge diagnostic facilities, the nations can also rank among the top locations for high-end diagnostic services, serving a larger section of the population. Also, customers of medical services are increasingly concerned about maintaining their health. Future demand for health-care services is anticipated to increase due to factors such as advancing income levels, an aging population, rising health awareness, and shifting attitudes.

19.30 Conclusion

Despite the fact that Medical Value Tourism has been negatively impacted by COVID-19, it is anticipated to recover over the coming months and then continue to develop quickly. Although nations can have sizable and expanding number of

JCI-accredited hospitals, standards still need to be raised in order to bring service levels up to line with international norms. For investors, this demand has produced fantastic opportunities. The majority of healthcare providers have been building new facilities to accommodate critical care or offer super-specialty services. Additionally, a number of significant hospital players are actively soliciting money for their expansion. Growth in the medical tourism industry is also opening up investment opportunities in institutions that provide paramedical and nursing personnel with training as well as cutting-edge diagnostic tools.

References

Anon (n.d.-a). http://www.medicaltourismassociation.com/en/for-governments.html

Anon (n.d.-b) Unit 10 HEALTH, MEDICAL AND WELLNESS TOURISM , Ignou Manual, 144–159

Anon (n.d.-c) Note on Health and Pharmaceutical Sector. Invest India

Anon (n.d.-d) Source: https://tourism.gov.in/sites/default/files/2022-08/usq%202223%20for%2004082022.pdf

Anon (n.d.-e) Unit 20: Tourism marketing 1: relevance, product, market research

Anon (n.d.-f). http://www.medicaltourism.com/blog/economic-benefits-of-medicaltourism/

Anon (n.d.-g) "SERVICES INDUSTRY" INDUSTRY REPORT, Nov, 2022 https://www.ibef.org/industry/services#:~:text=The%20services%20sector%20is%20not,has%20provided%20large%2Dscale%20employment

Aydin G, Karamehmet B (2017) Factors affecting health tourism and international healthcare facility choice. Int J Pharm Healthc Mark 11(1):16–36. https://doi.org/10.1108/IJPHM-05-2015-0018

Baloglu S, McCleary KW (1999) A model of destination image formation. Ann Tour Res 26(4):868–897

Beladi H, Chao C-C, Ee MS, Hollas D (2019) Does medical tourism promote economic growth? A cross-country analysis. J Travel Res 58(1):121–135. https://doi.org/10.1177/0047287517735909

Bookman MZ, Bookman KR (2007) Medical tourism in developing countries. Palgrave Macmillan, New York

Burns LR (2015) Medical tourism opportunities and challenges: Illustration from US-India trade. Int J Healthc Manag 8(1):15–26. https://doi.org/10.1179/2047971914Y.0000000091

Chen YYB, Flood CM (2013) Medical tourism's impact on health care equity and access in low- and middle-income countries: making the case for regulation. J Law Med Ethics 41(1):286–300

Cohen E (2012) Medical travel and the quality-of-life. In: Uysal M, Perdue RR, Sirgy MJ (eds) Handbook of tourism and quality-of-life research: enhancing the lives of tourists and residents of host communities. Springer Science+Business Media B.V, pp 169–191

Connell J (2006) Medical tourism: sea, sun, sand and […] surgery. Tour Manag 27(6):1093–1100

Connell J (2011) Medical tourism. CABI Publishing, Cambridge

Connell J (2013) Contemporary medical tourism: conceptualisation, culture and commodification. Tour Manag 34:1–13

Cook RA, Yale LJ, Marqua JJ (2002) Tourism: the business of travel, 2nd edn. Pearson Education Inc., New Jersey, USA

Crooks VA, Turner L, Snyder J, Johnston R, Kingsbury P (2011) Promoting medical tourism to India: messages, images, and the marketing of international patient travel. Soc Sci Med 72(5):726–732. https://doi.org/10.1016/j.socscimed.2010.12.022. Epub 2011 Jan 26. PMID: 21310519

Das R (2017) Medical marketing in promoting medical tourism in India. Elk Asia Pac J Market Retail Manag 8(3) ISSN 2349-2317 (Online). https://doi.org/10.16962/EAPJMRM/issn.2349-2317/2015

Doswell R (1997) Tourism: how effective management makes the difference 1st edition. https://doi.org/10.4324/9780080519463, eBook ISBN9780080519463

Eissler LA, Casken J (2013) Seeking health care through international medical tourism. J Nurs Scholarsh 45(2):177–184

Eurostat (2011) Population structure and ageing. Available at: http://epp.eurostat.ec.europa.eu/statistics_explained/index.php/Population_structure_and_ageing

Glinos IA, Baeten R, Boffin N (2006) Cross-border contracted care in Belgian hospitals. In: Rosenmöller M, Baeten R, McKee M (eds) Patient mobility in the European Union: learning from experience. European Observatory on Health Systems and Policies, Denmark

Goodrich G, Goodrich J (1987) Healthcare tourism-an exploration study. Tour Manag:217–222

Goossens C (2000) Tourism information and pleasure motivation. Ann Tour Res 27(2):301–321. https://doi.org/10.1016/S0160-7383(99)00067-5

Graburn N (1983) The anthropology of tourism. Ann Tour Res 10(1):9–33

Healthcare (2023a). India Brand Equity Foundation. Retrieved December 15, 2020 from https://www.ibef.org/download/Healthcare July-2019.pdf

Healthcare (2023b) Invest India. https://www.investindia.gov.in/sector/healthcare

Helble M (2011) The movement of patients across borders: challenges and opportunities for public health. Bull World Health Organ 89:68–72

Heung VCS, Kucukusta D, Song H (2010) A conceptual model of medical tourism: implications for future research. J Travel Tour Market 27(3):236e251

Horowitz M, Rosensweig J (2008) Medical tourism vs traditional international medical travel: a tale of two models. Int Med Travel J 3:30–33

Jeong C (2014) Marine tourist motivations comparing push and pull factors. J Qual Assur Hosp Tour 15(3):294–309. https://doi.org/10.1080/1528008X.2014.921772

John SP, Larke R (2016) An analysis of push and pull motivators investigated in medical tourism research published from 2000 TO 2016. Tour Rev Int 20:73–90. https://doi.org/10.3727/154427216X14713104855810. E-ISSN 1943-4421

Johnston R, Crooks VA, Snyder J, Kingsbury P (2010) What is known about the effects of medical tourism in destination and departure countries? A scoping review. Int J Equity Health 9:1–13

Kanagaraj C, Bindu T (2013) An analysis of push and pull travel motivations of domestic tourists to Kerala. Int J Manag Bus Stud 3(2):112–118

Kim SS, Lee CK, Klenosky DB (2003) The influence of push and pull factors at Korean national parks. Tour Manag 24(2):169–180. https://doi.org/10.1016/S0261-5177(02)00059-6

Lautier M (2014) International trade of health services: global trends and local impact. Health Policy 118(1):105–113. https://doi.org/10.1016/j.healthpol.2014.07.004

Lee K (2000) The impact of globalization on public health: implications for the UK Faculty of Public Health Medicine. J Public Health 22(3):253–262. https://doi.org/10.1093/pubmed/22.3.253

Loveluck CH (1991) Service marketing. Prentice Hall, Englewood Cliffs, N.J

Lunt N (2015) International patients on operation vacation: medical refuge and health system crisis. Int J Health Policy Manag 4(5):323–325. https://doi.org/10.15171/ijhpm.2015.56

Lunt N, Smith R, Exworthy M, Green S, Horsfall D, Mannion R (2011) Medical tourism: treatments, markets and health system implications: a scoping review. Directorate for Employment, Labour and Social Affairs, OCED, Geneva. https://www.oecd.org/els/health-systems/48723982.pdf

MacReady N (2007) Developing countries court medical tourists. Lancet 369:1849–1850

Mattoo A, Rathindran R (2006) How health insurance inhibits trade in health care. Health Aff 25(2):358–368. https://doi.org/10.1377/hlthaff.25.2.358

Mohammad BAMA-H, Som APM (2010) An analysis of push and pull travel motivations of foreign tourists to Jordan. Int J Bus Manag 5(12):41–50

Musa G, Doshi DR, Wong KM, Thirumoorthy T (2012) How satisfied are inbound medical tourists in Malaysia? A study on private hospitals in Kuala Lumpur. J Travel Tour Mark 29(7):629–646. https://doi.org/10.1080/10548408.2012.720150
OECD (2012) Medical tourism treatments markets and health system implications, OECD, Available at: www.oecd.org/els/health-systems/48723982.pdf
Pafford B (2009) The third wave–medical tourism in the 21st century. South Med J 102(8):810–813
Pocock NS, Phua KH (2011) Medical tourism and policy implications for health systems: a conceptual framework from a comparative study of Thailand. Singapore and Malaysia Globalization and Health 7(1):12. https://doi.org/10.1186/1744-8603-7-12
Pourkhaghan Z et al (2013) Interaction of economic indicators and medical tourism industry. Int J Travel Med Glob Health 1(3):133–139
Ramírez de Arellano AB (2007) Patients without borders: the emergence of medical tourism. Int J Health Serv 37:193–198
Rangan VK, Thulasiraj RD (2007) Making sight affordable. Innov Technol Gov Glob 2(4):35–49. https://doi.org/10.1162/itgg.2007.2.4.35
Saker L, Lee K, Cannito B, Gilmore A, Campbell-Lendrum D (2004) Globalization and infectious diseases: a review of the linkages. Social, Economic and Behavioural Research: Special Topics No.3, World Health Organisation (WHO), Available from: www.who.int/tdr/publications/documents/seb_topic3.pdf
Sarwal R, Prasad U, Madangopal K, Kalal S, Kaur D, Kumar A, Regy P, Sharma J (2021) Investment opportunities in India's Healthcare Sector. NITI Aayog. Investment Opportunities in India's Healthcare Sector, NITI Aayog
Skountridaki L (2015) The internationalisation of healthcare and business aspirations of medical professionals. Sociology 49(3):471–487. https://doi.org/10.1177/0038038514535863
Smith RD (2004) Foreign direct investment and trade in health services: a review of the literature. Soc Sci Med 59:2313–2323
Smith RD, Rupa C, Viroj T (2009) Trade in health-related services. Lancet 373:593–601
Source: Ministry of Tourism, Market Research Division, Government of India, India Tourism Statistics (2022) https://tourism.gov.in/sites/default/files/2022-09/India%20Tourism%20Statistics%202022%20%28English%29.pdf
Turner L (2007) 'First world health care at third world prices': globalization, bioethics and medical tourism. BioSocieties 2(3):303
Uysal M, Jurowski C (1994) Testing the push and pull factors. Ann Tour Res 21(4):844–846. https://doi.org/10.1016/0160-7383(94)90091-4
Vidalis T, Kyriakaki I (2014) Cross-border healthcare: directive 2011/24 and the Greek law. Eur J Health Law 21(1):33–45. https://doi.org/10.1163/15718093-12341304
Walker JR, Walker JT (2010) Tourism: concepts and practices. Pearson Education, Upper Saddle River, NJ
World Tourism Organization (1995) Collection of tourism expenditure statistics, UNWTO Technical Manual, No. 2 World Tourism Organization
Yoon Y, Uysal M (2005) An examination of the effects of motivation and satisfaction on destination loyalty: a structural model. Tour Manag 26(1):45–56. https://doi.org/10.1016/j.tourman.2003.08.016

SPRINGER NATURE

GPSR Compliance

The European Union's (EU) General Product Safety Regulation (GPSR) is a set of rules that requires consumer products to be safe and our obligations to ensure this.

If you have any concerns about our products, you can contact us on ProductSafety@springernature.com

In case Publisher is established outside the EU, the EU authorized representative for:

Springer Nature Customer Service Center GmbH
Europaplatz 3
69115 Heidelberg, Germany

The manufacturer's authorised representative in the EU is Springer Nature Customer Service Centre GmbH, Europaplatz 3, 69115 Heidelberg, Germany. If you have any concerns regarding our products, please contact ProductSafety@springernature.com

Printed and bound by CPI Group (UK) Ltd, Croydon, CR0 4YY
30/09/2026
02225318-0012